HANDBOOK OF CHILD AND ADOLESCENT OUTPATIENT, DAY TREATMENT AND COMMUNITY PSYCHIATRY

HANDBOOK OF CHILD AND ADOLESCENT OUTPATIENT, DAY TREATMENT AND COMMUNITY PSYCHIATRY

Edited by

Harinder S. Ghuman, M.D.
Associate Professor of Psychiatry,
Medical Director of Child and Adolescent Outpatient
Services at Walter P. Carter Center, Department of Psychiatry,
University of Maryland School of Medicine,
Baltimore, Maryland

and

Richard M. Sarles, M.D.
Professor of Psychiatry and Pediatrics,
Director of Child and Adolescent Psychiatry,
University of Maryland School of Medicine,
Baltimore, Maryland

Handbook of child and
adolescent outpatient,

USA	Publishing Office:	BRUNNER/MAZEL
		A member of the Taylor & Francis Group
		325 Chestnut Street
		Philadelphia, PA 19106
		Tel: (215) 625-8900
		Fax: (215) 625-2940
	Distribution Center:	BRUNNER/MAZEL
		A member of the Taylor & Francis Group
		47 Runway Road
		Levittown, PA 19057
		Tel: (215) 269-0400
		Fax: (215) 269-0363
UK		BRUNNER/MAZEL
		A member of the Taylor & Francis Group
		1 Gunpowder Square
		London EC4A 3DE
		Tel: +44 171 583 0490
		Fax: +44 171 583 0581

HANDBOOK OF CHILD AND ADOLESCENT OUTPATIENT, DAY TREATMENT AND COMMUNITY PSYCHIATRY

1 2 3 4 5 6 7 8 9 0

Printed by Hamilton Printing Co., Castleton, NY, 1998.

A CIP catalog record for this book is available from the British Library.
    The paper in this publication meets the requirements of the ANSI Standard Z39.48-1984 (Permanence of Paper).

Library of Congress Cataloging-in-Publication Data
Handbook of child and adolescent outpatient, day treatment and community psychiatry/[edited by] Harinder S. Ghuman and Richard M. Sarles.
    p. cm.
    ISBN 0-87630-874-4 (alk. paper)
    1. Child psychiatry. 2. Adolescent psychiatry. 3. Community mental health services for children. 4. Community mental health services for teenagers. I. Ghuman, Harinder S. II. Sarles, Richard M. (Richard Milford), 1935–   .
RJ499. H329   1998
618.92'89–dc21

                                                                98-18544
                                                                CIP

ISBN 0-87630-874-4

Contents

PART 6: OTHER COMMUNITY-BASED PROGRAMS

Contributors

BRUNO J. ANTHONY, Ph.D.
Associate Professor
Director of Maryland Center for Attention
    Disorders
Department of Psychiatry
University of Maryland School of Medicine
Baltimore
Maryland

REGINA CICCI, Ph.D.
Speech-Language Pathologist and Learning
    Specialist
University of Maryland Medical Systems
Baltimore
Maryland

LANCE D. CLAWSON, M.D.
Director
Child and Adolescent Psychiatric Services
Lowdoun Healthcare
Leesburg
Virginia

JEFFREY S. DANFORTH, Ph.D.
Assistant Professor
Eastern Connecticut State University
Department of Psychology
Willimantic
Connecticut

ANDRE P. DERDEYN, M.D.
WOHDAN Professor and Chief
Division of Pediatric Psychiatry
Arkansas Children's Hospital
University of Arkansas
Little Rock
Arkansas

LOIS T. FLAHERTY, M.D.
Clinical Associate Professor of Psychiatry
University of Pennsylvania School of Medicine
Philadelphia
Pennsylvania
and
Adjunct Associate Professor of Psychiatry
University of Maryland School of Medicine
Baltimore
Maryland

LAURENCE W. FORD, M.Ed.
Diagnostic and Prescriptive Teacher
The Forbush School
The Sheppard and Enoch Pratt Hospital
Towson
Maryland
and
Educational Consultant
Maryland Center for Attention Disorders
University of Maryland Medical Systems
Baltimore
Maryland

HARINDER S. GHUMAN, M.D.
Associate Professor of Psychiatry
Medical Director of Child and Adolescent
    Outpatient Services at Walter P. Carter Center
Department of Psychiatry
University of Maryland School of Medicine
Baltimore
Maryland

JASWINDER K. GHUMAN, M.D.
Assistant Professor of Psychiatry
The Johns Hopkins University School of
    Medicine
and
Director of Infant and Preschool Psychiatry
    Clinic
Kennedy Kreiger Institute
Baltimore
Maryland

JOHN J. GIBBONS, Ph.D., L.C.S.W.C.
Clinical Assistant Professor
Director of Family Therapy Training
University of Maryland School of Medicine
Baltimore
Maryland

SUSAN B. GLASSMAN, Ph.D.
Director of Adjunctive Therapies
Foundation Behavior Health
Doylestown
Pennsylvania

MARSHA GORTH, L.C.S.W.C.
Assistant Coordinator
Child and Adolescent Outpatient Services at
    Walter P. Carter Center
Department of Psychiatry
University of Maryland
Baltimore
Maryland

MOHAMMAD HAERIAN, M.D.
Clinical Associate Professor of Psychiatry
University of Maryland School of Medicine
Baltimore
Maryland

JACQUELINE HAIMES, M.D.
Assistant Professor of Psychiatry
The University of Illinois
Chicago
Illinois

KEVIN HARRISON, M.D.
Clinical Assistant Professor
Director, Child Day Hospital
Department of Psychiatry
University of Maryland School of Medicine
Baltimore
Maryland
and
Consultant Psychiatrist
The Sheppard and Enoch Pratt Hospital
Towson
Maryland

EILEEN HASTINGS, R.N.C., L.C.S.W.C.
Deputy Director
Division of Community Psychiatry
and
Program Director at Walter P. Carter Center
    Outpatient Services
Department of Psychiatry
University of Maryland
Baltimore

NOREEN J. HERBERT, R.N.
Nurse Administrator
Mental Hygiene Administration
University of Maryland School of Medicine
Baltimore
Maryland

STEVEN L. JAFFE, M.D.
Professor of Psychiatry and Behavioral
    Sciences
Emory University School of Medicine
Morehouse School of Medicine
and
Director
Child and Adolescent Services
Charter Peachford Hospital
Atlanta
Georgia

MARK JENNINGS, M.D.
Assistant Professor
Division of Pediatric Psychiatry
Arkansas Children's Hospital
University of Arkansas for Medical Sciences
Little Rock
Arkansas

ILENE JOSEPH, L.C.S.W.C.
Clinical Director
Early Childhood Behavior Services Childhaven
St. Louis
Missouri

PARAMJIT T. JOSHI, M.D.
Director of Clinical Services
Associate Professor of Psychiatry
Division of Child and Adolescent Psychiatry
Johns Hopkins Medical Institutions
Baltimore
Maryland

BURTON LOHNES, Ph.D.
Director of Education
The Forbush School
The Sheppard and Enoch Pratt Hospital
Towson
Maryland

MICHAEL LONGO, M.A.
Director
The Narrative Project for Crisis Intervention
Belmont
Massachusetts

ROBIN J. MOGUL, M.D.
A Senior Fellow in Child and Adolescent
    Psychiatry
Emory University School of Medicine
Atlanta
Georgia

ROBINSON J. MUNOZ-MILLAN, M.D.
Assistant Professor of Psychiatry
Director, Infant Study Center
Department of Psychiatry
University of Maryland School of Medicine
Baltimore
Maryland

CHARLES OSEROFF, M.D.
Medical Director
The Children's Guild, Inc.
Baltimore
Maryland

SHERIDAN PHILLIPS, Ph.D.
Associate Professor
Department of Psychiatry and Pediatrics
University of Maryland School of Medicine
Baltimore
Maryland

RICHARD M. SARLES, M.D.
Professor of Psychiatry and Pediatrics
Director of Child and Adolescent Psychiatry
University of Maryland School of Medicine
Baltimore
Maryland

KRISTEN SCHMIDT, Ph.D.
Fellow in Prevention Science
Prevention Research Center
Department of Mental Hygiene
The Johns Hopkins School of Hygiene and
   Public Health
Baltimore
Maryland

STEPHEN L. SOFFER, Ph.D.
Post-Doctoral Fellow
Division of Adolescent Medicine
University of Maryland
Baltimore
Maryland

ERIC P. VAN SCHOOR, Ph.D.
A group analyst and staff psychologist at
   University of California
Davis
Sacramento
California

MARK D. WEIST, Ph.D.
Associate Professor
Director of Center for School Mental Health
   Assistance
Department of Psychiatry
University of Maryland School of Medicine
Baltimore
Maryland

Preface

In the past, both editors were involved with the inpatient treatment of children and adolescents and had the opportunity to publish *The Handbook of Adolescent Inpatient Psychiatric Treatment*. Since the publication of this book in 1994, there has been a massive shift in health care, particularly from inpatient care toward treating children and adolescents in non-hospital, community ambulatory settings. This change in service delivery has been driven primarily by economic pressures. Insurance companies and managed care organizations have not only restricted access to hospitalization and limited length of stays but they also have sharply reduced reimbursements for treatments. State and federal policies for inpatient treatment and reimbursement have followed similar trends.

Mental health planners have attempted to develop programs to deal with this trend of restricted inpatient care, shifting treatment of children and adolescents to home and community settings. Some of these new programs are well planned, others are hastily planned and implemented. As new programs have developed new terms have been added to the lexicon of ambulatory and community psychiatry including "family preservation initiatives," "wrap around services," "umbrella services," and "in-home services." The emphasis on treating children and adolescents in their home and community is, according to health planners, primarily to strengthen the family and community bond and to decrease family dependence on others to take care of its problems. Reducing costly treatment modalities such as inpatient care is clearly a driving force for such community treatment.

The pitfall to this community approach, however, is that there is a population of chronically and severely disturbed children and adolescents, and highly stressed parents, often lacking adequate personal and family resources, who may not respond to these new less restrictive, less costly community approaches which potentially may lead to an unsafe and dangerous situation for the child, adolescent, family, and community.

The increase in violence toward children and adolescents, and violence and suicides by children and adolescents raises many troubling issues for structure and safety and demands that these children be closely monitored. The new trend of treating children and adolescents in their home and community challenges mental health professionals to be more creative, knowledgeable, and experienced in their ambulatory community psychiatry work. With that in mind, the purpose of this book is to provide comprehensive and up-to-date information regarding child and adolescent outpatient, day treatment, and community psychiatry. The book emphasizes practical knowledge through clinical case illustrations and explains various strategies in a detailed fashion.

The book has six sections. Section One deals with general issues related to administration, staffing, training, and collaborative aspects of outpatient work. It is divided into four chapters. The first chapter presents a historical view of ambulatory treatment and provides a summary of the types of settings and services offered. Contemporary issues and challenges pertaining to clinical, financial, and training aspects are discussed in detail from an administrative point of view. This chapter also describes how milieu treatment and a team approach can be applied to an ambulatory setting. In recent years ambulatory services have placed increased emphasis on specialty clinics. Chapter 2 describes the essentials of setting up specialty clinics, including administrative and financial aspects, staffing patterns and procedures, and how to integrate training and research in such a clinical setting. Recently, there has been a trend toward privatization of community mental health centers. Chapter 3 addresses transitional issues related to privatization. This chapter describes administrative structure, staffing patterns, staff recruitment and orientation, stages of staff and team development, and the role of the team leader and medical director. It also discusses the problems encountered in service delivery, such as the need for home- and community-based services instead of traditional office-based services. Chapter 4 deals with training in ambulatory settings, because in university and university-affiliated clinics there are often many professionals in training including child psychiatry fellows, general psychiatry residents, psychology interns, and social work, medical, and nursing students. The role of the training director, chief resident, faculty/attending, and supervisors, and the financial aspects of training, a didactic curriculum, and trainees' expectations and anxieties are all looked at in this chapter. Collaborative aspects of work with pediatricians as well as training general pediatric and behavioral pediatric residents is also discussed.

Section Two addresses assessment aspects of outpatient work. Chapters 5, 6, and 7 examine the psychiatric assessment of infants and preschool children and parent-child interaction, school-age children, and adolescents and their families. These chapters describe the evaluation process including essentials of history taking, examination techniques, formulation, and treatment planning within the developmental level of the youngster. Chapter 8 addresses psychological evaluation and assessment. The various behavior ratings and self reports used in assessment of children and adolescents are discussed in addition to the various tests to assess cognitive, neuropsychological, personality, emotional functioning, and academic achievement, and their strength and limitations. Chapter 9 is devoted to speech and language evaluation and describes various components of a language system. A description of various speech and language disorders, indications for evaluation, and the assessment procedure and treatment techniques are included. Chapter 10 focuses upon forensic community child and adolescent psychiatry describing the history of the juvenile court and the psychiatrist's role in the juvenile court pertaining to custody disputes, child abuse and neglect, and psychiatric evaluation in the forensic setting.

Section Three includes chapters (11–16) on common disorders of childhood and adolescence including Affective Disorder, Obsessive-Compulsive Disorder, Tics and Tourette's Disorders, Separation Anxiety Disorders, Attention Deficit/Hyperactivity Disorder, Conduct and Oppositional Disorders, Alcohol and Substance Abuse Disorder, Pervasive Developmental Disorders, and Learning Disorders. These chapters describe a historical perspective, diagnostic criteria, assessment, epidemiology, etiology, differential diagnosis, management, and course of the various disorders.

Section Four describes various therapeutic interventions. Chapter 17 is devoted to pharmacotherapy and describes the history of psychopharmacology and current use of stimulants, antidepressants, mood stabilizers, neuroleptics, clonidine, guanfacine, and beta-blockers in the treatment of psychiatrically disturbed children and adolescents. A discussion of indications, pretreatment workup, dosing regimen, ongoing medical monitoring, and adverse effects of these medications is included. Chapter 18 is on cognitive-behavioral therapy. Cognitive-behavioral therapy has become popular because the treatment program can be completed in a relatively short time, and this chapter describes a historical and theoretical background and commonly used cognitive-behavioral strategies. Chapter 19 describes individual psychotherapy and the use of play with children with a historical perspective, indications, goals, the process of play therapy, and the length of treatment. Chapter 20 focuses on individual psychotherapy with adolescents and addresses the need for such therapy, developmental issues affecting the adolescent-therapist relationship, and the psychotherapeutic process and techniques. Chapter 21, on behavior therapy with children and adolescents, presents a description of the theoretical underpinning of behavior therapy and common issues involved in behavior therapy, including the issue of the therapist's experience, patient and family resistance, family issues and resources, the therapeutic relationship, and ethical considerations. Chapter 22, regarding group psychotherapy with children and adolescents, includes a description of the historical background, models of group psychotherapy, setting, structure, group dynamics and processes, and the role of the therapist and co-therapist. Chapter 23, on interventions with parents and children, describes various models of family therapy and addresses the process and technique of intervention with families.

Section Five describes mental health services which are intermediate in level of intensity between inpatient and outpatient treatment. These services are of increased importance because of the restriction on inpatient treatment by managed care companies. These companies are often willing to fund day treatment services in place of inpatient care since day treatment is less costly. For some children and adolescents day treatment is appropriate as it provides the necessary structure, supervision, and activities during the day without uprooting youngsters from their homes. However, for children and adolescents with more serious disturbances and chaotic family situations, day treatment may not be optimal or enough. Chapter 24 discusses marketing and funding issues, staffing and administrative structure, physical facilities, and relationships to outside agencies. Chapter 25 describes the patient population and treatment approaches in a day hospital, and differences between children's and adolescents' programs, limitations of day hospital, and various treatment interventions, rules, structures, and daily schedules. Chapter 26, on day school for emotionally and behaviorally disturbed children and adolescents, discusses funding issues and various models of day school programs and their advantages and disadvantages. Included are detailed descriptions of educational programs, intake procedures, courses, support services, discharge, and potential pitfalls.

The last section of the book presents various aspects of community-based programs. Chapter 27 concerns mental health services in the school and describes historical and theoretical background, administrative and program developmental issues, and examples of clinical practice in the school. Chapter 28 is devoted to home- and community-based care and describes a hospital diversion program, including the use of systemic narrative therapy. The therapeutic nursery is discussed in Chapter 29 and there is a description of a delivery model for mental health services to preschoolers, including underlying principles and function. The final chapter, Chapter 30, addresses issue of foster care and describes reasons for placement, risk factors associated with foster care placement, specialized foster care programs, psychiatric problems, psychological development of children in foster care, and the role of the child and adolescent psychiatrist.

The aim of this book is to provide a guide to the more experienced practitioners of child and adolescent mental health and to child and adolescent psychiatry, psychology, social work, and nursing trainees, along with current knowledge and practical examples of the delivery of contemporary ambulatory psychiatric care for children, adolescents, and their families.

Acknowledgments

One of us (H.G.) would like to acknowledge a number of individuals who made significant contributions to his personal and career development and whose help was indispensable to the conception of this book. These teachers include Drs. John Romano, E. James Anthony, Roy Mendelsoln, Donald Saidel, and, lastly, but, importantly, co-editor, friend, and mentor Richard Sarles. R.S. would like to acknowledge his co-editor, colleague, and friend, without whom this book would have never been conceptualized or completed.

We both appreciate and acknowledge the support of Dr. John Talbott, Chairman of the Department of Psychiatry, Dr. Fred Osher, Director of Community Psychiatry, and Ms. Eileen Hastings, Deputy Director of Community Psychiatry, all at the University of Maryland School of Medicine for providing not only leadership in community ambulatory psychiatry but also for their personal interest in the care of children and adolescents.

We wish to express our deep appreciation to all our contributors for their hard work and enthusiasm. Michelle Titus and Ginger Hayslip were especially helpful in transforming chapters from various contributors into a final coherent whole. We thank Ms. Natalie Gilman, past editorial vice president and Brunner/Mazel, Inc. for supporting the production and publication of this book. We wish to thank the staff at Taylor & Francis, including Lansing Hays, Anthony Wahl, Stephanie Weidel, and Elisa Heisman, for their insightful suggestions and expertise in orchestrating the final editing and publishing phases of the book.

We are very grateful and appreciative for the support of our friends and family, especially our wives, Jaswinder Ghuman and Lois Sarles, and our children, Avniel Ghuman and Kristen and Karen Sarles who have provided understanding, support, tolerance, and inspiration.

Part 1

Ambulatory Services: Clinical, Administrative, and Training Issues

Ambulatory Services for Children and Adolescents: Historical View, Definition, Present Issues, Challenges, and Solutions

Harinder S. Ghuman, M.D. and Richard M. Sarles, M.D.

HISTORICAL PERSPECTIVE

The history of assessment and treatment of mental disorders in children and adolescents extends over centuries. It is misguided to seek origin simply in terms of recognizable modern specialization, and rarely justifiable to claim primacy of theories, interventions, or publication (Parry-Jones, 1994). Practitioners and theorists as far back as medieval times have been struggling to define childhood and adolescence mental disturbances, find underlying reasons for the disturbances, and determine how best to treat them and in what kind of setting. The following two historical anecdotes illustrate some of the major problems facing contemporary child and adolescent psychiatry.

Johann Weyer is considered as the first "psychiatrist" who practiced medicine in the 16th century. His interest turned from general medicine to the study of individual human behavior, particularly the study of women who had been accused of witchcraft. It may be that he was not only the first psychiatrist but also the first child and adolescent psychiatrist to suggest careful evaluation and care of children and adolescents. He described a case of a 10-year-old girl who had supposedly existed for over a year without food or drink. Weyer moved this child and her sister to his home to live with his family. After a period of close observation, Weyer concluded that the child's behavior represented an unconscious desire to malinger. His writing reflects his recognition of the importance of the therapeutic relationship and careful examination and observation, and that the needs of the individual rather than the rules of the institution must be given primary consideration (Mora, 1967).

In 1799 Citizen Bonaterre reported in the *Journal des Debats* the discovery of a "wild" boy in the woods of the Department of Aveyron. The "wild boy" was brought to town and placed in the hospital of Saint-Afrique and later transferred to Paris as a result of the public's curiosity and excitement in seeing a true human savage untainted by society's vices. He was examined by Pinel and diagnosed as an incurable idiot and not a true *homo ferus*, or savage man. Pinel referred to him thereafter as the Pretended Wild Boy of Aveyron to distinguish the wild children as a special species of human.

Itard, a student of Pinel, begged the National Institute for the Deaf and Dumb, where the boy was housed, to let him try out his pedagogical theories on the boy. The directors agreed and Itard labored for five years and taught the boy to dress himself, take care of bodily functions, and even to read simple words and do easy calculations, but he was unable to teach him to speak. Pinel had diagnosed the boy as an idiot and incurable whereas Itard said he was a wild boy untouched by civilization's teachings. Apparently, truth was somewhere between the two. Although Itard could not teach the boy to speak his efforts started a movement toward the training of the deaf and dumb and the mentally defective (Winkler & Bromberg, 1939).

Several issues from these two cases are still relevant to the contemporary practice of child and adolescent psychiatry including the debate of nature versus nurture in etiology, the need for specialists and sub-specialists, how much effort and expense to put into treating a difficult case, in what kind of setting one should treat a patient, and whether one should attempt new or unpopular means of treatment. The evolution of treatment of psychiatric patients, including children and adolescents, has gone through difficult and tumultuous times influenced by ignorance and the religious beliefs of society, the impact of psychiatric patients' behavior on society, and, at times, society's outright rejection and neglect of psychiatric patients. In general the role of economic factors and administrators has not been that obvious until recently but it is safe to conclude that human greed is as old as human beings and has contributed significantly to both the progression and the regression in the practice of psychiatry.

AMBULATORY CHILD AND ADOLESCENT PSYCHIATRY: DEFINITION, SETTINGS, AND SERVICES

Contemporary ambulatory child and adolescent psychiatry includes mental health services offered to children, adolescents, and their families in outpatient settings—school, day hospital, after school programs, and in-home services. Ambulatory settings range from the individual practitioner's private office to large programs with various components and multidisciplinary staff. It is important for the organization and the staff to have full knowledge of the mission and a clear understanding of the priorities of the program, the line of authority and role of the individual staff, and the relationship with various inter- and intradepartmental programs, outside agencies, and competing or parallel programs.

The spectrum of settings include: (a) individual practitioner's office, (b) group practice with same speciality staff or as part of a multi-speciality group, (c) university-based program, (d) general or psychiatric hospital-based program, (e) community mental health center, (f) managed care clinic/program, (g) specialty program, (h) services offered through other specialty settings such as pediatrics, adolescent medicine, or ob-gyn, (i) school-based mental health program, (j) day special education school, and (k) day treatment (hospital).

These ambulatory settings offer combination of mental health services to children, adolescents, and their families including: (a) diagnostic and evaluation services which include individual psychiatric assessment, psychological and educational testing, family assessment, medical assessment (lab, EKG, vital signs), and referral for physical and neurological examination if necessary; (b) general treatment services including individual psy-chotherapy, medication, family therapy, and group therapy; (c) day hospital services with emphasis on providing structure and supervision through a milieu approach in addition to traditional therapies to stabilize and manage acutely disturbed children or adolescents; (d) special education day school to provide long-term individualized special education and treatment services including various therapies and medication in a therapeutic milieu; (e) home-based interventions which usually include family therapy, parent skill training, behavior therapy, and case management; (f) school-based mental health services to provide brief evaluation, short-term supportive therapy, crisis intervention, education and consul-tation to staff, and referral for more intensive and comprehensive services; (g) after school and summer programs to provide a therapeutic milieu with structured therapeutic activities and group therapy; and (h) specialized foster home and group homes which provide a su-pervised residential setting for children and adolescents with psychiatric problems who are unable to be managed in their own homes. These settings create a therapeutic milieu using behavior modification, structured activities, limit setting, group therapies, and individual counseling techniques.

CONTEMPORARY ISSUES, CHALLENGES, AND SOLUTIONS: ADMINISTRATIVE-FINANCIAL

Since the mid-1980s there has been increased emphasis, primarily driven by economic fac-tors, on delivering medical services in ambulatory settings. This shift has created opportu-nities for good programs to strengthen and expand ambulatory programs. In the past, most ambulatory child and adolescent programs were supported financially by adult and/or child and adolescent inpatient programs through cost shifting. This has become increasingly dif-ficult as a result of shrinking inpatient resources and regulatory constraints on cost shifting. Ambulatory settings are therefore under increased pressure to become financially indepen-dent and to be a revenue-generating source for the organization. To have a good program, the program needs to be on a sound financial footing, and to be financially successful, it is important to consider the following factors:

1   The program should be of high quality, comprehensive, flexible, provide conti-nuity of services, and be based on the needs of the community.
2   The program needs a strong referral base. To obtain this, it must develop ongo-ing dialogue and close communication with referral sources. Optimal marketing strategies directed toward referring professionals and the community are essential.
3   There is a need for high-quality, innovative, and financially sensitive clinical as well as administrative staff. There should be clear and reasonable expectations regarding productivity of a particular staff and monitoring mechanisms. Administrators need to be constantly monitoring number of staff and trainees required to do the work. Hiring extra staff without increasing the referral base can result in unnecessary tension and lowering of morale as well as financial loss. On the other hand not having enough staff also can result in staff burnout, poor or delayed response to patients' needs (resulting in an unsatisfactory customer and referral source), and financial loss.
4   Managed care has been and will continue to be in some form or other a ma-jor force in influencing types and settings of treatment. It is incumbent on providers to provide efficient, cost-effective care without compromising the essentials of good care. Managed care contracting requires even more efficient intake processes, billing processes, and follow-up of the patient.

5 For the foreseeable future, the health delivery system will remain in a state of flux. Individual practitioners as well as administrators of ambulatory programs will need to be on alert constantly to the rapid changes occurring in health care financing and have flexible contingency plans to respond.

6 There is a significant increase in regulatory as well as financial controls in all settings, including the private and public and academic sectors. These controls serve to safeguard optimum care to the patient, provide that care within reasonable financial means, and prevent fraud. During any transition, especially that noted in the current draconian change in health care financing, adversarial positions develop. Unfortunately, currently, service providers and funding resources seem to be involved in a tussle over money and who can beat the other by whatever means (sometime unethical and illegal), often ignoring the needs of the patient. Administrators of a good program must be careful that:

- services are created with the patients' needs in mind,
- charges for services are reasonable,
- all the billed services are provided, and
- the clinic adheres to all the regulatory controls. The administrator must watch how consciously and unconsciously the message regarding regulatory controls is delivered to the staff.

ADMINISTRATIVE–CLINICAL

Increased focus on ambulatory services for children and adolescents requires an evaluation of already existing programs, an identification of gaps in services and the development of new programs, and coordination of various services within and among systems and the community: all critical factors for optimal clinical effectiveness and fiscal viability. It is not uncommon that there are several clinics providing mental health services to children, adolescents, their families in a large university or hospital setting through various departments such as psychiatry, pediatrics, adolescent medicine, family medicine, nursing, and social work, and sometimes even within the department of psychiatry itself. Often there is little communication and coordination of services provided by these clinics as a result of turf disputes, discipline and financial issues, and sometimes just simply because of lack of vision and disorganization within the system. The following discussions presents suggestions to meet present and future challenges.

Often, the child and adolescent psychiatry program in a university setting, private and public hospital setting, or community mental health setting is part of a general psychiatry department which is directed by a general psychiatrist and supported by a non-clinical administrator. There are also clinics which are directed by non-psychiatrist clinical or non-clinical administrators. In such systems the same arrangement is often replicated at the level of child and adolescent programs.

The development and growth of the child and adolescent program depends on a number of factors including the mission of the program, the administrative structure and the quality of integration of various departments at the highest level, the mission and interests at the departmental level, the personality and interests of the departmental chairperson and other significant administrators, and the effectiveness of the child and adolescent psychiatry director in working with the department chairperson, other administrators, and the child and adolescent psychiatry staff, and the quality of that staff. In addition, financial factors often play the most important role in the development and growth of the child and adolescent program. It is beyond the scope of this chapter, however, to discuss *all* the variables effecting the development of a child and adolescent psychiatry program.

To have a successful child and adolescent psychiatry program, it is essential at the departmental level that:

1   There is a clearly defined administrative structure with one child and adolescent psychiatry director who oversees and coordinates all the child and adolescent psychiatry services in the system.

2   There is free and open communication between the department chairperson and the child and adolescent psychiatry director. The chairperson must be genuinely interested in the child and adolescent psychiatry program, be open to the suggestions and advice of the child and adolescent psychiatry director, and curtail any tendency to apply adult psychiatry solutions to child and adolescent psychiatry. At the same time the director of the child and adolescent psychiatry program needs to assertively represent the interests and needs of the child and adolescent program without making excessive claims that children and adolescent needs, services, and solutions are different from or take priority over adult psychiatric services.

3   If there are several departments involved in providing child and adolescent psychiatry services in a facility, then it is necessary for the departmental heads and coordinators of these services to communicate with each other to clarify issues regarding referrals and services provided to ensure a uniform standard of care and better utilization of services with minimal duplication.

At the child and adolescent psychiatry program level, it is important for clinical administrative staff in conjunction with clinical staff to assess carefully gaps, strengths, and weaknesses in the program as well as needs of the community served. Most child and adolescent ambulatory programs continue to lack any or have minimal services for substance abusing youth, severe conduct disordered children, and adolescents, including juvenile offenders and developmentally disordered children and adolescents. There is still a lack or shortage of after school programs, summer programs, home intervention services, and school-based mental health programs. The program needs to prioritize which services to develop and how to strengthen the services already present. The services can be strengthened by:

•   streamlining the intake process, including providing a single point of entry for the patient into various components of the program. This requires staff at the entrance level with excellent interpersonal skills and knowledge of the program. In addition, there is need for close communication between the staff at the entrance level and the staff at the various clinical settings.

•   if there is more than one clinic in the program, designating the clinics to (a) serve special populations (e.g., juvenile offenders, patients with attention deficit hyperactivity disorder, post-traumatic disorder), and/or (b) provide special services (e.g., home intervention services, case management services, special group therapies). This way one clinic can complement work of the other clinic instead of competing.

•   the streamlining and easy transferability of paperwork and data collection among various components of a program, greatly enhancing efficiency of the staff. The program needs to find a way to serve the patient at the various sites and bill for the services without going through the tedious process of opening new charts at all sites.

When deciding about new psychiatric services for children and adolescents, it is important for administrators to find out what is already available and determine if it is better to collaborate or compete with existing programs in the community.

ADMINISTRATIVE–TRAINING

Training of Trainees

The shift in service emphasis from inpatient to ambulatory settings and from long-term to short-term interventions, along with the creation of new and innovative ambulatory programs has presented challenges to training directors as well as trainees. Some of the issues and suggestions that have arisen are looked at in the following discussion.

Traditionally, the no-show rate for appointments in university or public outpatient clinics has been 30 percent to 40 percent and even higher for intakes. The trainee may not be able to see enough patients because of such a high no-show rate and may not pursue the patient vigorously because of time restrictions and lack of experience. Closer scrutiny of trainees' patient caseloads by their supervisors and the clinic director is necessary for the trainees to get optimal training experience as well as for the survival of the training-focused clinic. The clinic can organize in such a way that there is a block of time set aside when all the trainees and some of their supervisors are available to do a certain task—for example, diagnostic evaluations or providing psychopharmacological or other interventions. Overbooking of patients with availability of clinic staff in case all the patients show up is one method of assuring an adequate number of patients. In addition to the benefit of seeing an increased number of patients, this procedure provides better training experience as a result of its hands-on, live supervision from individual supervisors as well as feedback from other supervisors and trainees as a group. This kind of setting also provides team experience for the trainees, supervisors, and supportive staff.

As a result of the growth in new ambulatory programs, the trainees need to learn contemporary methods of interventions as well as how to provide services in new settings in addition to traditional interventions and settings. Home- and school-based interventions are examples of this. Many of these programs are new, in the process of development, and in the community. It is important that trainees get proper supervision, are provided necessary security and support, and are not used primarily to cover new services to save money. By the end of training, the trainees should be knowledgeable and experienced in various types of interventions including short-term, time-limited psychotherapy, cognitive therapy, behavior therapy, parent training, and group therapies.

In addition, contemporary child and adolescent psychiatry requires some cross-professional training. For example, it is useful for a non-psychiatrist clinician to have knowledge of psychopharmacology if the clinician is treating a patient who is on medication and a psychiatrist sees this patient once every two or three months. It appears that child and adolescent psychiatrists continue to underutilize behavior therapies and depend to much on medication whereas a combination of these interventions may be more effective in a number of patients. The trainees, especially child and adolescent psychiatry residents, should continue to be involved in long-term, intensive psychotherapy training experiences not only to provide therapy and understand human interactions but also to provide leadership and perform a supervisory role in the field (see chapter 4, Training in Ambulatory Settings).

The recent past and present atmosphere in psychiatry and medicine in general has left administrators, clinical staff, and trainees confused, demoralized, and insecure about the future. It is important that training directors and faculty provide realistic views of present problems and issues to trainees, instill a sense of direction and hope, and ask the trainees to uphold high standards of medical care.

Training and Retraining of the Staff

Contemporary child and adolescent psychiatry requires the clinician to posses sharp diagnostic skills, experience in short-term interventions, knowledge about how to use community resources, and the ability to provide all or at least some of the services in the community instead of the clinic. Most of the issues related to trainees discussed previously also apply to the staff. What makes it difficult and complex in dealing with training and retraining of clinical staff is that the staff is no longer in a trainee role, may have been practicing for some time in a certain fashion, and may identify themselves with a certain expertise. The program administrator needs to be sensitive to the staff and should provide a clear explanation of why a particular staff is being asked to change their mode of functioning, to provide a sense of that particular staff's importance to the program, to empathize with staff's feeling of confusion, anxiety, and loss of control, to provide clear directions how the staff can learn about the new role, and to provide time and money for retraining. Administrators who issue dicta often as a result of ignorance and their own anxiety, without following the above suggestions, frequently lose good workers and end up spending a lot of energy and time in hiring new staff. The staff can be trained and retrained through individual supervision, group supervision in a team meeting or team activity, attendance at the clinical conferences, or rounds and special workshops, for example. In addition, in the present managed care atmosphere the staff needs to learn the intricacies of preparing necessary paperwork and how to communicate effectively with the providers.

MILIEU TREATMENT AND TEAM APPROACH

The concept of milieu treatment and intensive teamwork traditionally has been applied to inpatient settings. With increased emphasis on treating highly disturbed children and adolescents in their often dysfunctional family settings and sometimes dysfunctional community, it has become essential to use milieu treatment and an intensive team approach to ambulatory settings. Milieu treatment is already playing a major role in day hospital treatment (for details see Glassman and Flaherty, this volume), special education day schools, group homes, after school programs, and summer programs..

Milieu treatment can be defined as a growth-promoting environment where corrective emotional experiences take place. Waltos (1994) described unstructured and structured elements of a milieu. The unstructured elements include shared vision regarding the philosophy and functions of the milieu. Gunderson (1978) described functions of the inpatient milieu as containment, support, structure, involvement, and validation. The structured elements include order and organization of the treatment team, multiple treatment activities, stability of staff assignments, and lower reliance on medication. In the present state of ambulatory care, one can visualize treating severely disturbed children and adolescents in a milieu which extends from an individual clinician's office to the clinic and into school, home, and community at large.

The "core" clinic treatment team members with the support of "associate" team members including teachers, mentors, department of social services' workers, and probation officers (if any) work together in providing containment, support, and structure to the child and family. The concepts of "umbrella" and "wrap-around" services are relevant in providing structure to the outpatient milieu. Outpatient milieu treatment has become more important for clinicians who are spending a great portion of time in the homes of highly disturbed families with more than one child or family member having emotional problems. They have to create a hospital-like environment without the benefit of all the services available in the hospital. It is essential that these home intervention teams involve intensive teamwork including frequent rounds regarding the patients' conditions, sharing knowledge and responsibility for each other's patients, and working in pairs in dangerous communities. The intensive teamwork requires clear role definition for each team member, clear directions, and close communication. These teams have to be highly mobile to be effective. The "core" team members need to meet regularly with "associate" team members to assess the child's progress, improve communication, and plan future strategies. Jellinek (1994), in writing about designing the outpatient milieu, emphasized the importance of setting reasonable expectations based on clinical judgment that integrate a developmental approach.

To create a therapeutic milieu and a growth-promoting and corrective emotional experience, ambulatory care administrators have to be concerned not only about the quality of clinical staff but also the security of patients and staff, the physical setup, the quality of supportive staff, and the availability of vans and other transportation, among other factors.

SUMMARY

Ambulatory treatment of children and adolescents is growing rapidly. There is emphasis on treatment of children and adolescents in their natural home, school, and community environment instead of clinic-based treatment. Managed care demands short-term interventions. Administrators of ambulatory services need to be sensitive to these demands yet also carefully address financial, clinical, and training aspects of ambulatory care.

REFERENCES

Gunderson, J. G. (1978). Defining the therapeutic process in psychiatric milieu. *Psychiatry, 41*, 327–335.

Jellinek, M. S. (1994). The outpatient milieu. *Journal of American Academy of Child and Adolescent Psychiatry, 33*(2), 277–279.

Mora, G. (1967). History of psychiatry. In A. M. Freedman & H. I. Kaplan (Eds.), *Comprehensive textbook of psychiatry*. Baltimore: Williams & Wilkins.

Parry-Jones, W. (1994). History of child and adolescent psychiatry. In M. Rutter, E. Taylor, & L. Hersov (Eds.), *Child and adolescent psychiatry: Modern approaches*. Oxford: Blackwell Science Ltd.

Waltos, D. H. (1994). Nursing services: Coaching the patient to improved mental health. In H. S. Ghuman & R. Sarles (Eds.), *Handbook of adolescent inpatient psychiatric treatment*. New York: Brunner/Mazel.

Winkler, J. K., & Bromberg W. (1939). *Mind explorers*. New York: Reynal & Hitchcock.

Chapter 2

The Specialty Clinic: A Bridge Between Research and Clinical Practice

Bruno J. Anthony, Ph.D.

The number of specialty clinics and programs focused on the behavioral and emotional problems of adults, adolescents, and children have increased over the past 10 years. In general, development of these clinics has been based on the notion that assessment and treatment decisions are best made with a consistently applied theoretical framework, solid research findings, and documented treatment programs.

This growth has been fueled by several forces. First, there has been an explosion in information concerning a range of child and adolescent psychiatric disorders over the past 10 years. Recognition of the high prevalence of behavioral and emotional problems in youth under 18 years (17%–22%) and the importance of such problems to later functioning have heightened the significance of early intervention. Significant progress in defining and distinguishing psychiatric problems has been coupled with the development of better practices and instruments to assess them.

A second spur to specialty clinic development has been the growth in research into the psychological and pharmacological treatment of children and adolescents. This effort has produced targeted therapies for more circumscribed types of therapies which have begun to find their way to clinical practice. Treatment programs, protocols, and associated manuals and materials are appearing. However, as the following discussion shows, research findings often do not fit the needs of outpatient treatment. Specialty clinics provide an important setting to bridge the gap between research and practice.

A third factor leading to the increase in specialty clinics is their ability to attract patients to an outpatient program. Consumers are often unclear about how their particular constellation of symptoms falls into the general area of mental health problems. It is our experience that information provided by schools, the media, and by word-of-mouth is usually disorder-specific. Individuals tend to match the problems they or their children are experiencing to these templates and then look for help. The recent upsurge in interest in adult

Attention Deficit/Hyperactivity Disorder (ADHD) is an example of this pattern. Although, as with adult ADHD, self-diagnosis can often be inaccurate or misleading, the presence of a program offering specific help for these problems is a drawing card. The ability to attract a substantial numbers of patients with circumscribed problems enhances research efforts by allowing for more rapid collection of data. Finally, specialty clinics, containing well-investigated assessment methods and treatment protocols, make sense to health care administrators (in health maintenance organizations [HMOs], managed care organizations, and hospital and community clinics) who are looking for effective mental health care based on the most cost-effective dose and duration.

TYPES OF CLINICS

Specialty clinics are based on procedures and instruments developed in research-based programs often affiliated with university psychology and psychiatry departments. These programs are often integrated into an outpatient clinical service; however, because of their research emphasis, the methods may be more difficult to apply in a non-academic setting. Still, the procedures, particularly the assessment tools and manualized treatment protocols, provide a strong base for the development of specialty clinic programs that are sensitive to the realities and changing demands of clinical practice. The structure of these programs varies greatly from small enterprises involving one focused intervention to larger centers with a variety of functions.

The most common outpatient speciality clinics for children and adolescents have been developed to address specific mental health problems. Less frequently, programs are developed on the basis of particular therapeutic modalities (e.g., cognitive behavior clinics, psychopharmacology clinics). The following discussion looks at selected programs which focus on specific mental health problem areas. This discussion must not be construed to be exhaustive. Clinics devoted to Attention Deficit/Hyperactivity Disorder have been the most frequently developed because of the high prevalence of the disorder (3%–11% of school-age children), its debilitating effects on school and social functioning in combination with its frequently associated aggressive and learning problems, the relatively extensive amount of research generated on assessment of the problem areas, and the availability of effective treatment for the core symptoms. One of the most productive programs in terms of the development of assessment and treatment methodology has been the ADHD clinic at the University of Massachusetts Medical Center, developed by Russell Barkley and colleagues. Barkley's 1990 book and accompanying workbook provide a comprehensive guide to a biopsychosocial assessment of ADHD children and adolescents and carefully designed treatment modules involving parent training, family therapy, and social-skills and peer relationship training. Each module presents a structured, session-by-session description of goals and procedures.

Gordon (1993) also put together a practical book about setting up an ADHD speciality clinic. The Summer Treatment Program (STP) and the associated Saturday Treatment Program (SaTP) at the University of Pittsburgh Medical Center, pioneered by Pelham, is an innovative specialty service for ADHD children and adolescents. It involves an intensive eight-week summer program of assessment, evaluation, and treatment (stressing systematic reward-response programs, social skills training, strong parent involvement and training, and close medication management) carried out by a small cadre of professionals supplemented by a large group of paraprofessionals. The SaTP occurs biweekly during the school year to cement gains and enhance generalization. The STP boasts an extremely high satisfaction and completion rate (97%) and strong effects of the treatment package (Pelham & Hoza, 1996). This program has been used successfully in a variety of settings and, according to the developers, can be developed by mental health centers, school districts, and group private practices.

Kendall (1992) pioneered development of the assessment and cognitive-behavioral treatment of anxiety in children through the mechanism of the Child and Adolescent Anxiety Disorders Clinic at Temple University, a combination service provision and research program. The clinic involves an individually tailored but structured program of about 20 sessions divided among an educational focus, identifying and altering anxious cognitions, and gradual exposure to fear-producing events (Kendall, 1992; Kendall, Kane, Howard, & Siqueland, 1990). The program for latency-age children has developed a number of useful assessment devices as well as developmentally appropriate materials and innovative techniques (workbooks, stickers, and videotaped "commercials").

Another specialty clinic has developed group-based treatment packages for anxiety disorders also involving cognitive-behavioral techniques. Silverman and colleagues (Silverman & Kurtines, 1996), through the Child and Family Psychosocial Research Center at Florida International University, promote a "pragmatic" treatment approach that makes a great deal of sense for the development of speciality clinics. Their goal is to integrate and combine the most efficacious procedures and adapt them for practitioners' use. This process has produced a 10- to 12-week, exposure-based Group Cognitive Behavioral Treatment (GCBT) with separate sessions for youth and parents. The program has been applied to phobias, overanxious disorders, and post-traumatic stress disorder and focuses on a "transfer of control" model; contingency management skills are passed from therapist to parent and self-control skills from therapist to child. The group process facilitates the latter process through peer reinforcement and modeling.

Programs specializing in the treatment of mood disorders tend to integrate a variety of behavioral and cognitive behavioral approaches. Psychopharmacological interventions are employed; however, the equivocal effectiveness of antidepressant medication with children and adolescents has placed more emphasis on the development of effective psychosocial treatment. These programs vary in their use of individual, group, and parent/family, although most tend to use a combination of these modalities. Particular treatment interventions are linked with specific, empirically defined disturbances, and particular sets of interventions are selected based on the specific problems exhibited by the child or adolescent (Lewinsohn, Clarke, & Rohde, 1994; Stark & Kendall, 1996). Mood and motivational symptoms are approached with educational activities (e.g., emotional lability, self-monitoring), often in game formats, with goal-directed and pleasant events scheduling, emphasizing mastery, and with the development of coping skills.

Problem-solving and cognitive restructuring are used when the child's disturbance includes social dysfunction and negative thoughts, expectations, and self-evaluations. Parent training components are used commonly to educate, reduce conflict and improve communication, and develop a more structured home environment to support the child's attempts to cope with his or her mood-related difficulties. Specialty mood-disorder clinics have also begun to evaluate interpersonal therapy for depressed adolescents, using procedures derived from adult studies (Mufson, Moreau, Weissman, & Klerman, 1993).

FUNCTIONING

The following section provides suggestions on the administrative, service development, and teaching and research functioning of specialty clinics. Discussion will draw heavily on our experience with the Maryland Center for Attention Disorders (MCAD), a multidisciplinary program operating within the Division of Child and Adolescent Psychiatry of the Department of Psychiatry of the University of Maryland Medical System. The MCAD was founded in 1991 and has experienced growth, particularly over the last two years, in the number of referrals for evaluation, the number of patients in treatment, the size of the clinical and administrative staff, and in the research generated.

Administrative and Financial Aspects

Specialty clinics require a core group of individuals, with expertise and credentials in a particular area, to provide direction to the program and to "market the product." To distinguish them from more traditional approaches to outpatient care, specialty clinics tout a comprehensive approach to evaluation and treatment. For instance, the MCAD evaluation sequence involves an initial diagnostic interview with the patient's parents followed up by a family assessment, a review of educational history, and a psychiatric interview to discuss medication status and history. Information from all these interviews is combined with checklists and testing data to produce an accurate formulation and useful recommendations.

The director of the clinic should provide the overall direction; however, to best implement a multidisciplinary approach, coordinators, with specific training in particular aspects of program, should be identified. In the MCAD, we have coordinators for individual and family assessment and treatment, a medical coordinator, and an educational consultant. These coordinators are responsible for all care within their area which includes direct service, supervision, report writing, and community outreach. The latter function is particularly important. We have found it very successful to develop in-service programs in which several staff members present our coordinated approach to evaluation and treatment. Also, we encourage our coordinators to present separately to both lay and professional audiences in the area of their expertise.

The level of administrative support depends on the structure of the outpatient program within which the specialty clinic is situated. Patient volumes often do not justify the employment of full-time secretarial coverage; therefore, a sharing arrangement with other outpatient programs, housed within the same physical space, is the best alternative. Besides traditional functions of scheduling, telephone answering, communication, and word processing, support staff of a specialty clinic must also learn to computer-score assessment tools and, if appropriate, manage a database.

With the increasing influence of managed care, it is critical that a person within the support staff be trained in the intricacies of gaining authorization from insurance companies and an understanding of the structure of the sometimes complicated reimbursement schedules. This is particularly important for the specialty clinic whose structure often does not fit easily into reimbursement patterns of third-party payers. As an example, most insurance companies allow only one diagnostic interview session; therefore, other aspects of the evaluation must often be coded under other procedures (e.g., individual therapy, family therapy, psychopharmacological consultation). We have found it best to provide insurers with a written explanation of our evaluation procedures and their justification.

Staffing Patterns   It is our opinion that specialty clinics, whether university-based or not, work best when developed because of clinical/research interest by the participants, not only because of market pressures. Although part of the Department of Psychiatry, the MCAD operates like a free-standing outpatient clinic. Whereas many specialty clinics derive their clinicians from the graduate student population, who participate as part of their training and research duties, all of the work, except for administration of psychological/neuropsychological testing, is carried out by faculty and staff, many of whom participate, in part, to generate income. Depending on how the professional staff is reimbursed, the early development period of a specialty clinic may result in a low funds collected to time invested ratio. The interest of the specialty center staff and the rewards of multidisciplinary clinical work and research serve to maintain morale during the development period.

The MCAD began with a core group of clinicians who had worked extensively with ADHD children in inpatient and outpatient settings. Dr. Anthony, the director, has been an active researcher in the area of attention and its dysfunction prior to coming to the university. Others within the department were recruited to coordinate different aspects of the care of ADHD children: experienced family therapists (licensed social workers and psychiatric nurses) to assess family functioning and develop and implement a family-based treatment program as well as child and parent groups; a child and adolescent psychiatrist to perform diagnostic evaluations and follow patients for medication management; and, an educational consultant (special educator) to participate in psychoeducational evaluations and confer with school personnel, transmit the educational recommendations, and participate in school meetings.

Specialty clinics often concentrate on assessment. However, these functions tend to be labor-intensive and less adequately reimbursed, in large part, because of the staff time put into registering and scheduling patients, verifying insurance, and report writing. For a specialty clinic to survive, a strong intervention program must be developed quickly. A cadre of clinicians needs to be recruited who share the goals of the clinic and who are willing to implement more consistent and more structured types of therapeutic programs.

Procedures

Referral   A steady flow of referrals depends on several factors. First, the "product" of the evaluation must be viewed as professional and useful by both the referring source, those to whom the report is forwarded (e.g., schools, pediatrician, therapists), and the family. At our center, staff involved in the process jointly contribute to a report, adding sections to a template available to all on a common computer directory. The production of a comprehensive report of an evaluation is often time-consuming; however, we have experienced very positive response to our reports and they have served to generate referrals. Second, referrals are stimulated by direct community outreach. We cannot emphasize this fact too much.

As noted previously, we encourage the professional staff to speak to a wide range of audiences. The MCAD group has presented research findings and clinical workshops to mental health professionals at conventions, grand rounds, continuing education programs, and special conferences. We also provide in-service presentations to school groups. We work closely with local self-help organizations, serving on advisory boards and providing informational presentations to lay audiences. Finally, we make ourselves available to the media. Working within a university/hospital setting is an advantage since media outlets often contact these sources first.

Assessment   Evaluation services are usually an important part of a specialty clinic. Given the goal of a comprehensive, relatively standardized, multidisciplinary approach, the clinic usually offers an assessment sequence that involves several types of evaluation interviews, standardized checklists and self-report instruments, and psychological testing. Specialty clinics often entail a team approach in which several staff are involved in the evaluation of a patient and the family. To promote integration, the assessment process is best served by including a team meeting for all concerned to discuss ongoing cases and prepare for new ones. In the MCAD, evaluations occur during one morning per week (8:30 a.m.– 12:30 p.m.) which begins with a 60-minute team meeting. For the next three hours, the team meets with several families, each of which may be at a different stage in the evaluation process.

Evaluation usually involves three to four visits: a parent interview to discuss presenting problems and developmental history, two further visits to complete the family and psychiatric interviews and psychological testing (if required), and a final wrap-up session in which results and recommendations are conveyed. We have found this structure to be the most time-efficient because all staff are at work for most of the morning and communication is enhanced. Moreover, we found that trying to squeeze the entire evaluation into one morning was quite taxing on the child and the family. In addition, the structure proved the most conducive for teaching purposes.

One of the advantages of specialty clinics is the ability to expand on traditional notions of evaluation. Clinics tend to administer a standard assessment protocol, collecting the same data in the same way for most patients who enter the program. This consistent practice ensures that relevant information is gathered from all patients and allows for more confidence in the diagnostic process. Collecting a wide range of data on individuals and their families is particularly important in evaluating comorbid conditions. In addition, it permits the development of a database which can be used for program evaluation as well as research purposes. Although becoming more prevalent, standardized assessment is still a rare commodity in outpatient treatment. The assessment protocol for the MCAD is presented in Table 1.

The use of well-normed, standardized information-gathering tools is an important aspect of the specialty clinic. As noted in this chapter and others (see chapter 8, Psychological Assessment) there are a growing number of well-developed instruments, both self-report and ratings by respondents (parents and teachers), for both broad and specialized assessment. Moreover, computer scoring of these instruments is also increasingly available, reducing the scoring burden which previously discouraged the use of such instruments. We mail out questionnaires and checklists for the family and the school in the information packet and ask parents to bring the completed forms to the first session. We have found it extremely helpful and time-efficient to be able to refer to this information during the interview. These instruments can then be re-administered after set amounts of treatment to assess effectiveness. As an aside, we have rarely encountered objections from families to the burden of completing standardized instruments, a concern often raised by practitioners.

Specialty clinics usually employ structured or semi-structured diagnostic interviews to provide a complete survey of symptomatology. Although the questions are often overlapping with information requested in the checklist and questionnaires, we find that, often, the latter questions are not understood by parents and answers change with further explication. There are several structured interviews available; however, complete administration tends to be lengthy and somewhat awkward. Specialty clinics must weigh these factors

Table 1 Assessment Protocol: Maryland Center for Attention Disorders

	Children/Adolescents	Adults
Ratings by Others	• Child Behavior Checklist (CBCL; Achenbach, 1991a) • CBCL Teacher Report Form (Achenbach, 1991b) • Disruptive Behavior Checklist • Home Situations Questionnaire (Barkley, 1991)	• Parent's Rating Scale (Wender, 1995)
Self Report	• Revised Children's Manifest Anxiety Scale (Reynolds & Richmond, 1985) • Child Depression Inventory (Kovacs, 1992) • CBCL Youth Self Report (Achenbach, 1991c)	• Wender Utah Rating Scale (Ward, Wender, & Reimherr, 1993) • Patient's Behavior Checklist for ADHD Adults (Barkley, 1991) • Self-Rating Symptom Checklist for ADHD Adults (Barkley, 1991) • SCL-90-R (DeRogatis, 1975)
Medical/ Developmental	• Developmental Factors (Barkley, 1991)	• Medical History, Developmental History, Physical Complaints Checklist (Barkley, 1991)
Interview	• Semi-structured Parent Interview • Semi-structured Family Interview	• Semi-structured Interview
Testing	• Continuous Performance Tests (visual and auditory) • Digit Cancellation Test • Wide Range Assessment of Memory and Learning subtests (Verbal Learning, Story Memory, Finger Windows, Sentence Memory) • Wisconsin Card Sorting Test • Wechsler Intelligence Scale for Children-3rd Edition subtests (Arithmetic, Vocabulary, Digit Span, Coding, Block Design, Symbol Search)	• Continuous Performance Tests (visual and auditory) • Letter Cancellation Test • Wechsler Memory Scale subtests (Logical Memory, Verbal Paired Associates, Visual Memory Span) • Wisconsin Card Sorting Test • Wechsler Adult Intelligence Scale for Adults-3rd Edition subtests (Arithmetic, Vocabulary, Digit Span, Digit Symbol-Substitution, Block Design)

against the requirements of such interviews for the publication of studies in which accurate diagnosis is a critical feature.

Some of these instruments, particularly the DICA-R, have been made more user-friendly and allow the option of using only certain diagnostic modules. Also, specialty clinics have produced their own structured interviews which concentrate on the particular disorder such as the Anxiety Disorder Interview Schedule for Children and Adolescents (Silverman & Albano, 1996). We have followed the option of crafting our own parent interview based on one used in the University of Massachusetts ADHD clinic (Barkley, 1991) which most efficiently serves our purposes. We also include a semi-structured family assessment interview in our evaluation sequence.

We feel strongly that changes in a child's or adolescents behavior, cognitions, and feelings will not be successful unless we take into account family structure, conflicts, and discipline practices. Besides gaining valuable information on the process of conflict within the home as well as intervention targets, this assessment begins to reframe individual problems within a family context and avoid taking a blaming, accusatory stance toward the patient.

TREATMENT

Research-based specialty programs have tended to be focused on a few treatment modalities, particularly behavior-modification and cognitive-behavioral techniques, and have tended to study non-referred populations displaying problems of mild severity and relatively uncomplicated presentations. Moreover, the resulting manualized treatment protocols have been quite restricted in their focus using a "one size fits all" approach that does not take into account the palatability of the procedures for parents and children (Jensen, Hibbs, & Pilkonis, 1996). Treatment in specialty clinics needs to build on outcome research yet modify these protocols to make them feasible, sensible, and palatable. The specialty clinic must focus on multiple modalities of treatment and multiple domains of functioning, incorporate the family's input, and, in general, tailor the treatment to specific clinical and developmental needs of the child and family.

The necessary "remodeling" of research-based interventions is illustrated by the development, in our center, of a program for families consisting of parallel parent and child groups. The program included modules on behavioral management, social skill training, and self-control drawn from several sources. However, we found that we could not implement the program in as structured a manner as devised. Participating parents were in substantial distress at the beginning of the program and first needed to establish a positive and supportive bond with the therapist and among themselves. Therefore, we included several sessions at the beginning of the program to build group cohesion. We also had to modify the child group structure. Our center frequently enrolls children with comorbid mood, anxiety, and oppositional problems and significant social difficulties, who have failed in treatment elsewhere. These difficulties forced a reduction in the nature and extent of the training. These experiences have led us to rely less on group treatment for young ADHD children.

Although research-based treatment packages are valuable starting points in outpatient treatment, it is usually inadvisable to simply follow a set program. In fact, some research suggests that adhering too closely to a treatment manual can reduce clinical effectiveness (Henry, Strupp, Butler, Schacht, & Binder, 1993). Rather, the major components of the treatment protocol need to be kept in mind along with those aspects of the person and family which may influence effectiveness and modifications in the protocol which minimize these obstacles. In this vein, individual modules of treatment packages can be used within outpatient therapy in a flexible manner.

TEACHING AND RESEARCH

The structure of a specialty clinic provides an ideal setting for training. Given the multidisciplinary/coordinated approach, trainees gain a rapid exposure to a variety of perspectives on a field. We gradually integrate trainees into the assessment sequence of the clinic, first requiring that they sit in with an experienced clinician before they carry out the particular assessment themselves. From the beginning, however, the trainee takes on administrative responsibility for a case, ensuring coordination among the different assessment components as well as pulling together the written report. In university-based clinics, trainees carry the major treatment burden. In outpatient settings in which patient selection does not ensure a homogeneous group with reduced co-morbidity, treatment tends to be more complex and require more experience. We carefully choose the cases that trainees are allowed to handle alone. However, they are immediately involved in group and family work as co-therapists.

The use of standard assessment protocols allows for the development of a database which can form the basis for research efforts within the clinic. The development of such a database requires the cooperation of clinicians in collecting the information. This cooperation is often difficult to achieve as clinical demands increase and therefore must be consistently reinforced. It is important to provide summaries that have clinical relevance and involve the staff in presentations and publications based on the findings.

CONCLUSION

Specialty clinics focus the efforts of professionals with substantial experience and interest in a particular mental health arena to provide more efficient and effective assessment and intervention and to increase understanding. They have the potential to bridge the gap between research-based programs and mental health practitioners by adapting the sometimes rigidly constrained methods developed in the clinical laboratory to take account of developmental changes, the timing and pacing of interventions, individual differences, and patient palatability—issues important to clinical practice with children, adolescents, and families. Specialty clinics also provide excellent opportunities for the training of clinicians in techniques to improve implementation of treatment programs and resulting therapeutic effects. Although not demanding absolute adherence to a protocol, their use of a limited set of interventions and the availability of large numbers of children and adolescents with a particular problem allow for more monitoring and training to promote treatment integrity. It is our opinion that the combination of experienced staff and well-developed methods leads to more effective and judicious assessment and intervention. In addition, the presence of a circumscribed common area of attention and well-defined procedures increases multidisciplinary interaction and collaboration and fosters research efforts.

Specialty clinics still represent a small part of outpatient mental health services. However, the continued increase in focused assessment devices and interventions facilitates the growth of such programs. Moreover, if developed well, they provide a solid, well-tested alternative to approach the large changes in mental health systems and reimbursement as well as increasingly sophisticated and empowered consumers.

REFERENCES

Achenbach, T. M. (1991a). *Manual for the child behavior checklist/4–18 and 1991 profile*. Burlington, VT: University of Vermont, Department of Psychiatry.

Achenbach, T. M. (1991b). *Manual for the teacher's report form and 1991 profile*. Burlington, VT: University of Vermont, Department of Psychiatry.

Achenbach, T. M. (1991c). *Manual for the youth self-report and 1991 profile*. Burlington, VT: University of Vermont, Department of Psychiatry.

Barkley, R. A. (1990). *Attention deficit hyperactivity disorder: A handbook for diagnosis and treatment.* New York: Guilford Press.

Barkley, R. A. (1991). *Attention-deficit hyperactivity disorder. A clinical workbook.* New York: Guilford Press.

DeRogatis, L. R. (1975). *SCL-90-R manual-II.* Towson, MD: Clinical Psychometric Research.

Gordon, M. (1993). *How to operate an ADHD clinic or subspecialty practice.* DeWitt, NY: GSI Publications.

Henry, W. P., Strupp, H. H., Butler, S. F., Schacht, T. E., & Binder, J. L. (1993). Effects of training in time-limited dynamic psychotherapy: Changes in therapist behavior. *Journal of Consulting and Clinical Psychology, 61,* 434–440.

Jensen, P. S., Hibbs, E.D., & Pilkonis, P. A. (1996). From ivory tower to clinical practice: Future directions for child and adolescent psychotherapy research. In E. D. Hibbs & P. S. Jensen (Eds.), *Psychosocial treatments for child and adolescent disorders* (pp. 311–340). Washington, DC: American Psychological Association

Kendall, P. C. (1992). *Coping at workbook.* Ardmore, PA: Workbook Publishing.

Kendall, P. C., Kane, M., Howard, B., & Siqueland, L. (1990). *Cognitive-behavioral therapy for anxious children: Treatment manual.* Ardmore, PA: Workbook Publishing.

Kovacs, M. (1992). *Children's depression inventory.* San Antonio, TX: Psychological Corporation.

Lewinsohn, P. M., Clarke, G. N., & Rohde, P. (1994). Psychological approaches to the treatment of depression in adolescents. In W. M. Reynolds & H. F. Johnston (Eds.), *Handbook of depression in children and adolescents* (pp. 309–344). New York: Plenum Press.

Marten, P. A., Albano, A. M., & Holt, C. S. (1991). *Cognitive-behavioral group treatment for adolescent social phobia with parent participation: Therapist's manual.* Unpublished manuscript, State University of New York at Albany.

Mufson, L., Moreau, D., Weissman, M. M., & Klerman, G. L. (1993). *Interpersonal psychotherapy for depressed adolescents.* New York: Guilford Press.

Pelham, W. E. (1994). *Children's summer day treatment program manual.* Unpublished manuscript, Western Psychiatric Institute and Clinic, University of Pittsburgh Medical Center, Pittsburgh, PA.

Pelham, W. E., & Hoza, B. (1996). Intensive treatment: A summer treatment program for children with ADHD. In E. D. Hibbs & P. S. Jensen (Eds.), *Psychosocial treatments for child and adolescent disorders* (pp. 311–340). Washington, DC: American Psychological Association.

Reynolds, C. R., & Richmond, B. O. (1985). *Revised children's manifest anxiety scale manual.* Los Angeles: Western Psychological Services.

Silverman, W. K., & Albano, A. M. (1996). *The anxiety disorders interview schedule for children-IV (child and parent version).* Albany, NY: Greywind Publications.

Silverman, W. K., & Kurtines, W. M. (1996). *Anxiety and phobic disorders: A pragmatic approach.* New York: Plenum Press.

Stark, K. D., & Kendall, P. C. (1996). *Treating depressed children: Therapist's manual for "ACTION."* Ardmore, PA: Workbook Publishing.

Ward, M. F., Wender, P. H., & Reimherr, F. W. (1993). The Wender-Utah Rating Scale: An aid in the retrospective diagnosis of childhood Attention Deficit Hyperactivity Disorder. *American Journal of Psychiatry, 150,* 885–890.

Wender, P. H. (1995). *Attention-deficit hyperactivity disorder in adults.* New York: Oxford University Press.

Chapter 3

Child and Adolescent Services in a Community Mental Health Center: Transition, Organization, and Staffing Issues

Eileen Hastings, R.N.C., L.C.S.W.C., Marsha Gorth, L.C.S.W.C., and Harinder S. Ghuman, M.D.

INTRODUCTION

Despite a growing awareness that traditional (office-based, by appointment) outpatient mental health services are not the treatment of choice for many of the increasing numbers of seriously emotionally disturbed (SED) children, they remain the primary psychiatric treatment delivered to this population. SED children are presented with multiple and complex problems that cannot be addressed adequately without intervening in the many systems in which the child lives. Since the 1980s, with the establishment of the Child and Adolescent Service System Program (CASSP), a National Institute of Mental Health (NIMH) initiative, this group of children has been defined and targeted as a priority by the public mental health sector. CASSP identified the need to develop a service system that focused on individualized treatment plans for these children with the family as a partner in the effort. Stroul and Friedman (1986) urged that outpatient programs develop flexibility in intensity, immediacy, and accessibility (both in location and hours) of services. Outcome data are needed to match consumers and problems to the appropriate type and level of care.

While many strategies have been successfully implemented in the treatment of seriously and persistently mentally ill adults, services to children have been slower to adapt to the changing needs of their consumers. In addition to lack of funding, the enormity of coordination between huge bureaucratic systems such as mental health, juvenile justice, schools and social services, has been an obstacle in moving ahead with the necessary reforms.

In this chapter, we describe the present structure and function of a recently privatized, traditional outpatient community mental health clinic (The Walter P. Carter Clinics) struggling with how to conceptualize and implement system change as a result of privatization and in preparation for Medicaid and Medicare reform. The clinic program described was a state-funded and governed agency which was privatized in January 1993 by the University of Maryland with which it had been affiliated. Privatization was the result of a state budgetary shortfall and was accomplished within a 90-day period from announcement to implementation.

Although the time frame was extremely short, the process involved significant alteration of some processes, procedures, and structure which had not been effective under the state system. Administrative and billing functions were completely revised and efficiency and effectiveness improved. Reduction of the clinical and support staff (from 71 to 36) led to an increase in caseload size from an average of 20 patients per C&A clinician to 30 patients per clinician and a demand for increased productivity. Many staff chose to remain with the state system, resulting in the hire of approximately 12 new employees. Two-thirds of the staff made the transition to the new system, but they experienced the loss of tenure, sick leave, and other benefits which many had earned over years of state service. Two of the four existing clinics were operated on a part- time basis for the first six months following privatization and were subsequently closed as a result of excessive overhead and decreased staffing.

The sense of loss by the staff, patients, and community was a tangible issue which required constant attention for the transition to proceed. Numerous meetings were held to address staff concerns about job security and benefits under the university. Community meetings took place in which state and university officials were present to address community concerns. Patients were reassigned as quickly as personnel hiring permitted with an effort to maintain stability with either their therapist and/or psychiatrist.

Despite some of the major administrative and structural changes that took place with privatization, the effect on the clinical service delivery system was limited. Under state auspices, the clinics were JCAHO-accredited and were licensed under the Code of Maryland Regulations (COMAR). While the mandate for the program is unchanged and the same regulations apply, the changing nature of health care and consumer need demands that clinical services adapt. Administration and staff struggled with major decisions around reorganization and redefinition of the clinical program.

The clinic program had been in existence since 1976 and evolved into a team-based treatment service. The clinic's consumer base consists of inner-city residents with multiple social and economic problems which complicate any presenting mental health issue. It was and is our belief that small, close-knit groups of multidisciplinary staff serving a specific population of children and adolescents is the most efficient, effective, and coordinated way to deliver a variety of mental health services. The team represents a variety of clinical and social perspectives which allow for more creative treatment planning. This model also provides peer support for staff who often are faced with complex and overwhelming clinical situations. It is important to place this team-based system within the larger context which follows.

ADMINISTRATIVE STRUCTURE

External Service System

The structure of a treatment program is extremely important to its ultimate fiscal and clinical success. The child and adolescent outpatient clinic service is embedded in a large inner-city community mental health center which serves constituents in the southern and southwestern part of Baltimore City. The program is affiliated with a teaching university hospital and is governed by a citywide core service agency (CSA) which coordinates public mental health services for seriously and persistently mentally ill (SPMI) adults and seriously emotionally disturbed (SED) children in Baltimore City. The Baltimore City CSA oversees seven public mental health "lead agencies" that together are responsible for the provision of all public mental health services within their respective catchment areas.

The Child and Adolescent clinic program is administratively under the University of Maryland Department of Psychiatry's Division of Community Psychiatry. This division consists of several components, the Program in Assertive Community Treatment (PACT) teams, an outpatient community mental health program, a large psychiatric residential and rehabilitation program, a psychiatric urgent care program, case management services for adults, an adult substance abuse program, and a specialized program for children ages 5 years and under at risk for emotional problems. The Division of Community Psychiatry is fiscally responsible to the CSA which oversees the distribution of state grant dollars to each lead agency in the city and monitors the fiscal and service operation of each lead agency's budget. The budgets of this division's programs are in restricted accounts outside the Department of Psychiatry's and hospital's budgets. The two C&A programs in this division report jointly to the Director of the Division of Community Psychiatry and to the Director of the Division of Child and Adolescent Psychiatry. This dual reporting can, and has, led to blurring of the lines of authority. The Department of Psychiatry is taking steps to address this potential for fragmentation by creating a new faculty position with responsibility to coordinate child psychiatric services throughout the department and hospital.

The mission of the clinics, as part of the Division of Community Psychiatry, is to deliver a wide range of mental health services for the residents of the catchment area who seek treatment. As part of a university hospital, teaching and research are also a part of our mission and commitment.

Internal Service System

The clinic program has an internal structure that has facilitated the accomplishment of its threefold mission. The outpatient program has two geographic sites which allow for easy access by most consumers. There are 1,550 active cases with approximately 21.3 percent of these (330) being children and adolescents.

There is a Program Director and Medical Director responsible for the overall clinical programming and administration of the clinics. Each site has a Clinic Coordinator who is a senior mental health professional who reports to the Program Director for the day-to-day management of the personnel and clinic sites. Each site has a multidisciplinary adult treatment team and a C&A treatment team administered by team leaders who are responsible to the Clinic Coordinators. The medical staff of the clinics are responsible for the clinical/medical treatment provided within the outpatient program. The child and adolescent service has a medical director who reports to the Program and Medical directors for programming of C&A services across both sites. An executive committee consisting of the Program Director, Medical Director, C&A Medical Director, Clinic Coordinators, and senior clinic psychiatrists meets weekly and makes administrative and programming decisions. The entire medical staff meets twice monthly with the Medical Director to discuss issues relating to clinical practice.

It has always been an advantage to have adult and child services coexisting within the same program. Families with multiple problems often require treatment of both the adults and children. Our structure has allowed close collaboration, coordination, and joint treatment of such families within the same physical setting.

CLINICAL SERVICES

The clinics were originally established as traditional office-based services where patients were expected to come for appointments. The range of services include evaluation/diagnostic services (psychiatric and psychological), outreach, crisis intervention, psychopharmacology, and a variety of therapies (individual, play, group, family, etc.). Individual and play therapy still represent the bulk of the treatment services provided. However, in the past few years group, family therapy, and parenting classes have increasingly been emphasized. Substance abuse treatment is now integrated into the C&A teams and several groups of varying ages are ongoing. Because exposure to substance abuse within the family is so pervasive in our patient population, a family group focusing on substance abuse has been established.

As Friedman (1996) noted in his discussion of mental health policy for children, there has been an increase in the rate and severity of mental disorders in children. Children are presenting for treatment at a younger age and the multiplicity of problems in the family and social environment contributes to the ineffectiveness of traditional services. Shorter hospital and residential treatment stays also contribute to the increase in the number of seriously ill children in the community. Clinic therapists have always acted as case managers for their patients, but this aspect of the treatment is now demanding more and more time, and often requires out of office interventions.

It was in response to this that we established the Child Mobile Team (CMT) which specifically targets patients identified by the C&A treatment teams who require more intensive psychiatric treatment and case management/wrap-around services. Maryland has implemented the psychiatric rehabilitation option which allows for reimbursement of off-site treatment services. This revenue generation potential has created important incentives for the delivery of off-site services and allowed for the expansion of this service. The team has been in existence since January 1995 and is still in its infancy in terms of size and program development.

We are planning to increase the staffing of the CMT and evolve it into a freestanding treatment team utilizing principles from the adult PACT team model (Burns & Santos, 1995) and the multisystemic approach of Henggeler, Schoenwald, Pickrel, Rowland, and Santos (1994). More specialization and expertise with conduct disorders and adjudicated youth are also needed. We can no longer fall back on the refrain, "This child is not appropriate for outpatient services." Our system is now accepting that these difficult to treat patients are our consumers and we are obligated to develop a system of care that can address the needs they present rather than blame the consumer and exonerate ourselves. This is our challenge.

TEAM STRUCTURE AND STAFFING PATTERN

C&A team size in the clinics varies from 5 to 12 permanent staff. All teams within the clinic are multidisciplinary with the four core professions (psychiatry, psychology, nursing, and social work) represented. Substance abuse staff from the Division of Community Psychiatry's substance abuse program work part-time in each clinic providing dual-diagnosis evaluations, treatment, and staff training on all teams. In the C&A service, the Child Mobile

Team utilizes a community support specialist (bachelor's- or master's-prepared counselor). Trainees from a variety of disciplines are regular members of the treatment teams. Psychology interns at the master's and Ph.D. levels, psychiatric residents, and master's-level social work students are placed for one-year rotations on each team.

As part of the collaboration with the Division of C&A Psychiatry, school-based mental health staff work some hours per week in the CMHC carrying a small caseload. This staff works primarily within the city schools in an innovative program providing primary, secondary, and tertiary mental health services in vivo. Working in the CMHC for a few hours per week has been instrumental in establishing closer bonds with the school system and in facilitating referrals for more long-term treatment.

CASELOAD SIZE

The size of clinicians' caseload is dependent on the service (adult versus C&A) and the nature of the team function (traditional outpatient services versus mobile case management/treatment). The CSA had set standards for adult and C&A services in both caseload size and productivity requirements by clinician and program. Caseload size for the C&A outpatient treatment teams is set at 1 clinician to 30 patients with an expectation of 18 to 20 hours per week of face-to-face clinical service per FTE. The caseload expectation for the CMT is 1:12 with the same direct service expectation (18 to 20 hours per week).

There are no CSA-established standards for the psychiatrists' caseloads. However, the Director of the Division of Community Psychiatry has set standards for all services using the baseline of 1:200 patients per FTE on the adult service. This has been the modal ratio established over years of practice. Goldman, Faulkner, and Breeding (1994) suggested an ideal of 1:225 as a "desired level of care" for psychiatrists in an adult CMHC. A ratio of 1:100 for the C&A service was set, taking into consideration the labor intensity of working with children and their families. Psychiatrists' clinical responsibilities consist primarily of conducting diagnostic evaluations and prescribing medications. However, the responsibility for clinical oversight of all treatment rests with the team physicians.

STAFF RECRUITMENT

Turnover in our program on all teams has been minimal. However, with the demand for increased productivity and new treatment strategies and the advent of managed care external reviews, a slight increase in turnover has been noted recently. Staff with solid clinical skills who are flexible and creative are desired to maintain clinical standards in light of fiscal constraints. The clinic program has used a "committee" model of recruitment for non-medical staff in which the program director, clinic coordinator, and team leader of the team where the vacancy exists interview all prospective candidates. The top two to three candidates are then interviewed by the team psychiatrist prior to a final decision which is collaborative. This method allows the candidate to meet the primary administrative staff and provides validation for the interviewers. We have found that poor personnel choices are less likely to occur with such an interview process. Faculty recruitment is a more lengthy process that involves department-wide participation because most faculty have split responsibilities. However, the key staff in the clinical program are a part of the process and have a voice in the decision.

PERSONNEL ORIENTATION

It has been our experience that this is an often overlooked aspect of the hiring process. In an organization as large and complex as ours, it is imperative that orientation occurs on multiple levels. The hospital conducts an orientation in several areas: benefits/compensation, hospital mission and values, personnel policies, and key operating procedures such as infection control, fire/safety, and so on. This process occurs within the first month of employment, usually in the first week.

It is left to the department and individual programs to orient the employee to policies and procedures at these levels. Minimal guidelines are given and the result is a varied experience from program to program. The clinic has evolved a fairly lengthy and detailed orientation conducted within the first two weeks of employment that is aimed at orienting the employee to the department/division context of the employee's position and to specific program policies and procedures.

New staff meet with other Division of Community Psychiatry program directors or their designees about the role of their program and interface with the clinics. Many clinic staff are involved in the program orientation through a series of meetings in which various aspects of the program are discussed. This includes support staff, clinical staff, and administrative staff. This process gives the new and old employees an opportunity for a mutually gratifying meeting activity.

STAGES OF STAFF AND TEAM DEVELOPMENT

Current outpatient treatment for child and adolescent mental health services is based on a community mental health model that was developed during the early 1900s to meet the needs of juvenile offenders. In 1915, Dr. William Healy and the Chicago Juvenile Court system became interested in studying youthful offenders so they might prevent these adolescents from developing into adult criminals. Dr. Healy formulated the idea of combining the disciplines of psychiatry, psychology, and social work to address the delinquency problem in a scientific manner. This study led to other demonstration projects in several other major cities conducted by the National Committee for Mental Hygiene through the Division on the Prevention of Delinquency. These projects are considered to be the origins of the early child guidance clinics.

"The psychiatrist had tried for years, without help, to handle a wide range of personality and behavior disorders, but the value of the threefold cooperation of the psychiatrist, clinical psychologist and social worker in the study and treatment of the child gradually won recognition" (Stevenson, 1934). The concept of teamwork stems from the early growth in child and adolescent services that suggests that the structure of the basic team may be considered from three angles: organic, functional, and emotional.

The organic structure is defined by the specific role of each of the team members. The functions of each member may vary or differ from one another and more directly effect the emotional structure. Attention to the personal and emotional life of the team cannot be minimized. Consequently, an ability to address tensions and unresolved conflict is critical to the internal structure of a highly organized group. A team that is well organized and harmonious will lessen the importance of individual tensions and allow for valuable discussions of problems that can be resolved within the team. Considering these factors, the team sets out to meet the program objectives through the shared task of serving a population of children and adolescents (World Health Organization [WHO], 1960).

The privatization of the Walter P. Carter Clinics in 1993 by the University of Maryland challenged the emotional life of the clinic staff. Although the delivery of services was uninterrupted, the impact on the teams was evident. In most instances, the treatment teams had existed for many years and were cohesive and well functioning. As a result of privatization, these teams were dismantled and new teams were developed that had to begin the long road back to smooth team functioning.

Prior to privatization, the child and adolescent team of one of the clinics consisted of two social workers, a psychiatric nurse, a consulting psychologist, a senior counselor, and a psychiatrist. The team was usually assigned one to two psychiatric residents. At the time we were privatized, only two social workers chose to continue with the program. Several new staff were hired: a psychiatrist, an entry-level social worker, and a part-time psychiatric nurse.

After privatization, the membership of the team gradually grew from 6 to 11 staff. The newest members of the team brought vitality and balance which initially resulted in a smooth transition and an ability to cope with the emotional upheaval of the change in governance. The first major change was the integration of school-based clinicians into the team. Clinicians were master's- prepared social workers who were primarily based in local Baltimore City schools as part of a school mental health initiative of the Baltimore City public school system and coordinated by the University of Maryland Department of Psychiatry. These social workers were only in the clinic for 8 to 10 hours per week and were unable to participate regularly in team meetings and functions. Initially, this was seen as an intrusion and burden to both the team and team leader. Coverage of cases, chart maintenance, supervision, and operational issues were, at times, problematic. The multidisciplinary approach was compromised because of the unavailability of these clinicians. Integration into the team took a much longer time, but these staff are now seen as a link with the school system and an asset to the team's work.

The second major change came with the addition of two psychology interns to each clinic team. The decision to add interns to the team was the result of fiscal changes in the Department of Psychiatry and an effort to support the training mission of the university. Interns are in the doctoral program and were expected to be in the clinic 16 hours a week providing direct clinical services. The team was asked to accept these trainees knowing that they would require more time and effort, as most of the interns were unfamiliar with community resources and the delivery of child and adolescent services in an urban community. Initially, the interns were viewed with some skepticism and animosity because of the additional time required to assist them. More importantly, it appeared that the familiarity and comfort of a small, well-coordinated team was being lost to the demands of an expanding program.

The interns were expected to meet the same standards of practice as the permanent members of the team. Initially, they were expected to cover any clinical emergencies that arose even during the time they were not scheduled to be in the clinic. This often proved unworkable and the team had to provide this backup for the cases assigned to the interns.

Clinical supervision of the interns was assigned to off-site supervisors who often were not familiar with the clinic patient population, community resources, or philosophy of treatment. These supervisors were not readily available to the interns outside the scheduled supervisory hour and, again, the team had to provide this backup. Supervisor signatures were required on all progress notes and treatment plans because of COMAR regulations, but this simple task became extremely difficult since charts are not permitted out of the clinic.

Interns were directly responsible to their training director who had to be consulted on numerous matters. This often caused tension among program directors. An example of such a dilemma occurred during a patient care monitoring conference when it became evident that the intern was uncomfortable working with a highly dysfunctional family and preferred to proceed with terminating services. The team encouraged him to consider other methods of engaging the family, but it became clear that he and his supervisor felt they had the power to make the final decision. Clarifying lines of authority and responsibility took over one year.

As we end the third year with the psychology interns, it has become easier to incorporate them into the team. For the most part, they have proven to be an asset to the multidisciplinary team and have made every effort to utilize this experience in a positive and productive way. In addition, as the permanent team members have become more confident and cohesive, it has been easier to incorporate trainees at each level.

Recently, a substance abuse counselor with dual training in addictions and child mental health joined the team. This change was met with resistance but on a more unconscious level. The team readily acknowledged the need for substance abuse expertise on the team, but did not seem able to integrate this aspect of care in their treatment. Several factors may contribute to this response. We suspect that the idea of children needing substance abuse services was still not widely accepted as most child and adolescent therapists have minimal training in this area. Additionally, the acknowledgment of the problem results in the therapist surrendering his or her authority and power to another colleague. Again, it became necessary for the substance abuse counselor to demonstrate his skill to be validated by the team.

The final change in the team was the departure of the medical director who had served as the team psychiatrist for approximately five years. This was seen as an individual loss and was unsettling to the team. The medical director was a knowledgeable and flexible individual with a solid understanding of child and adolescent services. The search for a medical director with a similar style and philosophy was important to the team. The hiring of a new medical director in 1994 led to some further changes for the team. Although the style was similar, the philosophy and expectations differed in that the level of professionalism and standards of practice were higher, with a view toward research and expansion of services.

ROLE OF THE TEAM LEADER

With the growth of the outpatient program, the responsibility and functions of the team leaders have dramatically increased. In many settings in the past, the role of "team leader" was traditionally assigned to the psychiatrist, but recently this position has more often been held by either a social worker or psychiatric nurse. In our program, non-medical staff have always held the position of team leader. The team leader's role is to implement program objectives, provide day-to-day administrative leadership, promote staff creativity and, recently, to function as a business middle manager with attention to morale, productivity, retraining, personnel management, and administrative priorities.

In view of the multidisciplinary approach, the team leader should have a good understanding of group dynamics and process. He or she must meet the multiple needs of both trainees and permanent staff. The careful selection and assignment of cases must be viewed with an eye toward the requirements of the program, needs, interests, and skill level of the staff and the length of time each trainee will be present in the clinic. Such a balance must be maintained to enhance harmony and cohesion. This task is often complicated by the regular rotation of trainees through the program. Consequently, the team leader must be sensitive to the ongoing needs of patients, trainees, staff. and administrators.

ROLE OF THE PSYCHIATRIST

The role of the child psychiatrist as medical director varies from clinic to clinic and largely depends upon how the clinical and administrative duties are assigned. In our program, the medical director's primary role is the provision of clinical leadership to the team while the team leader is responsible for day-to-day program and personnel management. With our model, role confusion and conflict or competition between the team leader and the medical director can lead to friction in teamwork. Therefore, it is essential that the medical director and team leader meet frequently to work out their differences, set priorities and tasks, and make plans for the team. It is critical that both the medical director and team leader have a genuine belief and interest in interdisciplinary collaborative work and mutual respect for each other.

The medical director's role in our outpatient clinic where duties are shared with a team leader is as follows:

- to provide clinical leadership by

  - making recommendation for further evaluation including use of various behavioral scales (CBCL, Connors, CDI, etc.) and medical workup;
  - making treatment recommendations and providing psychopharmacological treatment as necessary; and,
  - overseeing the quality of the treatment provided.

- to provide clinical supervision and teaching. The medical director is the clinical supervisor for the team leaders and provides clinical direction for all staff. He or she is directly responsible for and involved in the training of residents, psychology interns, and medical students which is accomplished in one-to-one supervision and in the team meetings. Time is set aside in the team meetings for the trainees to present a case in detail and to practice how to make biopsychosocial diagnostic formulations and to develop treatment plans. As the trainees' master diagnosis, they are asked to share their therapy/other treatment issues. Medical students learn from observing assessment interviews with a senior clinician or resident and attending team meetings. Monthly clinical case conferences or grand rounds with outside expert consultation is another method to help the staff enhance their knowledge and skills. The medical director has to keep in mind both the trainees' and clinic's needs. The program may need the trainee to provide medical coverage or provide a specific service while the trainee may desire the time for additional training activities. It is essential to set clinical and productivity expectations for trainees so that everyone is clear about the parameters of the trainees' role. The medical director and the team leader can then collaborate to provide a rich, varied, and comprehensive experience for the trainees.

- to provide support to the team leader and clinical staff. It is important that the medical director actively support the team leader's decisions, especially with psychiatry residents and medical students who may be more responsive to the medical director's authority. The medical director can assist the team leader in resolving interdisciplinary problems. The medical director needs to be aware of the strengths, weaknesses, and needs of the team, as well as of the individual clinicians, and take the lead in involving them in appropriate educational and training activities. The medical director should encourage staff interest in research, academic publication, and other creative activities to make the job more varied, interesting, and academically fulfilling for the clinician.

- to work with the program and division administration. It is important that the medical director meets regularly with the clinic program director and division chiefs. Attendance at various departmental activities such as faculty meetings and training committee meetings is essential. The medical director serves as a liaison between clinic staff and the administration and plays an important role in planning new programs. In many outpatient clinics, the child and adolescent clinic is part of a larger adult outpatient clinic. It is important for the medical director to be aware how the child clinic fits in the overall service delivery system and to educate the clinic administrator regarding child and adolescent psychiatry issues and to ensure these issues are recognized and addressed.

PROBLEMS ENCOUNTERED IN CHILD AND ADOLESCENT SERVICE DELIVERY

As noted earlier, the exclusive use of traditional modalities in child and adolescent work has come under scrutiny. The pressures of health care reform, limited dollars, and the increasing demands for immediate improvement call into question the efficacy of customary treatment. Trained in play, group, and family therapies, clinicians increasingly find themselves struggling to provide services to a population of severely disturbed children for whom these modalities are clearly not sufficient in themselves.

Managed care demands a re-examination of treatment services for youth. Understandably, therapists tend to resist changes that challenge the fundamentals of traditional clinical practice. For some, this has meant their departure from community mental health. For others, it may offer an opportunity to create new horizons.

A major factor having an impact on all child and adolescent programs is limited community resources. Clinicians must compete for services that are time-limited, costly, and questionably successful. Case management, advocacy, and coordination of resources traditionally have been solely the responsibility of the therapist. Although the clinician is expected to work independently, the team has become a vehicle for resolution, information sharing, and case consultation. Knowledge of each case allows for coverage, dialogue, and coordinated treatment. The incorporation of mobile case management services as part of the clinics' system of care provides additional support for the patient, family, and therapist. Intensive case management is a valuable tool which increases the flexibility of service delivery and expands the available range of service. Case management offers a unique opportunity to meet the patient and family in their environment and adapt services to the multiple needs of the family.

At times, the effort at collaboration between the case manager and therapist can be problematic. The use of case management requires the therapist to surrender some responsibilities to others, trusting that the case manager will meet the needs of the patient appropriately. However, fragmentation of care may occur if there is poor communication and lack of appreciation of the numerous demands placed upon both therapist and case manager. It is this difficulty in collaboration and inefficient use of time spent in communication that has led to the decision mentioned earlier to establish the Child Mobile Team as an independent treatment team that will be assigned full responsibility for the most difficult cases.

In fact, intra- and inter-program rivalry and competition has been more prominent in our program as a result, in part, of the administration's efforts to standardize policies and procedures across the Division of Community Psychiatry and the program.

CONCLUSION

Our system, while providing quality care by a very dedicated and committed staff, has an obligation and a need to move more quickly into a new era. The clinic program has undergone sweeping changes in the past three years since privatization, but we recognize that this was only the first step in a long process. Good intentions are less relevant in today's world where efficiency, quality, and results are the required elements of service providers. But we strongly believe that these elements are compatible with the "old fashioned" values which motivated staff to choose this career. It is the administration's responsibility to effect the necessary changes and to uphold these values. We hope to create a system with the needed flexibility in the areas of intensity, immediacy, and accessibility and that much of the current system can act as the foundation for the new system we must become. As we continue to move ahead in our evolutionary process, we must maintain our commitment to meet the needs of our consumers, staff, and community.

REFERENCES

Burnes, B. J., & Santos, A. B. (1995). Assertive community treatment: An update of randomized trials. *Psychiatric Services, 46*, 669–675.

Friedman, R. (1996). Mental health policy for children. In B. L. Levin & J. Petrolia (Eds.), *Mental health services: a public health perspective*. (pp 234–248). New York: Oxford University Press.

Goldman, C. R., Faulkner, L. R., & Breeding, K. A. (1994). A method for estimating psychiatrist staffing needs in community mental health programs. *Hospital and Community Psychiatry, 45*, 333–337.

Henggeler, S. W., Schoenwald, S. K., Pickrel, S. G., Rowland, M. D., & Santos, A. B. (1994). The contribution of treatment outcome research to the reform of children's mental health services: Multisystemic therapy as an example. *Journal of Mental Health Administration, 21*(3), 229–239.

Stevenson, G. S. (1934). *Child guidance clinics: A quarter century of development*. New York: Garland Publishing, Inc.

Stroul, B. A., & Freidman, R. M. (1986). *A system of care for children and adolescents with severe emotional disturbances* (Rev. ed.). Washington, DC: Georgetown University Child Development Center, CASSP Technical Assistance Center.

World Health Organization. (1960). *Child guidance centers*. Geneva: Palais des Nations.

Chapter 4

Training Issues in a Child and Adolescent Ambulatory Setting

Kevin Harrison, M.D, Harinder S. Ghuman, M.D., and
Richard M. Sarles, M.D.

Medical education is based on the premise that trainees learn best by participating, under supervision, in the day-to-day care of patients. Historically, most of this clinical education has taken place on inpatient services of teaching hospitals. However, currently, fewer patients are admitted to inpatient units, and those who are have significantly shorter stays as a result of the economic forces in health care. Current health delivery systems emphasize ambulatory care to minimize the number of inpatient stays to, in turn, reduce the overall cost of health care. As such, today's inpatient services offer a very different experience in clinical training than in the past. To keep abreast of the changing health care environment, education in ambulatory care settings must become a more important component of medical training in general. Child and adolescent psychiatry certainly is experiencing this trend as much as any other medical specialty.

The economic and educational mandate to make such a move in medical training is encumbered with a large gap between rhetoric and execution. This chapter examines issues that are not necessarily unique to ambulatory care settings, but which may be obstacles for optimal training experiences in child and adolescent psychiatry. The major focus is on the training of both general psychiatry residents and child and adolescent psychiatry residents in child and adolescent psychiatry. Many of the issues discussed in this chapter are also relevant to the instruction of psychology and social work trainees.

GENERAL CONSIDERATIONS

Training Requirements

Training in child and adolescent psychiatry requires learning to work in a team with other mental health professionals. Close, productive interaction with psychologists, social workers, and other health professionals fosters this team building. Such collaboration provides an educational context in which trainees can learn from peers and colleagues.

The Accreditation Council for Graduate Medical Education (ACGME), through the Residency Review Committees (RRC) of each medical speciality, sets the training requirements to ensure that each program produces competent specialists. The ACGME mandates that a psychiatry residency program demonstrate that it provides an educational experience of such caliber as to ensure that its graduates possess sound clinical judgment and significant knowledge about diagnosis, treatment, and prevention of all psychiatric disorders and the common medical and neurological disorders that relate to the practice of psychiatry. This requisite knowledge includes an understanding of the biological, psychological, social, economic, ethnic, and family factors which influence physical and psychological development in infancy, childhood, adolescence, and adulthood. Skills include experience and competence with all age groups. The choice of the methods applied to achieve this educational and experiential learning goal is flexible enough to allow individual programs to create experiences that fit their resident population and clinical site availability.

Trainees in child and adolescent psychiatry fellowship must complete PGY I-III requirements in general psychiatry, plus two years training in an accredited child psychiatry program. The child fellowship program must offer a well-supervised and well-balanced experience with inpatients, outpatients, and consultees, as well as provide a formal educational experience. While there are guidelines for the amount of time to be spent on inpatient or acute care settings, outpatient and consultation requirements are less clearly defined. "Work with outpatients must include evaluations and an adequate experience with psychodynamic therapy, including work with some children and adolescent patients for at least a year's duration" (ACGME, 1995). However, this requirement is becoming ever more difficult to fulfill in today's health care reform movement.

Psychology programs leading to a doctoral degree require a minimum of the equivalent of three full-time academic years of graduate study. Doctoral programs in clinical, school, and counseling psychology include systematic intensive training in the application of psychological principles and skills to human problems. This field training is generally graded in intensity and responsibility, and is offered sequentially through practicum and internship experiences (American Psychological Association, 1986). The specific structure and sites of these experiences vary with the specialty. Practicum training is field experience, usually taken for academic credit, often on campus. Practicum training should begin as early as feasible in a training program, and choice of facilities should be based primarily upon their quality and relevance to the training objectives of the program. The minimum practicum experience is 400 hours, of which at least 75 hours is in scheduled supervision, and at least 150 hours is in direct service. The practicum is intended to prepare the student for the internship and is prerequisite to it.

The nature of the psychology internship, its locus, the populations served, the experiences provided, and other relevant considerations vary with the graduate program's training model. Internships in clinical psychology require a full-time experience for one calendar year. School and counseling psychology internships require a full-time experience for either the academic or calendar year. Internship sites should conform to all relevant American Psychological Association guidelines. It is common for psychology internship programs to have a consortium, in which a group of administratively independent sites pool their resources. Although it is not expected that every intern will receive training at every site in the consortium, an intern should receive training at more than one site and have potential access to all sites.

Social work training includes two years of academic curriculum and field placement to obtain a master's degree. In addition, two additional years of supervised work are required before the licensing examination to obtain a L.C.S.W. can be taken.

There are several other types of professionals and paraprofessionals who may be working in an ambulatory child and adolescent psychiatry setting, with a variety of education and training backgrounds—nurse practitioners, lay counselors, case managers, and family therapists, for example. Turf wars, unclear roles and responsibilities, wide differences in background and experience— all present potential pitfalls in establishing training and working alliances. Supervised, active collaboration among mental health personnel in the treatment of patients will provide the best possible care while exposing all involved to diverse learning experiences.

Ambulatory Training Sites

As the shift to training in ambulatory care settings becomes more pronounced, the creative resources to provide needed services soars. Different, and less expensive means of delivering mental health care are often more varied than the types of professionals and paraprofessionals who work in them, so that there is no longer a university-run mental health clinic where trainees practice their clinical knowledge. But now there are managed care offices, private offices, school mental health clinics, pediatric clinics, community clinics, partial hospital programs, after school programs, home care, and therapeutic nurseries. Working conditions are inevitably becoming more diverse, but some basic preconditions, presented in the following discussion, must be kept clearly in the forefront to provide for the best patient care and training experience.

Safety

Trainees are frightened enough of their formidable responsibilities and fragile self-confidence, so adequate backup and supervision are musts. This may entail easy availability of security, access to mobile phones, and working with others or only when other personnel are in the immediate vicinity. No trainee should be put in a position where his or her safety, or that of patients, could be compromised.

Physical Location

A sense of comfort with the intimate work space, the provision of privacy, and the convenience of a well-equipped office—all provide for ease of work and a professional tone. "All residents must have offices adequate in size and decor to allow them to interview patients in a professional manner. The facility must also provide adequate and specifically designated areas in which residents can perform basic physical examination and other necessary diagnostic procedures" (ACGME, 1995). For most trainees the acquisition of one's own office is a significant milestone on the road to becoming a professional.

Resources

Resources such as a library, audiovisual equipment, observation rooms, playrooms, conferences rooms, and computers set the appropriate tone for educational pursuits.

Working Conditions

The working environment is affected by many things and will greatly affect one's attitude. In a survey by Marriage and Halasz (1991), lack of support from colleagues or administration, political infighting, organizational dysfunction and lack of leadership, excessive demands and workloads—all rank high in unhelpful training experiences.

Balance of Training Variety and Travel

A balance between providing the needed variety in a training program, and the demands of traveling to numerous sites is an important issue. It is unlikely that most training programs are able to access the full range of necessary training experiences at only one or two sites. With the shift to increased ambulatory training comes a need for trainees and faculty to become more ambulatory themselves, and in doing so, time is added for travel, in addition to the ever-increasing demands for direct patient care.

GENERAL PSYCHIATRY RESIDENTS' TRAINING IN CHILD AND ADOLESCENT PSYCHIATRY

The training of general psychiatry residents in child and adolescent psychiatry is naturally different from the training of child and adolescent fellows. This is a result largely of time constraints within the training program. Of equal importance is the support of general psychiatry for training in child and adolescent psychiatry. Equally important, too, is the level of interest or motivation on the part of residents in working with children, and the residents' lack of experience and resultant anxiety in dealing with children and their families. External factors such as how well an outpatient clinic is organized, how clear expectations for the residents are, and who is providing the teaching and supervision to the residents are critical factors.

General psychiatry residents often express concerns about having too many or too few cases, not receiving concrete and practical guidelines from supervisors, not having certain types of experiences (e.g., family therapy) and not being provided with training in dealing with a child in crisis. Supervisors are often concerned about insuring that the resident meet training requirements, obtain information that is unique to child psychiatry (e.g., developmental and school histories), overcome resistances to seeing younger children, under-diagnosing, and completing paperwork. To ensure that general residents have an optimal training experience, their progress must be closely coordinated and followed by both general and child residency training directors. Unfortunately, in some programs, general psychiatry resident training in child and adolescent psychiatry is given little emphasis which often leads to inadequate or outright bad experiences. This not only affects patient care, but can deter residents from pursuing fellowship training in child psychiatry secondary to their unsatisfactory experience.

Issues such as when in training a resident should begin child training, whether to set aside a block of time specifically for child training, or to extend it over a longer course, and whether to make the focus more ambulatory or inpatient requires careful consideration. As general psychiatry residents are often required to evaluate children in an emergency room setting early in their training, it is critical to provide them with education, supervision, and support, otherwise the experience could be traumatic, leaving the resident with a lack of confidence and enthusiasm in dealing with this population. As general psychiatry residents have less experience and perhaps less interest in dealing with a pediatric population, they are likely to require tighter supervision and nurturance than child and adolescent fellows. It is useful for residents to observe experienced clinicians performing interviews with a variety of age groups, and have their first few evaluations directly observed by a supervisor, rather than their being "thrown to the wolves." In an ambulatory setting with general residents, the establishment of a diagnostic clinic in which the residents participate as a group with direct faculty supervision and mentorship can make for easier scheduling, make faculty involvement far more efficient, and create a more collegial atmosphere.

It is important to establish clear expectations regarding how child training time will be divided among the variety of possible activities. For example, in a training program in which a general psychiatry resident spends eight hours a week for one year in a child training rotation, the resident could have two hours allocated to diagnostic evaluations including supervision, one hour each for long-term and short-term therapy, one hour for family therapy, two hours for psychopharmacology cases, and one hour for supervision. Multidisciplinary team meetings as well as experiences participating in other disciplines' assessments may also be incorporated. An expectation for the number of diagnostic workups to be completed, the range of age groups and psychopathology, and types of interventions should be emphasized. General psychiatry residents are often reluctant to see young children merely because of inexperience and opportunity. For example, in our clinic, one resident was resistant to seeing children under 10 years of age. With close supervision and support, he was assigned a 5-year-old with depression and encopresis. The resident developed an excellent relationship with the child and her family, the child improved considerably over time, and the resident's fears were replaced with a newfound confidence in working with the younger child.

CHILD AND ADOLESCENT PSYCHIATRY RESIDENCY TRAINING

Administrative Structure

Training Director   "The residency program in child and adolescent psychiatry must be under the direction of a fully trained child and adolescent psychiatrist who is Board certified in child and adolescent psychiatry or who possesses suitable equivalent qualifications as determined by the Residency Review Committee. The person shall devote at least half-time to the training program, including clinical teaching activities" (ACGME, 1995). The exact role of the training director often varies for each program, and may be solely as training director, but more commonly is in combination with other duties. The training director should have a comprehensive understanding of all aspects of the training program, but ideally with as little direct intervention with training issues as possible so as to allow the trainees a certain sense of autonomy to aid in their own professional and personal growth.

The training director should be available to mediate conflict, delegate responsibility, spearhead advancement in training, and interface with other academic and medical administration on behalf of the program. Management and leadership skills of the training director and others responsible for conducting a training program is of equal importance to clinical and teaching abilities. The child psychiatry trainee can derive a boost of morale and confidence from the fact that the training director's goal is the trainees' assuming leadership in the mental health field. In contrast, whenever a training director infantilizes trainees or creates prolonged subservience, the training program falls short of the ideal of optimal professional and personal growth of trainees.

Chief Resident   Many training programs choose a chief resident to serve a "middle-management" role, being a representative to the administration on behalf of the trainee group, as well as disseminating information and dealing with issues of concern from the administration to the resident group on a day-to-day basis. This can be a difficult role to carry out as it lacks the power and authority of a regular faculty member, but requires power and authority greater than the usual resident. It is common for the chief resident to shift the pendulum between peer group and administration, looking for a comfortable and productive medium. Most problems arise when a chief resident cannot be flexible enough to wear both hats, and he or she allies with one group to the exclusion of the other.

It is not unusual in larger programs with their variety of training sites to have co-chief residents sharing duties. In fact, this may even be preferable considering the number of responsibilities they may have in addition to their regular clinical and academic obligations. While in some medical specialties the role of chief resident requires an additional year, with child and adolescent psychiatry, where five postgraduate years have already been invested, the additional year is not common. However, there are often some additional stipends or other "perks" to reward the chief resident for his or her toils and troubles, over and above the education the chief resident receives in administration.

The role of the chief can be most pronounced in an ambulatory setting, where the structure and support of an inpatient setting is not present. Assisting junior residents with basic office management skills, assigning patients and monitoring caseloads, troubleshooting problem areas, and providing emergency backup are just some of the duties a chief can be called on to perform. Chiefs can be an excellent and pragmatic resource for all trainees. They can prevent minor problems from progressing up the chain-of-command, and serve as a buffer in various conflicts where someone may just need a chance to ventilate. As leaders of the resident group, they can set the tone for other trainees. By anticipating morale problems, they can assist in intervening before acting out becomes the coping strategy. By encouraging camaraderie and the ability to work and play together, an example is set that will be invaluable in the years to come. Effectively representing the practical concerns the trainee group experiences in the ambulatory setting can better induce change from administration. While decisions for training may make sense in the abstract and sound good on paper, it is not until they are put into practice that difficulties may emerge. With so many new training issues coming to the forefront as ambulatory care receives a higher priority, the role of the chief as intermediary in deciphering the problems and relaying them back to the administration for reworking is heightened.

Faculty/Attending   "The faculty must include a total of at least three full time equivalent, fully trained, child and adolescent psychiatrists in the child and adolescent psychiatry residency program" (ACGME, 1995). It is inevitable that faculty or attendings will have developed their own philosophies about childhood disorders and their treatment during professional growth, possibly restricting a trainee's experience. It is not only essential for trainees to update their knowledge base and maintain flexibility with the changing care patterns that are emerging, but to have instructors who have this flexibility themselves, and who are motivated to stay on the "cutting edge" of new information in child and adolescent psychiatry. By maintaining a diverse group from multiple disciplines, the trainee can gain awareness of different styles to approach treatment issues in the ambulatory setting.

Supervisors   Supervision, along with didactic teaching and self-directed learning, form the essential triad of a training experience. In fact, 75 percent of respondents to Mrazek's and Prugh's investigation (1980) described supervised psychotherapy with children as the most useful experience in their training, which, from most current trainees' experience, still holds true today, although "supervised psychotherapy" is not as prevalent today as "supervised treatment."

A supervisor's role is to monitor and contribute to both the clinical work and the personal and professional growth of the trainee. Ongoing, weekly supervision of a specific outpatient case, or a number of cases, demonstrates to the trainee how an experienced child and adolescent psychiatrist will view, organize, and deal with an unfolding case. It provides a focal point from which to distill the mass of data into a sensible treatment plan.

But although supervised psychotherapy has been a critical skill and central expectation of what a child psychiatrist does in practice, it is no longer as central in the modern child psychiatrist's repertoire. The contemporary child psychiatrist is a diagnostician, medication manager, consultant, or supervisor of other mental health clinicians. An inherent problem is that to perform these duties satisfactorily, a foundation in psychotherapy is essential. Supervisors are needed, then, who can incorporate a strong foundation in psychotherapy with the demands the contemporary child psychiatrist faces. Obtaining the cases to learn these skills in the managed care environment is often problematic.

In the ambulatory setting, supervisor case presentation remains an issue, although a very valuable method. Even with the ease of technology, it can be cumbersome to use videotaping to present cases. This may be caused by equipment security precautions secondary to theft, the necessity for signed releases, and/or confidentiality issues from wary parents sensitive to having their family's private issues aired to the public. It is not uncommon for patients to "play to the camera" during videotaped sessions, and thus present an inaccurate version of themselves. Audiotaping, in contrast, may be a less cumbersome way of detailing information but it is not widely used. Using a one-way mirror is a less intrusive way to supervise therapy, but few supervisors and trainees have the luxury of timing this together, and scheduling the extra time needed to process the session.

Another supervisory technique is to have the supervisor present in the room with the trainee during the therapy session. This can be very distracting for the patient and clinician, but probably the most enlightening of all the methods of supervision. Supervision that uses one-way mirrors and audiovisual equipment, as well as direct observation of interviews done by senior faculty, seems to be underemphasized in most programs, and an increased emphasis in these training procedures in the outpatient setting is generally highly valued by trainees.

Given the number of supervisors a trainee will work with during training, it would be surprising if some interpersonal difficulties did not arise from time to time. How these are dealt with can have a significant impact on a trainee's experience. It is ideal to allow the supervisor and trainee to work them out together which provides an educational experience in itself. However, there are sometimes inflexible personalities involved, and to let the problem fester can lead to acting out. The training director must be aware of the concerns from both trainee and supervisor, and monitor closely the progress of resolution. Sometimes direct mediation or change of supervisors is necessary. A trainee's frequent conflicts with different supervisors reflects a likely problem with that trainee, but it is certainly possible for multiple complaints to be registered regarding a particular supervisor. Unless the administration is willing to address such problems actively, significant morale difficulties and mistrust within the training program may develop. It remains vital for trainees to review their supervisors periodically to provide feedback on the training program and the styles, benefits, and problems that may be associated with a particular supervisor.

Support Staff   A major complaint of trainees, as well as health professionals in general, is the burdensome and time-consuming demands of record-keeping, billing, phone contacts, obtaining and sending reports, and the various other "unbillable," non-clinical time that is necessary in any clinical setting. Many trainees become demoralized by finding themselves thrust into a myriad of clerical duties which they see as distracting from clinical activities. This is often not what they expected when going into the health care field, with idealistic notions of directly interfacing with and helping patients, without having to go through many, if any, bureaucratic hassles. Obviously, the maturation of the trainee must include casting aside some naive notions such as these, and developing an understanding of the balance between clinical and administrative duties. Having support staff in the ambulatory training setting to assist trainees in their administrative tasks is important. It affords quality of services, a professional atmosphere, and streamlining of duties. However, performing these tasks is an important learning experience in itself, allowing a trainee to understand the bureaucracy and appreciate the responsibilities involved, and, also, not to misuse the support staff.

FINANCING AMBULATORY CARE TRAINING

A variety of barriers confront the development of more and better programs in ambulatory care training. Financing is only one of them, but it is at the core of the problem. Dramatic changes in health care financing and delivery systems, along with diminished federal support for clinical training, threaten academic child psychiatry's attempts to increase faculty commitment to research and education and reduce the likelihood that the field will continue to attract sufficiently qualified residents into its training programs (McKelvey, 1990).

Issues of financing are a primary problem slowing the growth of training in ambulatory care for multiple reasons:

* Training in ambulatory care settings may actually increase operating costs. Overhead expenses for utilities, office space, support staff, and so on increase with the number of trainees. Outpatient, resident-run clinics typically serve indigent populations that are usually on medical assistance or sliding-scale/no-pay schedules, often with few monetary benefits distributed to the academic institution. Currently, most states are facing the change of medical assistance patients to managed care programs, which may further jeopardize training programs.
* When education is introduced into an ambulatory care setting, costs go up but revenue may decline as productivity suffers, because trainees are less efficient, at least in their early training, and have a much slower turnaround time in patient care. Trainees are less experienced dealing with utilization review and advocating for services from insurers for their patients. There is little, if any, incentive for trainees to see patients over their expected caseload to meet training requirements. In fact, in many training programs where strict adherence to productivity is not enforced, it is to the advantage of the busy trainee to have patients "no-show."
* Ambulatory settings do not generate as much revenue as inpatient care. Yet the role of the hospital in the care of patients has been altered by incentives from payers to reduce lengths of stay by expanding services provided before admission and after discharge. Unfortunately, these expanded services are not always included as training opportunities. Instead there is competition between managed health care and alternative services for the available and most cost-efficient treatment provider. Increased managed care, increased competition from proprietary hospitals, and reduced inpatient benefits all contribute to the

steady erosion of ambulatory teaching facilities' ability to generate significant revenues to pay for child and adolescent psychiatric training.

• As consumers, patients are faced with assuming an increasingly larger part of their health care payments in the forms of increased insurance premiums, co-payments, denied coverage, and self-payment. Thus, they are more likely to want only the best treatment services and may be less willing to accept care by trainees in the ambulatory care setting. As a result of the need for training programs to stay competitive with non-training ambulatory settings, and still meet the demands of financing training, there is an increased emphasis on the service expectations of the trainee. No training occurs without service. Still, the amount of service assigned to the trainee must be limited so that clinical duties do not smother didactic and supervisory opportunities. The "service versus training" dilemma exists in all training programs, and the resident group often calls attention to any imbalance to the training committee. Institutions and organizations contributing stipends to a training program often have their own reimbursement for services rendered from managed care or some type of strictly controlled insurance program. Obviously they certainly have a need to ensure reasonable productivity to pay for their investment in training. Unfortunately, many managed care companies do not reimburse for trainees to see their patients, or they will only cover diagnostic evaluations and pharmacotherapy which leads to a restricted opportunity for trainees to see a variety of cases, including either short- or long-term therapies.

There is currently a controversy in today's mental health care delivery systems over whether child and adolescent psychiatrists should be expected to learn psychotherapy. Since many psychiatrists are not being reimbursed for these services in practice, some argue, training should be focused on those skills that are currently the "bread and butter" of managed care child psychiatry—that is, evaluation and medication management. Others argue definitely not, as there are more than enough available experiences in most training programs to learn psychopharmacotherapy and diagnosis. To be a truly well-rounded psychiatrist, however, one needs to have an ongoing experience with a patient, to understand the issues of transference and countertransference, and to recognize growth and change. No more important is this than in the field of child and adolescent psychiatry, where the need is to understand the various complexities of development, which can be best understood through long-term psychotherapeutic experiences with a variety of patients, in all age groups, and their families,. Not only is this crucial in the maturation of a trainee's clinical abilities, it is critical in providing them with the skills to provide future supervision to other mental health workers who may be providing therapy to their patients.

Creative ways to have psychiatry trainees see long-term cases include billing at a lower rate—that is, billing for the amount an insurance reimburser would pay to a paraprofessional or professional of lesser training and/or having trainees see patients in residential treatment, special education settings, or other areas where children have been referred for long-term care with mental health services.

Finances are of paramount importance for training programs which are under pressure to reduce size, require more hours of reimbursable service, and even lower stipends. These economic constraints can adversely affect recruitment into the field, thus potentially decreasing the availability of child and adolescent psychiatry services provided to underserved populations that generally depend on trainees for their care. Financial issues seem to be of increasing importance to the trainees themselves, too, as most have significant debt from educational loans, little capacity to save as a result of the high cost-of-living in the areas where most programs are located, and a weariness of living a life of near-poverty proportions throughout their many years of schooling. Moonlighting, or trainees working jobs outside their regular duties, continues to be a common and excellent means of supplementing incomes of trainees, though presenting both benefits and problems of its own.

Besides its economic benefit, moonlighting offers the trainee practical experience in dealing with issues such as self-employment tax, malpractice, billing, licensing, and other such domains that may be taken for granted during training. Moonlighting provides outside experiences not always available in a training program and exposes the trainee to job opportunities following training. Although strictly forbidden by the Residency Review Committee, the outside work can interfere with the training experience as well as causing excessive hours to cut into study and outside reading time, and limit the self-learning that is crucial in the field. Some residents may even "double-dip" or moonlight during times when they are expected to be on duty for their training program. They may fatigue themselves so that they cannot provide a high quality of service during their regular workday. Most training programs are flexible enough to realize the financial constraints of their trainees, but the training program cannot allow outside experiences to disrupt the required training needs. Sometimes training programs can offer moonlighting availability within their own system, which is an ideal way to allow extra income for the trainees and provide supervision over their experiences. Trainees can be very adept at finding funding and educational resources that may even be beneficial for the training program. A key point here, as in much of life, is to not to get stuck in one extreme or the other. Training programs that work with the trainee on their needs will demonstrate empathy, promote loyalty, and allow training programs to oversee their trainee's performance.

DIDACTIC CURRICULUM

Child and adolescent psychiatry is no different from other fields of medicine, in that its practitioners continue to add to the database of information needed to practice in this specialty. As we do so, we must determine what is important to continue to teach, and what can be de-emphasized to make way for the new. Unfortunately, there is no reliable way to ascertain this. One could argue that teaching the old, as well as the new information we continue to gain, is optimal. But the limited period of time (two years of training) is the predicament that training programs face.

Mrazek's and Prugh's survey of practicing child psychiatrists (1980) highlighted the strengths and weaknesses in child psychiatric training by identifying a well-supervised psychotherapeutic experience and exposure to a variety of clinical problems in multiple settings to be the two most valuable aspects of professional development. Didactic experiences were rarely felt to be helpful. A decade later, a survey of psychiatry residents by Dech, Abikoff, and Koplewicz (1990) revealed that outpatient experiences, diagnostic assessments, child development, psychopharmacology, family therapy, and academic courses were felt to be the most important components to emphasize in the "ideal" training program. Major deficits identified in didactic teaching were the lack of emphasis on parental counseling regarding child behavior management; lack of awareness in the literature of developmental aspects of childrearing, special situations such as divorce, stepfamilies, foster care, and death, to name a few; and substance abuse education specific to children and adolescents.

Trainees today appear to continue to be ambivalent about didactics in their training experience. Although some learn from passive reception of information, an active role in learning generally makes a more lasting impression. In the ambulatory care setting, active participation in learning can be accomplished in several ways. Interdisciplinary team meetings which are patient-focused can provide time when trainees and senior clinicians can teach one another about specific topics. Grand rounds and clinical case conferences are also excellent forums for the sharing of clinical material with peers and faculty and they present a commonality in grappling with technical and personal aspects of child treatment. We advocate requiring trainees to do more teaching themselves, not only of their colleagues, but of other health professionals. "See one, do one, teach one" is still an axiom that child and adolescent psychiatry trainees should not disregard.

We do not propose a total cessation of didactic teaching. This would be in direct conflict with ACGME guidelines for approved training programs. However, rather than trying to teach all the facts a trainee must know to be a good child and adolescent psychiatrist, we suggest emphasizing the areas that are necessary to master, and direct trainees to the resources where they can access necessary additional information. This process would not only help trainees know what is deemed important, but it would provide the mechanism to help them promote their own self-learning. Obviously, this proposal assumes that trainees bring with them the lifelong commitment to continuous reading and learning. The best teachers are trainees who teach themselves.

TRAINEE EXPECTATIONS AND ANXIETIES

Trainees rely on their training program to provide them with what they need to know to become self-sufficient and competent health care providers. In turn, the trainee becomes the barometer of what is and is not working, and can be crucial in realigning or even redesigning a training program. The goal of a program is to meet the needs of the trainees as outlined by the residency review committees of the ACGME, and allow them to provide feedback and effect the changes that keep a program advancing in the field. Besides trainee perceptions and satisfaction, faculty interest and expertise, available funding and patient population, and hospital and community needs are important factors that will influence the content of the training program.

One major issue that contributes to trainee satisfaction is clinical case load. This can be a problem, with either too few or too many patients to see. The ideal clinical load is hard to define, for good reason. Learners are all different. Some trainees can learn best from prolonged and frequent in-depth contacts with five or six patients. Others learn best from having a broader experience with a greater caseload of 20 or more. To accommodate the learning needs for each trainee in the ambulatory setting while fulfilling the service obligations, a balance of longer-term, in-depth therapy and short-term, diagnostic and psychopharmacology cases should be required. In addition, hours of care per week rather than number of cases per week with the required balance can help prevent resentment among trainees and staff.

In an inpatient setting, trainees have a captive audience. This is not so in the outpatient department, where competition for patients is keen, and no-show rates can be very high. Scheduling problems with parents' work and children's school schedules often present difficulties. Providing a quality control mechanism to ensure that the ambulatory patient is receiving quality care, as well as having some method to make the patient accountable for missed appointments should be considered.

Trainees rightfully question how they can be exposed to new therapeutic approaches and other advances if their instructors, themselves often trained a generation earlier, retain an allegiance to skills and priorities currently out of synch with today's treatment modalities. Clearly it is the responsibility of the division director and training director to ensure that the faculty are retrained and maintain skills and knowledge current with treatment modalities. Another solution is to have teachers who are involved in research and more likely to be appraising critically both traditional and "cutting-edge" approaches. An appreciation of the value of empirical investigation and critical awareness of methodological principles can be developed as trainees are taught how to understand the limitations of particular studies. Development of sufficient understanding of principles of research to be able to discriminate between contradictory results of differently designed projects is a goal. While this has long been appreciated, it is not adequately communicated to trainees. Part of the reason lies in the resistance of some trainees to research, and the inevitable brick wall that materializes at the mere mention of the word. If the field of child and adolescent psychiatry wishes to produce psychiatrists who are clinicians/scientists, then training programs will have to devise unobtrusive ways to offer increased research exposure during training.

There is a relative unavailability of some types of training experiences in just about every program. Group therapy, behavior therapy, cognitive therapy, and substance abuse treatment are some of the more commonly neglected areas reported by trainees. How to provide adequate training in all these areas, not just in didactics, but ongoing clinical experiences, remains a challenge for most training programs. As trainees are often dealing with families with unyielding psychosocial problems and limited resources, attention must also be given to improving the management and leadership competence of trainees to enable them to look at the "big picture" and the impacts on community systems. Trainees also express a need for greater medical knowledge and the skills to make more sophisticated medical differential diagnosis and to know when to make an appropriate referral. Perhaps this can be done in ambulatory pediatric clinics where general pediatrics, psychiatry, neurology, and other specialties could serve side-by-side. Not only would such an experience offer trainees a broader medical education, it would allow for greater exchange of ideas and exposure to normal development, and perhaps overcome some of the misconceptions of mental illness that our colleagues in other areas of medicine still possess.

BEHAVIORAL PEDIATRICS

In university-based or affiliated sites, it is not uncommon for trainees and staff in various disciplines to work together. All ACGME-approved pediatric training programs in the United States must provide two months of training in behavioral pediatrics sometime during the three-year residency training program. Behavioral pediatrics is defined as a subspecialty within pediatrics which deals with behavioral and developmental problems of children and adolescents. Developmental problems could include mental retardation, cerebral palsy, and pervasive developmental disorders, including autism, for example. Behavioral pediatricians must complete a three-year general pediatric residency program and then must complete a three-year developmental and behavioral pediatric fellowship.

Behavioral pediatricians deal with patients encompassing a broad range of psychopathology, however, in general, they deal with the high-frequency, low-acuity disorders such as ADHD, LD, enuresis, encopresis, simple fears and phobias, and perhaps mild dysthymia. Most behavioral pediatricians limit themselves to these conditions and usually quickly and appropriately refer complex diagnostic and treatment cases to child psychiatrists or child psychologists. Behavioral pediatricians often may offer counseling but seldom wish to provide ongoing psychotherapy.

A major problem for behavioral pediatricians is that theirs is not an approved ABMS subspecialty, and thus lacks a RRC setting standards for curriculum and clinical rotations. Therefore there is a wide diversity in the orientation and training in the various fellowship programs in developmental behavioral pediatrics throughout the country. Some programs focus on developmental issues, others have a research orientation, and still others are more clinically based. All fellowships have a requirement of at least one full year of research.

In an ambulatory child and adolescent psychiatry setting one could envision pediatric residents and/or behavioral pediatric fellows participating with mental health professionals in the diagnosis and treatment of children and adolescents. Independent work with patients presenting with the full spectrum of mental health problems could be difficult for a pediatrician or behavioral pediatrician because of the lack of adequate training and experience in the diagnosis of psychopathology and the treatment of emotionally disturbed children and adolescents. Nonetheless, behavioral pediatricians and/or general pediatric residents could certainly profit from the experience of seeing children representing the full spectrum of *DSM-IV* psychopathology; the focus of the experience would be, however, on the recognition of various diagnostic entities in the general pediatric setting and the appropriate referral procedures.

Thus, the high-acuity, low-frequency disorders such as psychosis, OCD, or major depression could be included in their diagnostic experience but would be excluded from their management/treatment experience. In contrast, the high-frequency, low-acuity disorders such as ADHD could appropriately be diagnosed and treated by the pediatrician. It must be kept in mind that the average pediatrician sees one patient approximately every 10 to 15 minutes in a busy office practice. Thus, the ability to diagnose and adequately treat these high-frequency, low-acuity disorders should be the focus of the educational experience in the ambulatory mental health setting.

An additional benefit for the ambulatory child and adolescent psychiatry setting from having trainees from various disciplines is the capacity to provide a telephone consultation service to pediatric practitioners in the community. Also, a good working relationship with pediatricians in the community can significantly enhance referrals to the child psychiatry ambulatory setting thereby assuring adequate diagnostic and treatment resources for the community.

CONCLUSION

Training child and adolescent psychiatrists in the ambulatory setting is of primary importance today. While many barriers challenge the development of more and better programs in ambulatory training, they are not insurmountable. Financing training programs is a primary problem, and must be dealt with first. When funding problems are solved, issues such as educational philosophy, acceptance of clinical programs by patients, competition from private physicians, and managed care demands are more easily overcome. The education of specialists whose training emphasizes outpatient experience is in society's best interest. Public grants and appropriations should be earmarked to facilitate this training in ambulatory care. To encourage innovation in several options of financing the education of trainees should be actively pursued.

Training child and adolescent psychiatrists in the ambulatory setting will increase the visibility and accessibility of mental health professionals in the community, which can help generate assets other than increased funding. It can demystify the profession, teach others to be aware of the mental health of our children, and potentially improve recruitment. The ideal training program will convey a zest for inquiry, promote a proliferation of scholarship, and portray child and adolescent psychiatry as an intellectual discipline. In the ambulatory setting, sharing responsibilities, fostering independence, and trusting others to perform valued services for the children and their families seeking help, will help the trainee grow as a person.

REFERENCES

Accreditation Council for Graduate Medical Education (ACGME). (1995). *Special requirements for residency training in psychiatry.*

American Psychological Association. (1986). *Criteria for accreditation: Doctoral training programs and internships in professional psychology.* Washington, DC: the Author.

Dech, B., Abikoff, H., & Koplewicz, H. (1990). A survey of child and adolescent psychiatry residents: Perceptions of the ideal training program. *Journal of the American Academy of Child and Adolescent Psychiatry, 29,* 946–949.

Marriage, K., & Halasz, G. (1991). A 13-year follow-up of child psychiatry training. *Australian and New Zealand Journal of Psychiatry, 25,* 270–276.

McKelvey, R. S. (1990). The coming crisis in funding child psychiatry training. *American Journal of Psychiatry, 147,* 1220–1224.

Mrazek, D. A., & Prugh, D. (1980). Critical incidents in child psychiatric training. *Journal of the American Academy of Child and Adolescent Psychiatry, 19,* 311–319.

Part 2

Assessment

Chapter 5

Psychiatric Assessment of Infants and Parent-Child Interaction

Robinson J. Munoz-Millan, M.D.

INTRODUCTION

Infants and toddlers referred for psychiatric assessment generally present disturbances of development—whether delay or deviance—or specific symptoms such as failure to thrive or sleep or feeding disturbance. Some infants and their mothers are referred because of disturbance of the attachment process and some families are seen because the child displays symptoms suggestive of physical or sexual abuse. Toddlers are often referred because of disruptive behavior or depressed mood. Children with cerebral palsy or neurodegenerative diseases are usually sent by the primary physician to child neurologists or developmental pediatricians although occasionally they are seen by the child psychiatrist.

In these instances, the infant psychiatrist must determine whether a delay or disturbance of development is present, assess the behaviors of concern to differentiate between normative and abnormal behaviors given age and other variables, and evaluate the parent-child and family relationships to rule out abnormal and aggressive patterns. Furthermore, the infant psychiatrist must give an opinion about etiology and prognosis, and make recommendations for treatment. The evaluation cannot be done by one specialist alone. A multidisciplinary team including social workers, psychologists, speech and language pathologists, and physical therapists collaborates with the child psychiatrist in carrying out the evaluation and eventually treatment as needed.

The conceptual structure of the evaluation is not unlike all psychiatric evaluations, although it is adapted to meet the specific characteristics and circumstances of infants and toddlers. The basic principles of the evaluation of very young children are based on the understanding that children are competent organisms biologically determined to develop in a systematic and progressive pattern. This pattern of development results from the unfolding of hereditary potentials interacting actively with the physical and social environment. Of these physical and social factors, the caregiving provided to the child by the principal caretaker(s) is of paramount importance for the cognitive and emotional growth of the child.

This caregiving environment—the parent-child relationship—is in turn under the powerful influence of cultural, social, political, and economic factors. Therefore, the assessment should address three levels:

- the biological, which encompasses the innate potentials and weaknesses related to the hereditary context of the child and family, as well as the infant or toddler's gestational and pediatric history;
- the parent-child relationship, including the interactional patterns and styles the infant and parent bring to the relationship and the emerging characteristics of the dyad; and,
- the sociocultural forces that shape and modify the previously mentioned realms.

These different domains may be examined separately, but the findings must be integrated in a comprehensive biopsychosocial formulation. For example, a three-year-old boy was referred because of irritability, hyperactivity, and a recent decrease in cognitive functions. The diagnosis of lead intoxication was readily confirmed by elevated lead levels in the blood, necessitating treatment to decrease the lead levels and environmental changes to prevent further exposure. However, an understanding of the mother's response to the child's symptoms was as important as the understanding of this etiology. A single mother, burdened by poverty, lack of social supports, and her own depression, had responded to the child's behavior with frequent reprimands and punishment, interpreting the symptoms to mean that the child was "dumb and evil... out to hurt me." She added: "He is just like his father, always after me." The father had physically abused her and was incarcerated for assault at the time of the evaluation. By the time of the evaluation the child had became increasingly clingy and the mother responded with angry withdrawal to his approach.

The comprehensive assessment of this case demanded an understanding of the dynamics within the mother-child dyad. The maternal perception of the child as dangerously aggressive, sharing with his father a propensity for assault, caused her to misinterpret the infant's clingy behavior as an attack, leading to her withdrawal behavior and thus preventing a more supportive response from her to the child's approach. Similarly, the mother's symptoms of depression decreased her tolerance for the child's symptoms and facilitated her withdrawal. The evaluation also needs to address the correlation between the social and economic stressors (single parenthood, poverty, lack of social support, inadequate housing) and the mother's use of aversive and punitive child rearing practices. A lack of understanding of these biological, psychological, and socioeconomic domains would not allow for the development of an informed and comprehensive plan of action.

A comprehensive evaluation needs to include a review of individual and family history, an examination of the child, an assessment of the parent-child relationship, and an assessment of the sociocultural circumstances of the child and family. The assessment can be divided into the following components:

- Clinical interview: This interview aims at a definition of the problem as seen and understood by the family, the family's expectations from the evaluation, and the establishment of an initial contract. An essential goal of the interview(s) is the establishment of a therapeutic alliance based on realistic goals for the evaluation. The interview should also review the developmental and pediatric history of the child, and the family's psychiatric and medical history.
- Developmental examination of the child: This examination assesses the developmental competencies of the child in four domains: gross motor, fine motor, language, and

social skills. The examination of the child also addresses temperament and patterns of self-regulation and of social interaction.

• Assessment of the immediate environment: This assessment focuses on the parent-child dyad overt interactive behaviors and on the parent's subjective representation of the child and of the relationship. It focuses on the dyad itself and on the parental contribution to the relationship. The dyadic relationship needs then to be understood against the context of the family structure and family dynamics.

• Assessment of the broader social environment: This assessment addresses social, cultural, and economic factors that determine the characteristics of the physical and social environment of the family and child.

CLINICAL INTERVIEW

Chief Complaint

Depending on the complexity of the history, the clinical interview can take two or three sessions. If possible it is important to interview all the caregivers the child has had, including grandparents, stepparents, foster parents, and other household residents, because part of the history may not be known to everyone. When feasible, data from birth records, pediatrician reports, and other resources may fill the gap. In some cases the social worker assigned by state agencies is the person most familiar with the child's history and can be an invaluable resource.

During the initial interview the clinician should offer the patient, family, and others accompanying the family an opportunity to discuss their concerns and worries. Of paramount importance is understanding what the family sees as the problem, what they believe its causes to be, and the expected outcome. It is important also to understand what family members imagine the evaluation to entail and what they expect from therapy. Often, this enquiry will elicit a view of the problem that is different from that of the clinician. The task, at this point, is not to "correct" the family's understanding of the condition, but to learn what factors have determined their point of view, such as lack of information, cultural style of viewing development and illness, denial, guilt, suspicion, and so on. The understanding of these factors will allow the clinician to search for a common ground on which to plan the evaluation, and also to modify the interviewing approach to address such factors. Empathy with the family's distress, acknowledgment of their view of the problem, and an approach that places the family in the role of a valuable partner in the evaluation process will facilitate the development of a therapeutic alliance and enlist the active participation of the family in the therapeutic process.

DEVELOPMENTAL HISTORY

The developmental history should cover those areas listed below.

Gestational History

This should include ages of the parents, length of gestation, medical or obstetrical problems (i.e., bleeding, toxemia, diabetes, etc.), and exposure to alcohol, tobacco, illegal drugs, medications, and so on.

Labor and Delivery

This should include characteristics and length of labor, whether spontaneous or induced, whether vaginal or cesarean, presentation, condition of child at birth (including Apgar scores), obstetrical complications, and so on.

Neonatal History

This should include weight, length and head circumference, length of hospitalization, complications such as jaundice, respiratory distress syndrome, and congenital abnormalities.

Developmental History

This should address the achievement of milestones in the four general domains: fine and gross motor, language, and social skills. This part of the evaluation should not be a rigid set of questions, unresponsive to emerging information. However, clinicians, particularly those in the process of developing skills in this area, should not be discouraged from using protocols and timetables as guidelines to a comprehensive evaluation. Unless the data will be used for research, there is no reason not to use instruments flexibly to elicit clinical data. Of particular help to the clinician can be the clear definitions of milestones and the criteria for pass and fail that most instruments offer such as the timetables developed by Capute (Johnson, 1993) and Denver II.

Pediatric History

This should include a history of immunizations, trauma, illnesses, surgery, previous treatment, and so on.

Family Medical and Psychiatric History

This component of the interview focuses on hereditary medical and psychiatric conditions present in the family (which may represent risk and predispositions in the child), and other medical history that may directly or indirectly affect the primary caregiving environment of the child. When possible the interview should include both the paternal and maternal sides of the family to avoid gaps in the data caused by informants' lack of information or denial.

DEVELOPMENTAL EXAMINATION OF THE CHILD

Because there are significant differences between the examination of neonates and other infants and toddlers, they will be described separately.

Neonatal Examination

The neurodevelopmental assessment of a newborn focuses on two main areas: the neurophysiological status of the central nervous system and the newborn's style of self-regulation and patterns of interacting with caretakers. The assessment of the neonate's neurodevelopmental status and degree of risk for developmental disabilities focuses on reflexes, tonus, cranial nerve intactness, and behavior. Because it is particularly difficult to diagnose developmental deficits in the neonate period, the goal of the assessment is to recognize those neonates at heightened risk for developmental deficits. Children at risk then can be targeted for specific follow-up interventions. Neurodevelopmental examination findings need to be integrated with a comprehensive assessment of the physical status of the neonate, and as stated in previous paragraphs, with a detailed gestational and perinatal history and family history regarding genetic, neurological, and developmental disorders.

Among neonate examination protocols, the Neonatal Neurodevelopmental Examination (NNE) developed by Allen and Capute (1989) is easy to learn, rapid (duration of 15 to 25 minutes), and selects children at heightened risk for developmental disabilities. When NNE findings are correlated with neuroimaging and EEG the predictive power is significantly enhanced. The second component of the examination, the assessment of the neonate style of self-regulation and of relating to the caretakers, focuses on the capacities for self-modulation of arousal levels, capacity for use of pertinent adult interventions to regulate inner states (amenability for soothing, focusing of attention, etc.), and the potential for progressively attuned interaction with the caretaker. It addresses the neonate's capacity to communicate needs and elicit appropriate caretaking behavior that ensures the neonate's survival and development. Such information can be used by the clinician to facilitate a parent-child interaction that is effective and mutually gratifying. Interventions based on these findings aim at the prevention of attachment deficits and other disorders of the parent-child dyad that ultimately interfere with the child's development.

A widely used examination routine for neonates is the Newborn Behavioral Assessment Scale (NBAS) developed by Brazelton (1984). The NBAS takes approximately 20 to 30 minutes to administer and two administrations are recommended (on the third day and ninth or tenth day after birth). The NBAS is designed to be used with infants between 36 and 44 weeks of gestational age. With the use of a set of nine supplementary items, the scale can be administered to premature and at-risk infants (born to mothers addicted to alcohol, narcotics, malnourished mothers, etc.). This is an examination that demands a rather lengthy training to meet rigorous inter-rater reliability norms. Further, an examiner needs to use the examination frequently to maintain skill levels.

The findings of the NBAS can be put to use to facilitate the establishment of a mutually gratifying and effective relationship between the neonate and the parents. The Family Administered Neonatal Activities (FANA) is a modified application of the NBAS in which the parents are involved in administering parts of the examination. The experience, facilitated by a clinician, can promote in the parents a sense of competence and increased adaptive behaviors, as well as an increase in realistic expectations regarding the infant's capacities (Cardone & Gilkerson, 1990).

Examination of Infants and Toddlers

The psychiatric examination can be divided into a developmental component and an interactive component. The developmental examination traditionally is divided into four domains: gross motor, fine motor/problem solving, language, and social skills. This examination is carried out in two formats that are complementary: clinical assessment and standardized testing. The clinical examination is carried out in the playroom as part of the play interview of the child. The parent(s) should be invited to participate in the interview and to intervene as they would at home. In those rare cases where the parents are actively and pervasively disruptive of the child, they can be invited, in a second interview, to observe through a one-way mirror. Some writers suggest that another clinician accompany the parents in the observation room to assist the parents in attending to relevant aspects of the child's performance and the child's response to the interviewer's interventions.

The examination focuses on the child's best performance and pays particular attention to the strategies the child uses to achieve said performance, including the use of parental assistance. Of particular importance are the appropriateness of the parental assistance in facilitating the child's problem-solving performance (as opposed to intrusiveness or task disruption), and the child's integration of this parental intervention with his or her own abilities. Of primary relevance is not only what the child can do, but, also, how the child accomplishes the task. While this section of the examination is criterion-based, it is important to compare the child's performance to age-appropriate norms. As a general point of reference the clinician may use standardized norms—such as those of Denver II which is a screening test, or the developmental scales developed by Caputo, published in the *Harriet Lane Handbook* (Johnson, 1993).

Regarding the different developmental domains, gross motor performance is generally the easiest to assess. Generally, parents recall relatively easily the motor milestone achievements and active children readily demonstrate their abilities. The assessment of language is more demanding, particularly regarding prelinguistic language where the parents need more assistance from the clinician to differentiate between levels of functioning. The parental report of the child's language developmental sequence is a necessary complement to the direct observation of the child. Further, many children are reluctant to speak in the examining room and in those cases the parental observations are even more crucial. Caputo (1978) developed the Clinical Linguistic and Auditory Milestones Scale (CLAMS) that monitors the language development of the child utilizing the parents' report. It defines with precision the language milestones and helps in the differentiation of deviant language forms such as echolalia or programmed speech from utterances with true communication intent. In those cases of delay or deviancy in speech and language development, the child psychiatrist can refer the child for more systematic assessment by a speech and language pathologist.

The second component of the examination is the systematic measure of the four developmental domains under standardized circumstances. In the multidisciplinary team this examination is generally done by the clinical psychologist. It aims at a comparison of the child's performance to the norm for children of the same age. For this segment of the assessment, the most widely used instrument is the *Bayley Scales of Infant Development-Second Edition* (BSID-II) (Bayley 1993). The administration of this instrument takes up to 60 minutes and is applicable to children between the ages of 1 month and 42 months. The BSID-II systematically measures current functioning but must not be construed as predicting future intelligence. A newer and promising instrument, the Infant Mullen Scales of Early Learning (Infant MSEL) is based on a neurodevelopmental model and examines selectively five subscales in the areas of visual, language, and motor competencies.

Assessment of Temperament

Temperament is a set of relatively stable, biologically based characteristics of the individual regarding reactivity and self-regulation that is of great significance in the parent-child relationship, defining its quality and tone. The match or fit between the temperament of the caretaker and that of the child influences the interaction of the dyad.

Assessment of the child's temperament is an important measure of the contribution of the child to the parent-child relationship. This assessment can be done either by direct observation or by obtaining information from the primary caretaker. Since direct observation calls for assessment of behavior under different naturalistic circumstances, it can be time-consuming and logistically difficult to carry out. On the other hand, data obtained indirectly from questionnaires can be distorted by the observer's bias. Yet for pragmatic reasons, questionnaires are used both clinically and in research. The Infant Temperament Questionnaire (Carey & McDevitt, 1978) and the Toddlers Temperament Questionnaire, (Fullard, McDevitt, & Carey, 1984) assess the nine categories used by Thomas and Chess in the New York Longitudinal Studies. Scoring is relatively easy and allows for classification of the subjects into four temperament categories: easy, difficult, slow-to-warm-up, and intermediate.

Assessment of the Immediate Environment

The child's immediate environment corresponds at one level with the parent-child dyadic interaction and this dyadic interaction needs to be understood within the wider context of the family. In some circumstances it is more appropriate to speak of the primary caregiver-child dyad, when it is not a parent who is the primary source of child rearing. The next paragraphs address the evaluation in traditional terms, understanding that the clinician may need to adapt the process to specific characteristics of the child and his or her immediate environment.

Assessment of the Parent–Child Dyad

As posited by Stern-Bruschweiler and Stern (1989) the interaction between infants and their caregivers can be understood as an objective behavioral interchange between the partners of the dyad, each of which is in turn influenced by his or her own internal representations. The parent-child interaction can be reviewed in terms of the observable events between them (analysis of the interaction) and an assessment of the parent's internal representations of the child. These representations include the expectations, assumptions, and perceptions that the parents bring to the interaction with the infant, whether to enrich or disturb the relationship. The knowledge about the internal representations of infants and toddlers is highly inferential given their limited capacity to report inner experiences. The internal representations of children have been studied by psychoanalytic means but will not be reviewed at this point.

Regarding parent-child relationships in infants and toddlers, Anders (1989) highlighted the importance of the patterns of regulation developed within the dyad. These patterns modulate the child's levels of stimulation and arousal. Under ideal circumstances they encourage emotional and cognitive growth. The properties of the relationship that mediate this regulation are synchrony, reciprocity, engagement, and attunement. The regulatory functions are mediated also by the affective tone of the relationship, whose dynamic characteristics are range, modulation, and attunement. The quality of regulation in the dyad can be classified as normal, over-regulated, under-regulated, or within various types of deviant patterns. Many protocols and instruments have been developed to address these features of the parent-child dyad. Two protocols will be reviewed, one examining the overt behavior within the dyad and one examining the parental internal representations.

Analysis of the Parent–Child Interaction   The Greenspan-Lieberman Observation System for Assessment of Caregiver-Infant Interaction during Semi-Structured Play (GLOS) (Greenspan & Lieberman, 1980) focuses on objective behaviors of the parent and the child. The assessment includes the rating on 53 parent and 43 child variables of 15 minutes of videotaped free-play between the parent and child. The instrument focuses on the quality of physical contact in the parent-child dyad, and on a series of contingent and non-contingent responses to behavior and affect of the dyadic partner. This instrument focuses on the objective behavior of the parent and child, and does not explore subjective parental perceptions.

Assessment of the Parental Representations   The content of parental representations of the child can be elicited by the clinician in psychodynamically oriented exploratory interviews. The analysis of this information not only illuminates the quality of the current parent-child interaction, but can also yield information on the origins of the parental representations in the parents' own histories. Such understanding can assist the clinician in designing psychodynamic therapeutic interventions. (Fraiberg, 1975).

Zeanah and Benoit (1995) developed the Working Model of the Child Interview (WMCI), an instrument to assess the formal aspect of the parental representation of the child. The instrument allows the clinician to classify the parental perception of the child within three major categories: balanced, disengaged, or distorted. These categories have shown promising correlation with the child's quality of attachment and with the presence in the child of clinical disorders including sleep disorders and failure to thrive. Further, the instrument allows for refined analysis of other aspects of the parent's perception of the child, including richness of perception, flexibility of representation, coherence, and affective tone. It also studies the intensity of involvement, the degree of acceptance of the child, the caregiving sensitivity, and the parental subjective experience and response to the child's difficult behavior.

Assessment of the Family   A study of the parent-child dyad needs to be placed in the context of the total family. Because of the traditional central role of mothers in child rearing, the direct and indirect results of the presence of the father and his participation in caregiving are too often ignored. Research on the father's role as social support for the mother suggests that her effectiveness as a parent can improve as a result of his participation. The effect of the father's direct participation in caregiving is less studied but an important area of clinical information to be explored. The role of grandparents in terms of direct care or of support of the child rearing should be assessed in the evaluation. The corresponding negative effects of marital discord, intergenerational conflict, disintegration of the family, and actual absence of family members needs to be explored as well.

Assessment of the Broader Social Environment

The impact on the family of cultural, economic, and political forces is of paramount importance. The family's cultural background will shape its recognition and understanding of the problems leading to the evaluation. It is essential, then, for the clinician to understand the family structure, basic assumptions, and other characteristics of the cultural group to which a patient belongs as well as variations within this group. For example, within immigrant groups of recent arrival, the degree of acculturation represents an important source of variability in the way a family will react to the clinician's evaluation. Since the evaluation represents a view determined by the local culture's values, those families that are more acculturated may be more open to accept the clinician's formulation than those that may be at a earlier stage in adaptation to the new culture.

The clinician needs to be aware, also, of implications related to the social status of a family. Socioeconomic disadvantage, as illustrated in the case history at the beginning of this chapter, can be responsible for increased risk for physical illness such as exposure to lead in inner-city housing, increased risk for depression and substance abuse, and increased propensity for aversive and punitive child rearing practices.

Biopsychosocial Formulation

If the family has been an active and valued participant in the evaluation process, the final report and recommendations should not come as a surprise but as an integration of all the available data from which conclusions regarding etiology, prognosis, and treatment can be drawn. Some clinicians overemphasize the dynamics in the family and fail to provide the family with needed specific technical information. An opposite mistake is to become so technical that the impact of the report on the family is unattended. It is at this point that the infant psychiatrist knowledge of the incoming views of the family regarding the "problem" is useful.

During the evaluation, the family will have become progressively familiar with the professionals viewpoint and a common ground of understanding should have developed. However, often under the stress of facing a "final" report, the earlier views, fears, and defenses may reactivate. The psychiatrist needs then to deal with those views that detract from effective treatment. The interactions the psychiatrist had with the family during the evaluation, and the awareness of the interventions that facilitated the family's cooperation will allow for an informed selection of strategies to deal with the factors that interfere with adequate understanding of the conclusions and recommendations. Culturally determined views that do not interfere with adequate treatment must not be disrupted. It may be in the best interest of the child to coordinate medical treatment with practices determined by tradition and to tailor the recommendation to the characteristics of the family instead of demanding full agreement with a treatment plan that may appear meaningless or offensive to the family.

The results of the evaluation should be presented in a succinct but clear manner, free of jargon and hesitation. Degrees of certainty need to be described honestly and alternatives discussed with equanimity. Two circumstances should be considered indicators of a disturbed evaluation process. One of these circumstances is to be recognized when the family addresses the infant psychiatrist as an all-knowing expert whose advice they accept without questions. The narcissistic pleasure derived from this family response is short-lived. The unquestioning acceptance of the recommendations usually means that ambivalence and doubts are temporarily repressed and will re-emerge as the positive transference decreases. This re-emergence often takes the form of disgruntled dissatisfaction with the evaluation and evaluator, and a failure to carry out the recommendations.

Another indicator of a disturbed process is the situation in which the family questions every detail of the assessment and every step of the interpretation of findings. The process becomes circular and repetitive and regardless of extensive explanations there is no resolution but obsessive stagnation. In those circumstances, the psychiatrist must recognize that the impasses will not be resolved with increased information and more convincing tests and consultations. Instead, there is a need to explore the meaning of the obsessive circular-ity which is usually related to the anger and despair the family experiences regarding the findings. Unable to discharge the anger elsewhere, the family may direct their frustration at the psychiatrist or the team. It behooves the psychiatrist to address the basic feelings and conflicts and facilitate the family's coming to terms with the findings. It is the parents anguish that need to be addressed rather than the endless negotiations to negate the clinical findings.

CONCLUSION

Looking back at the different components of a psychiatric evaluation, it may seem like a monumental task, complex and difficult. However, the completion of an evaluation can be of significant help to the family and leave the clinician with the lasting satisfaction of making a positive contribution to the more optimal actualization of a child's potential.

REFERENCES

Allen, M. C., & Capute, A. J. (1989). Neonatal neurodevelopmental examination as a predictor of neuromotor outcome in premature infants. *Pediatrics, 83,* 498–506.

Anders, T. F. (1989). Clinical syndromes, relationship disturbances, and their assessment. In A. J. Sameroff & R. N. Emde (Eds.), *Relationship disturbances in early childhood.* New York: Basic Books.

Bayley, N. (1993). *Bayley scales of infant development. Second edition manual.* San Antonio, TX: Psychological Corporation.

Brazelton, T. B. (1984). *Neonatal behavioral assessment scale.* Philadelphia: J. B. Lippincott.

Capute, A. J., & Accardo, P. J. (1978). Linguistic and auditory milestones during the first two years of life: A language inventory for the practitioner. *Clinical Pediatrics, 17,* 847–853.

Cardone, I. A., & Gilkerson, L. (1990). Family administered neonatal activities: An exploratory method for the integration of parental perceptions and newborn behavior. *Infant Mental Health Journal, 11,* 127–141.

Carey, W. B., & McDevitt, S. C. (1978). Revision of the infant temperament questionnaire. *Pediatrics, 61,* 735–739.

Fraiberg, S., Adelson, E., & Shapiro, V. (1975). Ghosts in the nursery. A psychoanalytic approach to the problems of impaired infant-mother relationships. *Journal of the American Academy of Child Psychiatry, 14,* 387–421.

Fullard, W., McDevitt, S. C., & Carey, W. B. (1984). Assessing temperament in one to three year old children. *Journal of Pediatric Psychology, 9,* 205–217.

Greenspan, S. I., & Lieberman, A. F. (1980). Infants, mothers and their interaction: A quantitative clinical approach to developmental assessment. In S. I. Greenspan & G. H. Pollock (Eds.), *The course of life. Psychoanalytic contributions towards understanding personality development.* Bethesda, MD: National Institute of Mental Health.

Johnson, K. B. (1993). *The Harriet Lane handbook. A manual for pediatric house officers.* St. Louis: Mosby-Year Book, Inc.

Stern-Bruschweiler, N., & Stern, D. N. (1989). A model for conceptualizing the role of the mother's representational world in various mother-infant therapies. *Infant Mental Health Journal, 10,* 142–156.

Zeanah, C. H., & Benoit, D. (1995). Clinical applications of a parent perception interview in infant mental health. *Child and Adolescent Psychiatric Clinics of North America, 4,* 539–554.

Chapter 6

Psychiatric Evaluation of School-Age Children

Mohammad Haerian, M.D.

INTRODUCTION

The period between 6 and 12 years of age has been termed latency by psychoanalysts, age of "industry" by Erikson, "concrete operational stage" by Piaget (1952), and "school-age" by Chess and Thomas. Regardless of terminology, this period is characterized by a highly active interchange between the child and his or her environment, laying foundations for autonomy, learning social norms, developing the capacity for self-reflection, and the gradual attainment of morality.

Latency, according to psychoanalytic theorists, is the period of educability, pliability, and calm (Sarnoff, 1976). This can be achieved by a specific organization of ego mechanisms which enables the child to cope with his or her sexual and aggressive drives. These mechanisms include fantasy, repression sublimation, and reaction formation. The development of a rather harsh and rigid superego is another characteristic of this period.

As a result of the maturation of the central nervous system (CNS) and the consequent cognitive changes which occur, around age 6 or 7, the child enters the concrete operational stage. These changes play the central role in passage from pre-latency to latency and they are pivotal in development of autonomy, capacity for reasoning, problem solving, and moral development. It is no surprise then that the age seven in various cultures and different times of history has been considered a milestone marking a major shift in the child's capabilities (Shapiro & Perry, 1976).

The latency age may be divided into two periods, the first extending from 6 to 8 years and the second from 8 until 10 years (Bornstein, 1951). In the first period, "the ego still buffeted by the surging impulses is threatened by the new superego which is not only harsh and rigid, but still a foreign body" (p. 280). In the second phase the ego encounters fewer conflicts and the superego becomes less rigid. In addition, there is an increased maturation of cognitive functioning, a gradual shift from fantasy to reality, and a move toward independence. The child gradually moves toward peers and away from parents with the result of increasing independence. The school-age child also demonstrates improvement in reality testing and reasoning, which results in less reliance on fantasy and ushers in the gradual breakdown of the latency-age child's defense structure, namely fantasy, reaction formation, and repression. This process in part explains the confusion, fluidity, and instability of preadolescence and early adolescence years.

INTERVIEW

Although there has been a gradual decrease in the stigma attached to seeing a psychiatrist and, more importantly, to carrying a psychiatric diagnosis, it is still very difficult for some parents to seek help for their children. The parents go through a large array of informal and often unsolicited consultations with family members, friends, and church members. Many parents of children with obvious psychiatric disorders do not appreciate either the meaning or severity of their children's difficulties (Rutter, Tizard, & Whitmore, 1970). They may simply believe that the child is lazy, "he just doesn't want to do anything" or he eventually will grow out of it. Often problems of an unhappy child go unnoticed until he or she takes an overdose. Even in such cases, before contacting a mental health professional the family goes through a variety of consultations with family and friends (sometimes they try to keep the problem hidden from everyone) and homemade remedies. They may attribute the problem to too much sugar in the diet or lack of appropriate vitamins.

When the parents eventually consult a mental health professional, they are by then often frustrated and demoralized. Some may feel that they have failed as parents while others may blame the school or "bad friends," for instance, for their child's problems. Parents' attitudes toward the mental health professional are often ambivalent. On the one hand, they may see him or her (or expect him or her to be) as an omnipotent and omniscience person who would recognize and remedy the child's problem in no time. On the other hand, they may unconsciously wish the professional to fail because, after all, as the child's parents they were unable to prevent or remedy the problem and it is hard for them to accept that a stranger will be able to help their child. Parents also are often worried that they will be blamed for the child's problem. In addition, many parents do not have a clear understanding of psychiatric problems, the way psychiatric services are provided, and how they work.

Some children may be referred by social agencies or courts. In these cases, parents commonly are against the referral, they do not believe that there is a problem, and they often see the mental health professional as an agent of the court or government interfering with their private lives.

It goes without saying that only rarely does a school-age child ask his or her parents to be allowed to see a mental health professional. Children are often told that they will see a doctor or a therapist for various reasons. They know very little about psychiatry, and in fact have more misconceptions than their parents. Children frequently perceive that seeing a psychiatrist means that they are "psycho," "retarded," or other pejorative terms.

For all these reasons the psychiatric interview must focus on the social context and dynamics of referral as well as on the child. It is necessary to understand the dynamics of the process of referral, who is concerned, why are they concerned, and why now? In assessing children, a developmental approach is necessary because children behave differently at different ages. For instance, a behavior that may be appropriate at a certain age may be considered pathological several years later. Furthermore, there are certain stressors and vulnerabilities at different ages and there are predictable developmental tasks for different periods. For example, the toddler age is the time when children are most likely to be adversely affected by separation from their caregivers (e.g., hospital admission, entering preschool), and adolescence is the time that youngsters are subjects to periods of "the blues" and depression (Rutter, 1986). The clinician also must be aware of continuities and discontinuities in development, risk, and protective factors. Attention should be paid to major life events and transitions and how they have been experienced and negotiated by the child.

Data Gathering

The sources of data include an interview with parents, an interview with the child, a thorough mental status examination, medical examination, a school report, and observation of the child. (In some disorders like ADHD observation of the child in different settings often provides more information than clinical interviews.) Other sources of information when necessary may include psychological testing, educational assessment, speech and language evaluation, occupational therapy assessment, and laboratory tests and procedures (e.g., EEG, MRI, CT scan).

Interview with Parents

Most clinicians agree that it is most helpful initially to meet with the parents and obtain a clear and comprehensive history of the child's problems, reasons for seeking help at this time, past history, and medical and family history. However, some clinicians prefer to see the child alone initially with information about only the chief complaint from the parents in order to obtain a fresh, unbiased view of the patient. This approach can be particularly valuable when working with the adolescent patient. In the initial meeting with the parents the clinician should also inquire about the parents' expectations from the consultation and their feelings about it. Special attention should be paid to the dynamics of the process of referral. Since parents often feel guilty and may believe that they have failed or have caused the problem, it is essential to encourage the parents to express their concerns and talk about who initiated the referral and what they wish to get from consultation. After this initial phase the interviewer needs to move to more detailed and broad-based questioning.

Widely differing recommendations have been made about the best way to obtain accurate information. Some advocate a non-direct approach, letting the parents set the tone and talk freely about whatever they feel is significant. The assumption is that eventually their thought processes will lead them to talk about clinically significant materials. Others suggest a series of standard questions followed by nonspecific probes. Cox reports that systematic questioning is usually superior to less structured approaches(Cox, 1994). In the initial interview, however, the parents should be allowed to talk freely about their concerns. Often parents who cannot talk about the problems in their own terms feel that they have not been understood. Whether one takes a non-directive approach or asks systematic questions, often flexible, probing questions are necessary to clarify the answers. It is important to ask parents for examples of the child's behavior to help differentiate between what actually happened and what the parents felt happened.

When asking parents about the child's symptoms, the interviewer should inquire about the time that they first noticed the problem. Depending on the nature of the symptoms, parents' recollection and their accuracy varies. For example, the parents may clearly remember when the child set a fire whereas they may differ about the beginning of the child's depressive symptoms. It is important to get a clear picture about the evaluation of the symptoms from the time they were first noticed until the present. The interviewer should inquire about frequency, duration, and intensity of the symptoms and the impact on the child's relationship with peers, siblings, and school performance.

Although the effect of temperament on the child's behavior is relatively modest (Hubert, Wachs, Peters-Martin, & Gandour, 1982) it is often useful to explore about the child's temperament during infancy and toddlerhood by asking specific questions about the child's adaptability, adjustment, and capacity for self-soothing and self-regulation. Other areas of inquiry include school history, academic performance, hobbies, relationship with peers and family members, fears, phobias, separations, and traumatic events. Developmental milestones should emphasize motor and speech development and social development such as eye contact, social smile, and separation anxiety.

The parents should be asked to describe their child in their own words, including the child's likes and dislikes, quality of mood, capacity for compromise and negotiation, ability to postpone gratification and impulse control, and whether he or she can be trusted as well as whether he or she can trust others. Additionally, is the child a leader or a follower, is he or she secure in relationships, is he or she friendly, warm, demonstrative, cold, indifferent?

The family history should inquire about the presence or absence of major psychiatric disorders, alcohol and drug abuse, learning disabilities, and abnormal personality in the family members, including maternal and paternal grandparents, aunts, and uncles.

It is always valuable to understand parents' feelings about what they are describing. To achieve this, the interviewer needs to be sensitive and able to communicate in a language well attuned to feelings. A warm tone of voice and responsive facial expression are probably important in leading the informant to feel understood (Shapiro, 1969). Warmth may be conveyed by tone of voice, smiling, nodding, and brief expressions of interest and approval (Breed, 1972) (adapted from Cox, 1994).

Brown and Rutter have shown that with the use of these interviewing techniques, sensible, reliable, and valid information about various aspects of family life and relationships can be obtained from a single interview with one parent (Brown & Rutter, 1966). Areas of inquiry should include family activities, relationship with the extended family, social activities, marital relationships, possible tensions, and arguments and quarrels. It also is important to inquire about the extent to which the children are drawn into family arguments.

Interview with the Child

In most instances, the child is not even aware that his or her parents have already contacted a child psychiatrist. This is because of parents' anxiety and defensiveness about their decision and more often because of the fact that they simply do not know what to tell the child. Although it is important to avoid giving cookbook answers regarding this issue to the parents, one point should be made clear: honesty is the best policy. Parents may talk with the child about his or her difficulties at school, or his or her irritable and angry mood, or loneliness and inability to make friends (or whatever the problem is). They should emphasize that they have made many efforts to understand what is wrong and to help him or her with his or her problems but they have not been successful in doing so. Now they are seeking help from someone who specializes in helping children with these kinds of problems. The child should be told that he or she will have one or more visits with this doctor and the purpose is for the doctor to get to know him or her and to understand why he or she is having these problems. The child should be told that the doctor will be able to help the child and his or her parents to cope with these problems better.

The timing of this explanation is important: with school-age children, several days notice is helpful. This will help the child to think about the upcoming visit with the psychiatrist and give him or her the opportunity to ask his or her parents any questions. With very anxious and fearful children, three to four days wait may be too long as the visit may become another source of worry for the child.

The Office Setting

School-age children can be interviewed directly. Occasionally, however, it may become necessary to engage the child in some kind of game or play activity to "break the ice" and/or elicit information that otherwise is difficult to obtain directly. The setting of the office and choice of toys therefore becomes important. One should remember that the main purpose of the interview is to gather information in a systematic fashion in order to arrive at a diagnostic formulation. The way the interview is conducted and to a lesser extent, the office setting will help or hinder gathering information. The direct and indirect message to the child should be that the interviewer is trying to understand his or her problems. Having many toys in the office or beginning the interview with a game or play activity without any reference to the reasons for evaluation will make the child confused and often misled. Having emphasized that, it is prudent to have the following materials in the office:

- a variety of writing and drawing materials
- a selection of bendable toy human figures of different age, race and occupation
- hand puppets
- a dollhouse
- toy cars and trucks
- a variety of games and puzzles. The games may include both games of skill and chance and those which encourage both competitive and noncompetitive activities. A simple game of skill like checkers not only can reveal the child's cognitive style and problem-solving strategy, it also may reflect the child's ability (or lack thereof) to follow rules, to accept defeat, and so on. A time-consuming game or a game that requires intense and long periods of concentration like chess should be avoided.

The first contact usually occurs in the waiting room. The clinician should go to the waiting area, greet the parents, and rather quickly turn to the child, bending down to reach the child's eye level. The clinician should introduce himself or herself in a brief, pleasant, and casual way and state that he or she and the child are going to his or her office. The warm, pleasant, and reassuring conduct of the clinician during this brief initial contact is important in instilling a sense of trust and safety in both parents and the child.

Once in the office the clinician should move quickly to clarify why the child thinks he or she is seeing the clinician and to allay the child's fears. It is helpful to ask the child what he or she has been told by his or her parents about the visit and what type of doctor the clinician is. The clinician should tell the child clearly why he or she thinks that the child is there and what to expect from the interview and that no injections or other medical procedures will take place. He or she may say to the child, "I already have met with your parents, they have shared with me their concerns about your problems, and now I would like to hear from you." Usually, because an immediate barrage of questions about emotionally charged issues makes children very uneasy, it is usually best to begin with some rather neutral questions concerning topics such as social activities, hobbies, grades, and sports activities. If the child is aware of his or her problems, it would be helpful to ask him or her to describe them and explain his or her understanding of them. Although it is important to be flexible, it is equally important not to jump from one topic to another. Once a topic like a symptom of depression has been begun, it is best to continue until all the necessary information is gathered. If in his or her answers the child brings up an important issue the clinician may reassure him or her that they will return to that subject.

In inquiring about different symptoms the clinician should always ask for examples to make sure that the child and the clinician are talking about the same thing. The clinician should inquire as to what extent the child's symptoms are interfering with his or her social and academic functioning and how bothersome they are (ego syntonic versus ego dystonic). In the case of behavior problems (externalizing problems) the interviewer should ask about frequency and the setting in which those behaviors occur. For example, if the presenting problem is fighting the clinician would like to know how often it occurs, what precipitates the fights, whether it happens more at home, school, or in the neighborhood, and whether the child acts alone or in the company of his or her peers.

Open-Ended, Closed, and Leading Questions

Open-ended questions are those which offer a broad range of answers, while closed questions often require a limited set of responses. For example, if the child has just admitted stealing, an open-ended question would be, "tell me more about that" and a closed question would be "when was the last time you stole something?" Open-ended questions allow for expression of emotions and usually provide more data. Closed questions may be used to fill in the gaps in the information provided by open questions. A leading question is one that directly suggests its answer. For example, in the case of the child with a stealing problem, "I guess it made you feel guilty, didn't it?" would be a leading question and leading questions have no place in psychiatric interviews.

MENTAL STATUS EXAMINATION

Appearance

This part relies on the interviewer's power of observation. How a child of this age is dressed is more reflective of the parents' attitude. Whether he or she is tidy and neat or sloppy and dirty, however, reflects both the child's behavior and parental attitude. The examiner should pay attention to the child's height, weight, gait, and skin condition. Extremes of height and weight may suggest a metabolic condition. A dry skin with brittle hair may be indicative of hypothyroidism and presence of cafe au lait may suggest neurofibromatosis. Abnormalities of gait and toe walking may suggest cerebral palsy or fetal alcohol syndrome.

Behavior

How does the child relate to his or her parents and the examiner? Does he or she easily engage in conversation or does he or she need time to warm up to people? Does he or she have adequate eye contact? Is he or she cooperative or defiant? Is he or she curious? Does he or she explore the office or does the child appear very inhibited, sitting rigidly in the chair?

Motor Behavior   The examiner should pay attention to the child's level of activity. How impulsive is he or she? Does he or she get into everything or is he or she able to sit and follow the conversation? Does the child maintain interest in a task or does he or she get bored easily and move from one toy to another? Does the child respond to limits?

Speech and Thought Processes

Attention should be paid to the form, rate, rhythm, and content of speech. A number of psychiatric conditions may produce abnormalities in the form of speech. The slowness of speech in the depressed child with psychomotor retardation, pressure of speech in an anxious or manic child, the wooden quality of autistic speech are all examples of abnormalities of form of speech.

Speech content abnormalities may included neologism, incoherence, and poverty of content that may occur in schizophrenia and flight of ideas which occurs in manic children. Attention should also be paid to phonological problems such as stuttering and cluttering. (See chapter 9, Speech and Language Evaluation).

Thought Disorder   Thought disorder refers to problems in the logic of thinking and difficulty in understanding some comments or the overall thread of the conversation. Formal thought disorder consists of the following symptoms: illogical thinking, loose associations, incoherence, and poverty of content of speech. According to Caplan (1990), illogical thinking and loose associations are reliable, valid, sensitive, and specific measures of formal thought disorder in children with schizophrenia compared to normal children. Incoherence occurs rarely in middle-childhood schizophrenia and the poverty of content of speech which is a consistent finding in schizophrenic adults (Andreasen & Grove, 1986) occurs infrequently in schizophrenic children. Caplan et al. (1989, 1990) demonstrated that age seven years is the developmental cutoff point for illogical thinking and loose association in normal children. Illogical thinking may occur in normal children older than seven but it is very rare. Loose associations, however, are not found in normal children older than seven years of age. Certain aspects of thought disorder such as illogical thinking are found in childhood psychiatric disorders other than schizophrenia. Loose associations, however, seem to occur specifically in childhood schizophrenia.

Mood

A mood is a pervasive and sustained emotion that, when intense, colors a person's perception of the world (American Psychiatric Association [APA], 1994). Mood is used to describe one's psychological state in relation to environment. Mood is usually communicated through facial expressions, gesture, tone of voice, and general appearance. In exploring the child's mood the interviewer therefore should note whether the child looks happy or sad, does he or she sound angry or sullen? Does he or she appear anxious? The child may be asked to describe the way he or she feels most of the time. What kind of things make him or her happy, what makes him or her angry or sad? Has he or she ever been so sad that at the time he or she did not care about anything? (e.g., grades, parental and peer approval, consequences of behavior). Has the child ever thought that everyone would be better off if he or she were dead? Has he or she ever thought about ways of killing himself or herself? Has he or she ever tried? Is he or she thinking about it now?

Self Concept

A child may be asked to describe himself or herself. What do his or her friends like about him or her? What does he or she like about himself or herself? Is there anything that he or she may not like or, if possible, would change about himself or herself? What does the child think about his or her future? How does he or she see himself or herself 5 or 10 years from now?

Cognition

Usually during the interview, the clinician can get a rough measure of the child's cognitive ability, memory, attention, and fund of general information. The child's use of vocabulary and grammar is to some extent reflective of his or her degree of intelligence. His or her awareness of current events, whether some sports activities or world affairs, not only corresponds with his or her cognitive functioning but also reveals the child's interests and his or her attitude toward his or her environment as well.

Delusions

A delusion is a false personal belief that is firmly held in the face of contradictory evidence, and that is not held by other members of the individual's culture or subculture (APA, 1994). Delusions may be simple, complex, or systematized. They also can be categorized along different dimensions such as bizarreness, degree of individual's conviction of the reality of his or her belief, his or her level of preoccupation with the delusion, and so on. Children's tendency to blur the distinction between fantasy and reality and their inability to fully utilize logical reasoning makes it very difficult to ascertain delusions in children before age five years. By the same token delusions manifest themselves differently at different ages. Overall delusions are relatively rare before age 10. They tend to be simple, unsystematized, and centered on disturbances of identity.

Hallucinations

A hallucination may be defined as any perception which a) occurs in the absence of appropriate stimuli, b) has the full force and impact of the corresponding real perception, and c) the person has no voluntary control over. Hallucinations range from simple and unformed like shapes, shades, and sounds to very complex, organized, and well-formed perceptions like voices and figures. They may occur in one or more sensory modalities such as auditory, visual, kinetic, olfactory, or tactile. They may have an affective overtone or may be totally unrelated to the context of one's mood or thinking. Many consider hallucinations as strong evidence of severe psychopathology. However, considering the fact that hallucinations may occur naturally or may be induced in non-clinical subjects, one should caution against a psychopathology-based approach to hallucinatory phenomena.

Hallucinations may occur in Schizophrenia, Mood Disorders, and Dissociative and Post-Traumatic Stress Disorders. Hallucinations also occur in association with medical conditions such as some seizure disorders, alcoholism, head injury, and migraine. Other reasons for hallucinations may include sleep deprivation, sensory deprivation, and hallucinations related to stress or grief.

Hallucinations are difficult to ascertain in children prior to a certain level of language development. Nonetheless, hallucinations have been noted to occur in children as young as three or four years of age with or without major psychiatric disorders (King & Noshpitz, 1991). In general, hallucinations in children are often fluid and less complex in nature than those seen in adults.

Preschool children may experience visual or tactile hallucinations in reaction to acute anxiety or situational stressors. These hallucinations are usually transient, benign and of an acute onset and primarily occur at night. Such children commonly have tactile hallucinations of bugs crawling on their skin or clothes. Visual hallucinations may include insects and threatening animals. There is a similarity between these hallucinations and childhood animal phobias.

In contrast to these transient and acute hallucinations reported in otherwise healthy preschool and young school-age children, hallucinations in older children and adolescents are often more persistent and associated with psychopathology. They may occur in the context of schizophrenia and mood disorders and a wide variety of organic syndromes. Children may experience hallucinations as uncommon side effects of stimulants, aspirin, antihistamines, barbiturates, and decongestants.

Insight

Insight refers to one's ability to acknowledge his or her problems and accept responsibility for his or her behavior. The child may be asked why he or she is seeing you, what does he or she think has caused the problem, and how the problem may be solved.

Soft Neurological Signs

Although often suspected to indicate "organicity," soft neurological signs are often neurodevelopmental immaturities that usually disappear in time and are not pathognomonic of any specific disorder. Deficiencies associated with soft neurological signs may be in the areas of speech, gross motor coordination, and fine motor coordination. Some of the frequently observed signs are:

- Laterality: Handedness usually is established by age five years, footedness by age seven, eye preference by age seven or eight, and ear preference by age nine. To examine the child's preference you may ask him or her to look through a telescope, to write a sentence, and to kick a ball.
- Right/Left discrimination: The child should be asked to put his or her right hand to his or her left ear, and his or her left hand to his or her right ear. By age five children are able to identify right and left hands. At age six the child achieves ipsilateral orientation (i.e., left hand on left knee) and at age seven contralateral orientation is achieved (i.e., left hand on right knee).
- Heel to toe walking or hopping on one foot (usually achieved by age seven).
- Rapid alternating movements: Patting back of one hand with the middle finger of the other hand.
- Two-point discrimination: Ask the child to close his or her eyes. Gently touch the child's right cheek and back of his or her left hand simultaneously. The child should be able to perceive both stimulations.
- Extension test: The child stands, feet together, eyes closed and arms extended, and dorsi flexed for 20 seconds. In right-handed children the right hand is elevated but the right-handed children with learning disability tend to elevate the left hand.

PSYCHOLOGICAL TESTING

Psychological tests may prove a very valuable adjunct tool in the psychiatric assessment of children. The clinician, however, should be aware of the limitations of these tests, their utility, and the financial implications in that a routine battery of psychological testing including WISC III, Rorschach, and TAT usually costs between $800 and $1,000. These tests are usually reimbursed at 50 percent and are subject to a very strict scrutiny by managed care companies. Psychological tests by themselves cannot be relied upon as diagnostic tools but, taken in combination with other clinical and historical data, they may be quite useful in understanding the child's pathology (see chapter 8, The Process of Psychological Assessment).

Behavior Rating Scales and Checklists

Most rating scales are designed to obtain information on a predetermined set of items in terms of structured response categories. Benefits include:

- Rating scales are convenient and economical.
- They can be completed by diverse informants without specialized training.
- They can cover a wide range of data.
- They provide scores that are easy to analyze.

Limitations of rating scales include:

- Rigid adherence to a predetermined set of items.
- Rating scales compare individuals on predetermined dimensions.
- They are affected by the cooperation, knowledgeability, and candor of the rater (Achenbach, 1991).

The most commonly used parent rating scales for children are the Conners Parent Rating Scale (Conners, 1985) and The Child Behavior Checklist (CBCL) (Achenbach & Edelbrock, 1983). These rating scales have a teacher's version as well. We often find it very useful to ask parents to fill out CBCL independent of each other. The teachers are asked to fill out the teacher's checklist. The results, especially discrepancies between the parents, often point to a number of issues, including child's different behavior in different settings, parents' different perceptions of child's behavior, and others. There is a strong body of literature reviewing the validity and reliability of CBCL. As with other questionnaires, parents usually underreport their children's internalizing problems (e.g., fears, anxieties, depression) and over-emphasize their externalizing symptoms (e.g., behavior problems, aggressive behavior).

Structured and Semi-Structured Interviews

Some clinicians have a tendency to focus on a particular set of problems without giving adequate weight to the exploration of the full range of symptomatology. In the absence of a structured medical decision-making process, the clinician may find correlation between two phenomena, thus the presence of the first phenomenon may lead to the expectation that the second one exists as well. On the other hand, they may fail to see correlations that really exist (e.g., depression and conduct disorder).

To overcome these problems a number of interviews have been designed. Two basic strategies have been adapted from the adult interviewing literature. The first approach is called structured interview. These interviews consist of a fully specified set of questions from which the interviewer should not deviate. The burden of interpreting and understanding the question then is on the child. The interviewer is required only to know the rules governing when questions should be asked and can be performed with non-clinicians with relatively little training. The Diagnostic Interview Schedule for Children (DISC; Costello et al., 1984) and the Diagnostic Interview for Children and Adolescents (DICA; Herjanic & Campbell, 1977) are some of the best known examples of such interviews for children. However, the test-retest reliability of these interviews is usually low for one cannot be sure that what each child believes a question to mean is what the developers of the interview intended it to mean (Cox, 1994).

In a semi-structured interview the key question is provided for guidance, but the interviewer is expected to ask whatever question is necessary to determine whether a particular symptom exists or not. This approach is very close to a clinical interview but it ensures that all the issues that should be covered are covered. To administer a semi-structured interview the interviewer needs much more training. Another drawback of this approach is that one does not know exactly what questions have been asked.

The Kiddie-Schedule for Affective Disorders and Schizophrenia (K-SADS; Puig-Antich & Champers, 1978), the Child Assessment Schedule (CAS; Hodges, Klein, Fitch, McKnew, & Cytryn, 1981) and the Child and Adolescent Psychiatric Assessment (CAPA; Angold, Cox, Predergast, & Rutter, 1987) are examples of semi-structured interviews. The K-SAD does not have a good test-retest reliability, whereas the CASE and the CAPA both appear to be reliable (Hodges, Coals, & McKnew, 1989). Unfortunately, the structured and semi-structured interview schedules are time-consuming and often boring for the interviewer and patient. However, there is no doubt that they yield much more reliable information than unstructured clinical interviews. Those who have learned how to conduct a semi-structured interview often find that it greatly improves their interviewing skills and they often can call upon their experience in their daily practice.

Although use of these schedules may not be practical for every patient, particularly when the managed care companies authorize only one session for a psychiatric evaluation, in certain diagnostically difficult children it may become necessary and quite helpful to use them.

Brain Imaging Techniques

Brain imaging techniques can be divided into two broad categories:

- structural techniques to study brain anatomy and structure. These include Computed Tomography (CT) and Magnetic Resonance Imaging (MRI).
- functional/dynamic techniques to study brain metabolism and regional change in brain activity and neurotransmitter systems. They include Positron Emission Tomography (PET), Single Photon Emission Computerized Tomography (SPECT), and Evoked Response Potential (adapted from Harris, 1995).

CT scan techniques have been used to investigate children with a variety of neuropsychiatric conditions including autistic and schizophrenic children, those with Tourette's syndrome, and so on. Their usefulness, however, is to study structural and anatomical changes of the brain. They should be requested only when the clinician has a fairly valid reason to suspect organicity.

An EEG (electroencephalogram) is a non-invasive and inexpensive means of assessing cerebral functions. It can be an invaluable diagnostic aid in child psychiatry. Nonetheless, the clinicians need to understand the limitations of this procedure and its complexities because of the maturation of the central nervous system (CNS) throughout childhood and subsequent changes in the EEG. The most common reason for requesting an EEG in a child is when the changes in behavior and mental status raise the possibility of an organic cause (brain tumor, petit mal, partial complex temporal lobe). Another major reason to ask for an EEG is to find out whether the child has a seizure disorder. EEG studies have been used in a variety of other disorders such as learning disabilities, tic disorders, ADHD, autism, and conduct disorders. The use of an EEG in these disorders is more as a "soft" sign of cerebral dysfunction and of questionable utility and value.

PSYCHIATRIC FORMULATION AND TREATMENT PLANNING

The psychiatric formulation is the synthesis of all clinical findings. A comprehensive psychiatric formulation provides an integration of biological, psychological, and social factors that contribute to the development of the problem. The biological factors include genetic predisposition, temperament, the child's biological endowment such as intelligence, and any medical condition that may contribute to the problem. Psychological factors refer to the child's coping and problem-solving skills, interpersonal relationships, defense mechanisms, and perception of self and others. Social considerations include one's status in society, and the child's relationships with peers, family, and significant others.

Treatment Planning

Treatment planning involves determining appropriate and feasible interventions for the child's and family's problems identified in the case formulation. A comprehensive treatment plan should address all aspects of the child and family in a biopsychosocial format. For instance, a child with ADHD living with a single mother in a crowded inner-city housing project will need many interventions which may involve different social agencies, school personnel, and a child psychiatrist. The therapies may include psychopharmacology, individual psychotherapy to help the child with his or her poor coping and problem-solving skills, behavior modification for poor impulse control, and parental counseling to help the mother manage the child's behavior. Another child with a similar diagnosis may need a totally different set of services.

CONCLUSION

The period between 6 and 12 years of age is characterized by significant changes in cognitive functioning and the defensive structure of the child. Children at this age are capable of having insight into their behavior and can give a reasonable account of their problems. Interview with the child, preferably a structured interview, is the major source of information. Comprehensive history with attention to the child's temperament, peer relationship, school history, and evolution of behavioral problems is essential. Assessment of family dynamics is equally important. Psychological testing, educational assessment, and neuropsychological testing are often necessary to rule out learning disabilities and to assess the child's coping and problem-solving skills. Use of EEG and brain imaging techniques helps to rule out organic conditions such as seizure disorders and tumors which may present with psychiatric symptoms. A biopsychosocial approach to evaluation remains the essential in formulating the child's diagnosis and his or her treatment needs.

REFERENCES

Achenbach, T. M. & Edelbrock, C. S. (1983). *Manual for the Behavior Checklist and Revised Child Behavior Profile*. University of Vermont, Department of Psychiatry, Burlington, VT.

Achenbach, T. M. (1991). Clinical data systems—Rating scales and interviews. In R. Michelals, (Ed.), *Psychiatry* (vol. 2, chap. 23). Philadelphia: J. B. Lippincott.

American Psychiatric Association. (1994). *Diagnostic and statistical manual of mental disorders* (4th ed.) *(DSM-IV)*. Washington, DC: the Author.

Andreasen, N. C. & Grove, W. M. (1986). Thought, language and communication in schizophrenia: Diagnosis and prognosis. *Schizophrenia Bulletin, 12*, 346–356.

Angold, A., Cox, A., Prendergast, M., & Rutter, M. (1987, 1991b). *The Child & Adolescent Psychiatric Assessment (CAPA)*. This unpublished interview can be obtained from the Developmental Epidemiology Program, Duke University Medical Center, Box 3454, Durham, NC 27710.

Bornstein, B. (1951). On latency. *The Psychoanalytic Study of the Child, 6*, 279–285.

Breed, G. (1972). The effect of intimacy: Reciprocity or retreat. *British Journal of Social & Clinical Psychology,11*, 135–142.

Brown, G. W., & Rutter, M. (1966). The measurement of family activities and relationships: A methodological study. *Human Relations, 19*, 241–263.

Caplan, R., Foy, J. G., Sigman, M., & Perdue, S. (1990). Information processing deficits of schizophrenic children with formal thought disorder. *Psychiatry Research, 31*, 169–177.

Caplan, R., Guthrie, D., Fish, B., Tanguay, P. E., & David-Lando, G. (1989). The kiddie formal thought disorder rating scale (K-FTDS): Clinical assessment reliability and validity. *Journal of the American Academy of Child and Adolescent Psychiatry, 28*, 208–216.

Costello, A. J., Edelbrock, C. S., Dulcan, M. D., Kalas, R., & Klaric, S. H. (1984). The NIMH diagnostic interview schedule for children (DISC): Final report. *National Institute of Mental Health*, Bethesda, MD.

Cox, A. D. (1994). Interviews with parents. In M. Rutter, E. Taylor, & Hersov, L. (Eds). *Child and Adolescent Psychiatry* (pp. 34–50) Oxford: Blackwell Science Ltd.

Harris, J. (1995). Assessment, diagnosis and treatment of developmental disorders. *Developmental NeuroPsychiatry, Volume II*, New York: Oxford University Press.

Herjanic, B. & Campbell, W. (1977). Differentiating psychiatrically disturbed children on the basis of structured interview. *Journal of Abnormal Child Psychology, 5*, 127–134.

Hodges, K., Coals, J., & McKnew, D. (1989): Test-Retest reliability of a clinical research interview for children: The child assessment schedule. *Psychological Assessment, 1*, 317–322.

Hodges, K., Klein, J., Fitch, P., McKnew, D., & Cytryn, L. (1981). The Child Assessment Schedule. *Catalog of Selected Documents in Psychology, 11*, 56.

Hubert, N. C., Wachs, T. D., Peters-Martin, P., & Gandour, M. J. (1982). The study of early temperament. *Child Development, 53*, 570–600.

King, R. A., & Noshpitz, J. (1991). *Pathways of growth: Essentials of child psychiatry* (vol. 2, Psychopathology). New York: John Wiley & Sons.

Piaget, J. (1952). *The origins of intelligence in children*. New York: International University Press.

Puig-Antich, J., & Chambers, W. (1978). *The Schedule for Affective Disorders and Schizophrenia for School-Aged Children*. This unpublished interview schedule can be obtained from the New York State Psychiatric Institute, 722 West 168 Street, New York, NY 10032.

Rutter, M. (1986). The developmental psychopathology of depression: Issues and perspectives. In M. Rutter, C. E. Izard, & P. B. Reed (Eds.). *Depression in young people: Developmental and clinical perspectives* (pp. 3–30). New York: Guilford.

Rutter, M., Tizard, J., & Whitmore, K. (Eds.). (1970). Education: Health and Behavior. London: Longmans.

Sarnoff, C. (1976). *Latency*. New York: Jason Aronson.

Shapiro, D. A. (1969). Empathy, warmth and genuineness in psychotherapy. *British Journal of Social & Clinical Psychology, 8*, 350–361.

Shapiro, T., & Perry, R. (1976). Latency revisited. *Psychoanalytic Study of the Child, 37*, 79–105.

Chapter 7

Psychiatric Assessment of Adolescents and Their Families

Harinder S. Ghuman, M.D. and John Gibbons, Ph.D.

The purposes of the psychiatric assessment of the adolescent as delineated by the American Academy of Child and Adolescent Psychiatry (1995) are (a) to determine whether psychopathology is present and, if so, to establish a differential diagnosis; (b) to determine whether treatment is indicated; and, (c) if so, to develop treatment recommendations and plans to facilitate the family and adolescent's cooperative engagement in treatment.

PRIOR TO THE INTERVIEW

A majority of adolescents are brought to the outpatient clinic by their parents for psychiatric evaluation and treatment. Another group of adolescents are brought by their parents under pressure from various agencies including, for example, the Department of Juvenile Justice, Department of Social Services, or the school. There is a small group of adolescents who are self-motivated and who may come to the clinic on their own initiative and sometimes their parents may be resistant to the evaluation.

Before initiating the interview process, the clinician should be aware of who is interested in the evaluation, why the evaluation is desired now, what the reason is for the evaluation, and how the evaluation has been presented to the adolescent. Answers to these questions are important to understand and address before starting the evaluation to ensure the best potential for a beneficial outcome. A successful psychiatric assessment includes compliance with the recommendations. Depending on the responses to these questions, the evaluator can make a preliminary assessment of motivation, resistance, developmental/family crisis, acute/chronic situation, and expectation of the evaluation by the adolescent, the parents, and the referring agency (if involved).

Singh, Janes, and Schechtman (1982) reported that disagreements between the parent(s) and referring agency regarding the patient's problem(s) may play a significant role in the dropout of patients. For example, if an adolescent has been referred to the psychiatric clinic after a violent episode in school, does this adolescent or his or her family view the evaluation as a form of punishment by the school, as a way around legal consequence, or does the adolescent or his or her family view the evaluation as evidence of genuine interest in the welfare of the adolescent by the school staff. It is important that all the parties have a common understanding and agreement regarding need for the evaluation. Otherwise, there are chances that the clinic staff, the adolescent, and his or her family may go through the motions of the evaluation without any significant beneficial outcome.

APPROACH TO THE INTERVIEW

Often the parents of an adolescent call the psychiatric clinic and ask the intake worker how or what they should tell the adolescent about the psychiatric evaluation and what they should do if the adolescent refuses to come. The parents should be advised to be honest, up-front, and firm in their approach to the adolescent. They should let the adolescent know their concerns in simple and lay terms. Sometimes it may be helpful for the parents to explain problems to the adolescent in a family context, for example, explaining that they are seeking professional guidance because of their inability to resolve the problems. The parents should be advised against long explanations and back-and-forth arguments with the adolescent regarding the need for evaluation. At times it may be helpful when a close family member or a friend of the adolescent can be involved in the evaluation process. It may be helpful especially with older adolescents, to have the option to make his or her appointment and to see the psychiatrist alone, imparting some sense of control over his or her life. With the more resistant adolescent, the parents may seek assistance from juvenile services, home intervention services, and other agencies to bring an adolescent to the clinic. In the highly disturbed and dangerous adolescent, it may be appropriate that the adolescent be seen in the emergency room or inpatient setting in order to have a thorough assessment.

The question often arises, who should be seen first, the adolescent or the parent, and how many meetings are necessary to do a good psychiatric evaluation. Answers to these questions depend upon the developmental and psychopathological issues of the adolescent and the family as well as practical issues such as availability of the parents, financial limitations, managed care restrictions, and transportation. For example, the adolescent can be seen first if the adolescent has shown some ability to handle his or her affairs independently of the parent(s) and/or may be concerned as to how the parents will present the problems to the psychiatrist. This may be more relevant with older adolescents than younger ones. Some clinicians prefer to see the adolescent alone first to establish the initial therapeutic alliance, to evaluate the patient without the bias of the parental history. However, there are a number of adolescents who would rather depend on the parents to take charge of the evaluation and in these cases it is more appropriate to see the adolescent and parents together. There are parents who may be over-involved and desire to take care of everything for the adolescent; in these cases one may give the option to the adolescent to meet first. In all cases, whether the clinician sees the adolescent first or not, it should be made clear to everyone that the clinicians will be meeting with the parents sometime during the evaluation to get the history and information regarding the problem and to share the recommendations.

The number of meetings required to do a good psychiatric assessment varies depending on the adolescent and the family situation, as well as the clinician's experience and expertise. A minimum of two to three hours is required. This can be done either in one block of time or two to three one-hour sessions. There are advantages and disadvantages to both approaches. With disorganized or resistant parents or adolescents and when there is problem with transportation it is preferable to do the evaluation in a single block of time. This helps in decreasing the time spent on scheduling and rescheduling meetings, loss of interest, and patient dropout. By finishing the evaluation and having some recommenda-tions, the adolescent and the parents feel a sense of accomplishment and something to hold on to until the next assignment.

The benefit of seeing the adolescent and parent over a period of time is that it may give a complete picture of the adolescent and the parents. It is not uncommon when the adolescent and parent(s) come to the clinic for the first time that they may be anxious and distrustful of the clinician as well as experiencing increased tension among themselves. This may provide a false impression to the clinician of the adolescent and the parents. A clinician in training should spend the full allotment of time with the adolescent and the parents to obtain a complete picture of the situation and not succumb to the tendency to shorten the evaluation out of his or her anxiety related to a new and often difficult situation.

ISSUES OF CONFIDENTIALITY

The issue of confidentiality is particularly complicated with the adolescent patient. It is im-portant that the adolescent trust the clinician with his or her thoughts, actions, and feelings. Because the adolescent is living with and depending upon the parents, the clinician needs to gain the trust and support of the parents as well. The parents are often curious to find out what is happening in the clinician's meeting with the adolescent. This curiosity may be out of interest in the welfare of the adolescent, a tendency to control and intrude, a fear of the adolescent blaming the parents for the problem, and/or a fear of being left out. The experi-enced clinician should be able to identify the parents' need to know about their adolescent and determine how much information is divulged without losing the adolescent's trust.

Both the adolescent and the parents need to know that whatever the adolescent says to the clinician is confidential, but if the clinician finds out that there is a danger to the adolescent and/or someone else then the information will not be confidential and all the interested parties will be informed in order to provide safety to the adolescent and others. This statement can cover suicide risk, homicide risk, and physical and sexual abuse. The adolescent referred for evaluation often is engaged in drug and alcohol abuse, sexual acting out, and various other illegal activities such as stealing, robbery, and violence. The parents may have no information regarding these activities or may not know their extent. If the adolescent informs the clinician of these activities, the intensity and immediacy of these acting out behaviors should guide the clinician in regard to the issue of confidentiality. The clinician who promises "absolute confidentiality" is foolish and likely to create more problems rather than helping the adolescent and the parents.

Meeks (1986) suggested that the therapist state clearly that the adolescent's feelings are confidential and only the adolescent's actions will be considered for possible discussion with his or her parents, and then only if in the therapist's judgment the particular actions represent danger to self or others. Often these adolescents test the clinician as to how the clinician will handle this information in relation to the adolescents' parents and society in general. If there is no immediate danger to the adolescent or others from the adolescent's behavior, the clinician's approach should be to help the adolescent bring up these issues with the family and society so that the adolescent can integrate into the family and societal systems. These issues can be identified during the assessment and worked out during the treatment.

To develop a trusting relationship with the adolescent, the clinician and adolescent can discuss how the clinician should interact with the parents and outside agencies. The adolescent can be given the option to be present during the clinician's meeting or telephone contacts with the parents or other agencies. All the written information can be shared in a paraphrased transaction between the therapist with the adolescent.

HISTORY TAKING AND THE INTERVIEW

The clinician may start the evaluation procedure by meeting with the adolescent and the parents together. After introduction, the clinician explains the assessment process to them and emphasizes that the clinician is trying to get information from both the adolescent and the parents, and both parties will have enough time to explain their point of view to the interviewer.

The clinician can advise the adolescent that the first hour or so will be devoted to getting an early history from the parents. Although the adolescent may feel left out, it is useful for the adolescent to stay in the meeting. This process can enhance the adolescent's trust in the clinician by allowing him or her to hear what the parents tell the clinician, as well as seeing his or her parents' trust in the clinician with the information and care of their child.

It may help the adolescent feel less anxious during the session when the adolescent is interviewed alone by the clinician. The adolescent may also hear his or her family and personal history, in some cases, for the first time in his or her life. Often, positive things about the adolescent are brought to the attention of the adolescent and the parents. There are times when the adolescent and the parents start to realize the onset of the problems and loss of their positive feelings and closeness to each other. It is also interesting to see how the adolescent sometimes is able to refresh the parents' memories or is able to provide more accurate accounts of certain events.

The interviewer may use a semi-structured format to obtain and record the history. The format should start with identifying data of the adolescent and the informant, and include the chief complaint, the history of present and past illness, the family composition and history, the developmental and medical history, and the social and school history. In addition, it is useful to obtain school reports and results of the previous psychiatric assessment and or psychological testing if performed.

INTERVIEW WITH THE ADOLESCENT

General Considerations

In interviewing an adolescent, the clinician needs to consider the following:

• The clinician should follow the adolescent's lead—for example, if an adolescent is outspoken and upfront, the clinician can be more passive in approach and let the adolescent explain his or her situation. In other cases, the adolescent may only provide clues; in these situations the clinicians should actively pursue these clues. The astute clinician is also aware that there are some adolescents who minimize their problems and others who readily admit to or boast about their behavior to present a picture of being "tough and cool." The adolescent's parents, teachers, and significant others need to be contacted to confirm or dispute information provided by an adolescent.

• In relating to the adolescent, a respectful, flexible, empathic approach is always warranted. Countertransference must be constantly focused on especially with adolescent patients. The clinician's seductiveness with a patient of the opposite sex, over-identification with the adolescent or parent, anger and or fear toward a violent or acting out adolescent, and feeling hopeless and helpless with the depressed patient—all can be diagnostic, but must be addressed as well as contained.

• At the outset of the interview, it is important to inform the adolescent that he or she has the option to respond or not to the clinician's questions and that the adolescent's honest response is more important than getting a made-up answer. If the adolescent opts not to answer a particular question, the clinician should inform the adolescent that there is a hope and expectation that the adolescent will be able to talk about this question sometime in the future, either with the interviewer or another clinician when the adolescent may feel more trusting and comfortable.

• As adolescents are often developmentally more concerned about issues related to self-image, self-esteem, and dependency versus autonomy, the interviewer, being an adult, needs to pay special attention regarding these issues in relating to adolescents in general and an adolescent with multiple handicaps in particular. The adolescent may be concerned about being labeled as "crazy" or "psycho." If the evaluator senses excessive defensiveness, the evaluator may need to address this directly with the adolescent. The clinician may also need to approach the vulnerable adolescent tactfully by starting the interview with simple questions and gradually leading into more conflictual and difficult areas—for example, sexual relationships or issues of abuse. It is important for the clinician to be familiar with developmental issues of early, middle and late adolescence so that the clinician has a frame of reference in assessing a particular adolescent. An early adolescent is more likely to be action-oriented than verbal and the examiner may make use of some of the interview techniques used with children.

• Some parents may be overly concerned about what questions clinician will ask their teenager. The parents may be worried that they will be falsely accused of some wrong-doing or that, in the process of the evaluation the teenager may be exposed to new ideas or topics from which they have tried to protect their adolescent. The clinicians need to emphasize to the parents that the questions that will be asked are part of a standard comprehensive assessment. It can also be emphasized that everyone's opinion and point of view is important even though they may be divergent and conflicting.

• As the interview is time-limited, the clinician needs to strike a balance to allow sufficient time for the adolescent to describe difficulties in his or her own words and at the same time allocate enough time to assess areas of mental and developmental functioning.

Process and Content of the Interview

The clinician can start the interview by asking the adolescent more neutral, demographic questions such as age, date of birth, grade, name of school, home address, and family constellation. This often helps to alleviate some of the adolescent's initial anxiety related to meeting a stranger who is also a mental health professional. After this initial interaction, the adolescent may be asked his or her understanding of the reasons for the evaluation. It is not uncommon for the adolescent at this point to respond in a negative manner or to deny any reasons for the evaluation. It is important for the clinician to notice: (a) what the adolescent mentions first and what areas are easily discussed or difficult to handle or omitted, (b) the sequence of events discussed and affect associated with various themes and the interview in general, (c) major themes and how the interview moved, and (d) nonverbal communication including closeness versus distance from the examiner, eye contact, and facial and body gestures.

Next the clinician can explore: (a) the adolescent's relationship with parents, peers, and teachers, (b) family relationships, (c) school performance, and (d) other interests such as hobbies, sports, and music. Exploration of early memories sets the stage for further questions regarding these four areas during elementary, middle, and high school years. The clinician observes the adolescent's appearance, posture, attitude, psychomotor activity, speech and thought processes, content of thought, and perceptions.

During the entire interview various aspects of possible psychopathology must be addressed. Following are some of the areas of psychopathology that need to be assessed along with typical questions asked.

Affective Illness   Tell me how do you feel most of the time? How is your mood in general? Is it sad, happy, angry, mad, down? Does your mood change a lot or frequently? Do you have a lot of ups and downs?

How is your sleep? Do you have difficulty falling asleep and or staying asleep? What time do you go to bed? What time do you fall asleep? Do you wake up early in the morning?; if yes, how early?

How does the future look to you?Do you ever feel hopeless about your situation? Do you wish sometime that you were not born or alive? Have you ever wished you were dead? Have you ever tried to hurt yourself?; if yes how many times and how? Did anyone know of this? How did he/she/they respond? Are you having thoughts now about hurting yourself?; if yes, how? Do you feel safe?

How is your appetite? Have you lost or gained any weight recently?

Do you ever feel that you are superman or have special powers? Do you ever feel that your mind is running fast?

Psychotic Illness   Do you hear voices when you are alone?; if yes, do you recognize whose voice it is and what is said? Do the voices tell you to do things and do you do them? Are the voices helpful or frightening? When do these voices occurs? Is it at night before you go to sleep or as you wake up or during the day? Do you think these voices are real or that your mind is playing tricks on you? Do you think these voices are coming from inside or outside your head? Do you think people can read your mind? Have you thought the television or radio was speaking to you personally? Do you often feel that others are talking about you or plotting against you? Do you see things that are not there or that others do not see? When does this occur?

Disruptive Behavior Disorders   Are you able to pay attention to the teachers and class work? Do you often feel restless and unable to sit still in your class? When you are studying do you easily get distracted by sound or something going on around?

How are you getting along with your teachers, parents, and other students? Were you ever suspended or expelled from school?; if yes, how many times and why? Have you been involved in any fights?; if yes, how many? What is the worst you were ever hurt? What is the worst you ever hurt someone else? Have you ever hurt someone that he or she had to go to hospital? Do you have thoughts about hurting someone?; if yes, who and why? What is stopping you from hurting this person? Have you ever been arrested?; if yes, how many times and why? Have you ever been involved in stealing, fire setting, rape? How do you feel after you_____? Do you ever feel bad about your behavior even if you are not caught?

Drug and Alcohol Abuse   Many teenagers experiment with drugs and alcohol, do you drink or smoke marijuana or use other drugs?; if yes, how much and how frequently? What is your drug of choice? Do you drink or do drugs alone? Have you ever used needles? When was the first time you drank or tried drugs? Have you ever passed out or not remembered what you did? How do you get alcohol and or drugs?

Anxiety Disorder/ Phobia/ Obsessive-Compulsive Disorder   Do you ever experience excessive sweating, fainting, heart beating fast, or breathlessness? Have you ever been afraid to leave home alone and go places? Do you worry a lot about harm coming to you or your parents? Do you experience nightmares and bad dreams? Some people are scared of the dark, animals, or thunderstorms, are you scared of something?

Have you experienced the same thoughts coming to your mind over and over? Do you find it impossible to keep certain thoughts away? Do you ever find yourself doing things certain ways or doing things over and over like washing your hands, taking several very long showers, or checking the locks or light switch?

Cognitive Impairment: Orientation   In general, these questions can be incorporated into the initial part of the interview such as: What is your name and your birthday? What are your address and telephone number and how far do you live from here? Do you know what the name of this place is? What is the date today?

Cognitive Impairment: Memory

Short-term—Give digit span (4–7 digit forward and 4–5 backward)

Recent memory—Ask the adolescent to remember 3 words and test recall at 1 and 10 minutes.

Remote memory—Ask the adolescent about past events in the adolescent's life.

Cognitive Impairment: General Knowledge and Intelligence   Who is the President of the United States? Who is the vice president? Can you name the president just before the current president? Who was the first President of the United States? What important events are currently in the news?

Reading, writing and mathematic abilities are seldom formally tested in a clinical interview but if desired the adolescent can be asked to read a paragraph and explain the contents, to write a short paragraph, and to do multiplication and division problems.

Cognitive Impairment: Abstraction

Similarities—How are an apple and orange similar?

Proverbs—All that glitters is not gold.

Cognitive Impairment: Judgment   If there is fire in the theater, what will you do?

Cognitive Impairment: Insight   How do you understand the problem you have and what can be done to solve this problem?

The clinician should assess the adolescent's self-concept by investigating the adolescent's view of self, likes or dislikes, areas of strength, and sense of accomplishments or weaknesses. The adolescent's values, models for emulation or disidentification, sense of future, level of psychosexual development, capacity to tolerate anxiety or frustration, degree of psychological mindedness, and vulnerability to regression or impulsivity should all be assessed (Schowalter & King, 1991). The quality of object relations should be evaluated by asking about the adolescent's relationship with parents, siblings, peers, and teachers. Depending upon the adolescent's comfort level, the clinician can explore topics related to sexual relationships, intimacy, and sexual orientation.

DIAGNOSTIC FORMULATION

The comprehensive formulation is a summary of the various biopsychosocial factors which have interacted in the adolescent's life, resulting in development of the present psychopathology. The formulation should also describe how the clinician arrived at the present diagnosis or diagnoses, especially in relationship to symptoms and behaviors congruent with diagnostic criteria from the *Diagnostic and Statistical Manual of Mental Disorders (DSM-IV)* (American Psychiatric Association [APA], 1994).

DIAGNOSIS AND TREATMENT RECOMMENDATIONS

Every clinician must be familiar with the various diagnoses in *DSM-IV* (APA, 1994) and how to use the multiaxial system. It is important that the clinician identifies a primary diagnosis, if one is present, which addresses the presenting problem. In developing a treatment plan, the clinician should discuss interventions and treatment setting necessary to have a positive outcome. The adolescent who is suicidal, homicidal, or involved in heavy substance abuse may require inpatient, residential, or day hospital treatment rather than an outpatient setting. Recommendations should include the need for further testing (psychological, neurological, educational testing, etc.), psychotherapy and psychopharmacological interventions, and educational and vocational needs. The adolescent and his or her parents should be advised of diagnosis, prognosis, and treatment recommendations in a simple and straightforward fashion and should be given ample time to understand and assimilate the information, ask questions, and express their concerns and feelings. The adolescent's and family's strengths should be emphasized to provide a balanced view and hope. It is not useful to try to completely alleviate the parents' anxiety or guilt, but, instead, to bring it to an "optimum" level necessary for the parents to continue treatment (Ghuman, 1994). The adolescent and the parents must be involved in developing a treatment plan and have a good understanding of the various steps in the treatment process.

FAMILY ASSESSMENT

The psychiatric assessment of adolescents includes an assessment of the adolescent's social context. This includes his or her family, foster family, or other extended family members that he or she may be living with. The purpose of the family assessment is to provide the clinician with information regarding the scope and quality of the adolescent's relationships with significant others, gather data regarding symptomatology, and assess the adolescent's potential support system.

This assessment takes place within the overall psychiatric assessment of the adolescent. The goals of this assessment are to:

- ascertain how each family member understands or makes sense of the presenting problem(s)
- assess how each family member reacts to the stated problem
- assess the quality of the relationship of each parent or guardian with the adolescent, and
- obtain a family history of psychiatric problems, alcohol and drug problems, learning problems, and/or other family problems.

Haley (1987) suggested the following guidelines for the initial family session:

- social stage
- problem stage
- interaction stage, and
- problem-solving stage.

Social Stage

The initial contact with family members requires a rapport-building time. The clinician provides the family with his or her name and role. Conversation around pertinent aspects of the family's situation takes place with the clinician taking a central role. The parents' job, education, other siblings, or issues related to setting up the appointment or coming to the clinic are discussed. This stage sets a tone of conversation, with the clinician leading, allowing for rapport that will let the family develop a sense of comfort to tell their story. The clinician is sensitive to family members' levels of anxiety and ability to enter into a dialogue with him or her at this stage.

Problem Stage

Szapocznik et al. (1989) suggested that the definition of the problem by family members is diagnostic of the family's systemic view of themselves. Do family members wonder if they have anything to do with the problem? Do they suggest that the patient is the only one with the problem? Do they accept any responsibility for the problem? Do they wonder what they can do as family members to make things better? Do they absolve the patient from all responsibility and blame themselves? The clinician is careful at this point to assess the family's sense of anger or hopelessness. How many times have they been to other therapists? What do they think will come out of this attempt to make things different? The clinician assesses the contextual nature of the problem at this point. Where does the problem(s) happen? When is it most likely to occur? Whom is it most likely to occur with? When does it become most intense or absent?

Interaction Stage

The interaction stage has three components:

- assessment of family members' usual behavioral responses to the adolescent during the problem and at other times
- assessment of family members" reasoning or understanding of their behavioral responses to the adolescent, and
- an enactment (Minuchin & Fishman, 1981).

The first part is accomplished by tracking (Minuchin & Fishman, 1981) family members' typical ways of interacting with the adolescent. The clinician tracks behavior when he or she asks significant family members what they do when the problem happens. For example, when the 15-year-old son of a single parent comes home late, mother screams at him for not listening to her. The patient screams back at her and they argue for 10 minutes. The mother usually ends up crying and retreating to her room for the rest of the evening. Neither mother nor patient brings up the matter again until the adolescent does something else to anger mother. The clinician tracks each person's behavioral response and then, once a pattern is identified, asks the adult and patient how they learned the response and what they think of their response. Are they happy with it? What would they change about it? This question address the second component.

The clinician assesses the family's pattern of relationships with each other and the outside world. Is the adolescent closer to mother or father? Does he or she have a relationship with any adults? Does the family go to church? What are his or her relationships with peers like? Do the parents have outside relationships or do they stay at home most of the time? The last component is addressed when the clinician asks mother and son to talk about the identified pattern of interaction and what they want to do differently. This "enactment" assesses their ability to tolerate each other in a dialogue, and their potential for change. Adolescents experiencing symptoms are at a disadvantage in that their impulsivity or mood can be quite extreme which often makes any sort of dialogue difficult. Parents coming for an evaluation for their child are often quite angry and impulsive themselves, making any dialogue difficult.

Family therapists frequently work to create conflict in order to restructure family interaction patterns, moving family members past their usual symptom-maintaining patterns. However, this type of strategy is not always useful and could potentially be quite harmful during the evaluation stage with a family member who is hypomanic or with others who have a history of impulsivity and/or cognitive impairment.

Problem-Solving Stage

Assessment of the adolescent's social context identifies family interaction patterns in two categories: (1) patterns that promote change, and (2) patterns that promote stability or homeostasis. It is important the clinician explore both categories. Often, patterns that promote change are overlooked in our endeavor to diagnose but these patterns are crucial in the evaluation of adolescents and their families. This stage of the evaluation focuses on the clinician's feedback to the family as to the presenting problem. It is best presented to the family after a consultation with other examiners, a review of records, and any testing that be indicated. The problem-solving stage could have several components including further testing and evaluation with recommendations for individual or family therapy. These recommendations are given based on the clinician's hypotheses of how the adolescent's symptoms are related, in part, to changes in the adolescent's family structure.

Treatment follows from assessment of family interaction and is sensitive to developmental issues. Family assessment is a fluid process that engages both the adolescent and his or her parents or guardian in a dialogue with potential interventions aimed at supporting the adolescent's need for autonomy and the parents'/guardian's need for control and safety.

CONCLUSION

The psychiatric assessment of adolescents and their families demands a thorough understanding of the reasons for the evaluation and who is asking for evaluation. The clinician needs to involve and gain the confidence of both the adolescent and the adolescent's parents while paying particular attention to developmental issues of the adolescent. The assessment must include a thorough history and a complete clinical assessment of the adolescent for any psychopathology. The family assessment should include an appraisal of the quality of the adolescent's relationships, family dynamics affecting the adolescent's condition, and the support system. The assessment should lead to a comprehensive biopsychosocial formulation, multiaxial diagnoses, and treatment plan.

REFERENCES

American Academy of Child and Adolescent Psychiatry. (1995), Practice parameters for the psychiatric assess-
    ment of children and adolescents. *Journal of the American Academy of Child and Adolescent Psychiatry*,
    34, 1386–1402.
American Psychiatric Association [APA]. (1994). *Diagnostic and statistical manual of mental disorders* (4th ed.)
    (DSM-IV). Washington, DC: Author.
Ghuman, H. S. (1994). Evaluation and treatment process. In H. S. Ghuman & R. M. Sarles (Eds.), *Handbook of
    adolescent inpatient psychiatric treatment* (pp. 18–34). New York: Brunner/Mazel.
Haley, J. (1987). *Problem solving therapy* (2nd ed.). San Francisco: Jossey-Bass.
Meeks, J. E. (1986). *The fragile alliance*. Malabar, FL: Robert E. Krieger Publishing Company.
Minuchin, S., & Fishman, H. (1981). *Family therapy techniques*. Cambridge, MA: Harvard University Press.
Schowalter J. E., & King R. A. (1991). The clinical interview of the adolescent. In J. M. Weiner (Ed.), *Textbook
    of child and adolescent psychiatry* (pp. 74–77). Washington DC: American Psychiatric Press.
Singh (Ghuman) H., Janes C. L., & Schechtman J. M. (1982). Problem children's treatment attrition and parents'
    perception of the diagnostic evaluation. *Journal of Psychiatric Treatment Evaluation, 4*, 257–263.
Szapocnik, J., Muray, E., Scopetta, M., Rio, A., Hervis, O., Cohen, R., Rivas-Vazquez, A., & Posada, V. (1989).
    Structural family therapy versus child therapy for hispanic boys. *Journal of Consulting and Clinical Psy-
    chology, 57*(5), 571–578.

Chapter 8

The Process of Psychological Assessment

Bruno J. Anthony, Ph.D. and Stephen L. Soffer, Ph.D.

Psychological assessment has a long tradition in the mental health care of children and adolescents and remains a critical component of outpatient treatment, providing information for diagnosis and the development of appropriate interventions. Above all, psychological assessment is a process of exploration. The choice of assessment instruments and the interpretation of data are guided by hypotheses generated from the referral questions and background information and altered during the course of the evaluation, dependent on the results.

This chapter highlights the major evaluation instruments that are useful when working with children and adolescents in outpatient settings. Areas to be reviewed include cognitive assessment, personality evaluation, neuropsychological testing, and the objective measurement of behavior. The types of clinical questions psychological assessment can address and the process used to answer them will be discussed.

GOALS

Psychological assessment of children refers to a set of developmentally sensitive and empirically defined methods to collect information in a relatively objective manner—that is, in a systematic way under standardized circumstances which allow comparison between individuals. A set of standard instructions and stimuli does not guarantee an adequate assessment tool, however. Three characteristics must be met. First, the instrument must be reliable. That is, do you get similar results when you test a sample twice (test-retest reliability), use parallel forms of a test, compare different informants (inter-rater reliability), or compare different sections of the test (split-half reliability, internal consistency). The reliability estimates all involve correlational measures, and one strives to obtain values of .80 or higher.

The second key characteristic of an instrument is its validity. Although it may reliably measure a quality of an individual, the results may not co-vary with a behavior or outcome of interest. Therefore, in the development process, an adequate instrument must be shown to produce similar results to other measures assumed to tap the same construct (concurrent validity), to predict a future outcome (predictive validity), or to co-vary with other relevant events (construct validity). In general, validity is established when empirical evidence confirms that we can generalize from the particular evaluation instrument to make accurate inferences about an individual's behavior in other situations. Finally, an adequate instrument must possess a strong normative base with which to compare an individual's performance.

CAUTIONS

It is always important to keep in mind that psychological assessment contributes only one class of data to the understanding of children and adolescents. The material elicited should be utilized only in the context of other clinical information such as personal history, patterns of behavior, and a comprehensive, diagnostic interview. Psychological testing was never intended to provide absolute information. The use of psychometrically sound tests is not inherently good or bad, but there is potential harm when results are inappropriately applied to treatment recommendations, interpretation of behavior, educational placement decisions, and more globally, social policy. In this vein, the assessment of intelligence in children and adolescents is seen as essential by some, but as culturally biased and unrelated to actual life experiences by others. While this topic is too broad to be covered in this space, it should be noted that the real danger is in how the scores are used. Indiscriminate use of testing results, without careful evaluation of situation and current conditions, including cultural experiences, can lead to characterizing people into rigid "slots," which may influence life-affecting decisions.

Interpretation of assessment results is constrained by sources of error that result in inaccurate measurement. These sources can result from transient changes in the physical (e.g, hunger, illness), mental (stress, worry, depression), or motivational state of the child, and lead to variation in scores which is captured in the statistic standard error of measurement. This term refers to a range of scores, which is assumed to include the person's score unaffected by sources of error. Understanding this concept will avoid spurious conclusions about "changes" in functioning when scores differ within the standard error of measurement. The most common example of such misinterpretation involves interpreting differences of a few points in IQ scores as an improvement or decline in cognitive ability.

A complete presentation of the appropriate uses of psychological assessment is contained in the *Standards for Educational and Psychological Testing* (American Educational Research Association et al., 1985).

HISTORICAL PERSPECTIVE

Several trends spurred the growth of psychological assessment in children and adolescents. Educational concerns at the turn of the century led to the development of intelligence tests. The Binet-Simon Scale, introduced in 1905 to determine school placement decisions, was the first comprehensive test of intelligence and began the tradition of ranking of items according to difficulty, using specific instructions to ensure uniform administration, and deriving an overall age-equivalent score.

Educational issues continue to be the main impetus for assessment and the chief beneficiary of the results and recommendations. The emphasis on educational placement and programming was reinforced by the enactment of Public Law 94-142, which ensures the right to education for all persons, including handicapped children. Of most consequence to psychological assessment, it mandates procedural safeguards to ensure accurate classification and appropriate recommendations. Although school systems are mandated to provide evaluations, psychologists are sometimes called on to evaluate because the school does not feel the assessment is necessary, or it has a lengthy backlog of cases, or because parents desire an independent evaluation. The need for more accurate assessment of learning problems contributed to an increase in the importance of neuropsychological assessment of children. The convergence of behavioral neurology and psychometric assessment in clinical psychology led to the development of test batteries that provide information regarding brain damage and resulting deficits. The usefulness of neuropsychological batteries to localize brain damage in children was complicated by the fact that similar lesions in the mature and developing brain may result in far different patterns of test results and expectations for recovery. These concerns, coupled with the development of non-invasive, neurodiagnostic methods, resulted in the gradual de-emphasis of the use of neuropsychological tests for making inferences about brain lesions toward the development of precise descriptions of processing strengths and weaknesses.

The belief that children have more difficulty accurately reporting on their behavior and identifying and expressing their feelings and needs led to the widespread use of projective and observational techniques. The "projective hypothesis" states that, when faced with an ambiguous stimulus, the individual "projects" previous experiences and needs onto the situation. Tests based on this hypothesis have formed an integral part of personality assessment for more than 60 years in spite of continual criticism of their reliability, validity, and "unscientific" nature. Self-report personality inventories were developed to provide a more normative data-based method for personality assessment, but are mostly used with adolescents.

Finally, the increasing popularity of behavior therapy prompted the growth of a more empirical assessment of behavior to quantify behavior more accurately and to facilitate a close and direct relationship between evaluation and treatment phases. The major techniques of such assessment involve behavior rating scales, which ask an informant to indicate the frequency and/or intensity of a set of behaviors displayed by an individual and techniques of direct observation in naturalistic settings such as frequency of a child's aggressive acts, or rating the intensity of a panic attack.

THE EVALUATION PROCESS

The following sections delineate the components of a thorough outpatient evaluation. To evaluate a child adequately, a multi-method approach based on empirically validated measures is recommended. However, we do not recommend a "test battery" approach—that is, one in which the same set of tests is used for each assessment. Rather, the composition of an evaluation rests on the nature of the referral questions as well as the personnel, time, and resources available. There is ever-increasing scrutiny of psychological assessment by third-party payers who demand justification for each instrument used.

To interpret assessment data in an informed manner, the psychologist must be aware of the clinical status of the patient, the psychiatric history, educational history, family background, previous evaluations, and developmental and medical history. Sometimes, parents or referring clinicians will wish to have an "objective" evaluation—that is, one that is not "biased" by prior information. This is rarely an advisable course. As we move through

Background Information

Howie is a 10-year-old with a history of substantial hyperactivity, disruptive behavior at both school and home, and lack of academic progress. He lives with his father and 17-year-old sister, only seeing his remarried mother sporadically. His father reported that Howie spends a lot of time at home on his own. He has no friends and is teased unmercifully. These comments do not seem to affect him; they are like "water off a duck's back."

Howie was delivered at term, passed motor milestones at a reasonable rate but showed some awkwardness, diffuse hypotonia, and fine motor control problems. His speech development was delayed. At 3 years of age, his ears were drained of fluid, PE tubes were inserted, and he had a bilateral adenoidectomy. Ear infections continued; therefore, two years later, he had a left canaloplasty. His speech improved somewhat after these procedures. Currently his speech is rapid but intelligible. Howie has worn glasses since he was 3-4 years of age and there is evidence of an atypical macula.

A pediatric neurological consultation when he was 8 years old revealed a head circumference two standard deviations below the mean, mildly dysmorphic features, and other physical abnormalities suggesting the possibility of intrauterine influences. An MRI showed an imbalance of grey and white matter and features indicative of disturbances of myelination. One year later, an EEG showed the presence of mild disorganization and bilateral slowing of background rhythm. No significant asymmetries or definite epilptiform discharges were present.

Howie was started on a course of Ritalin at 3 years of age and switched to Dexedrine then Norpramin, then Cylert over the last year, all of which produced unwanted side effects. Howie is currently taking 60 mg of Ritalin per day. Teachers have remarked on Howie's ADHD behaviors and learning problems since he entered preschool. He has attended a special program for learning and emotional disabilities since the age of 4 years, needing a highly structured, self-contained program. Currently, his academic progress is at a standstill at about the 3rd grade level.

Figure 1   Background information for case example.

the evaluation process, we will make reference to a patient, Howie, whose background information is presented in Figure 1.

THE REFERRAL

The evaluation process begins with development of specific referral questions, which determine, in part, the components of the evaluation. Often, however, the referral source is not familiar with the type of questions that can be addressed or devises questions that are too broad. Therefore, it is often helpful to provide a form which lists possible issues which can be investigated within the realm of the evaluation (see Figure 2).

In Howie's case, the questions include, but are not necessarily limited to:

- What is his cognitive capacity and specific pattern of strengths and deficits?
- Relative to the his cognitive abilities, how well developed are his academic skills?
- How significant are Howie's behavioral difficulties and adaptive deficits when compared to same-age peers?

CHILD AND ADOLESCENT PSYCHIATRY SERVICE

REQUEST FOR PSYCHOLOGICAL/NEUROPSYCHOLOGICAL EVALUATION

Patient: _Howard Peters_   Date of Birth: _8-21-82_   Date of Request: _12-7-95_

Person Requesting Evaluation (include phone #/beeper #): _Dr. Roscoe (776-8867)_

Check Type of Evaluation Requested:

Cognitive (IQ) _✔_   Attention _✔_   Memory: _✔_   Speech/Language: __

Educational _✔_   Adaptive Functioning _✔_   Personality/Emotional: __

Neuropsychological __   Other: _____

Check Key Questions:

Verbal Comprehension _✔_   Verbal Reasoning _✔_   Verbal Expression _✔_

Visual Discriminiation _✔_   Spatial Understanding __   Non-Verbal Reasoning __

Serial Processing __   Attention _✔_   Planning/Organization _✔_

Memory _✔_   Fine Motor _✔_   Learning Disability _✔_

Thought Disorder __   Object Relations __   Ego Strength __

Depression __   Anxiety __

Other _____

Previous Testing: WISC-R 5 years ago: Verbal IQ of 91, Performance IQ of 85, and Full
                    Scale IQ of 84. Bender-Gestalt showed delayed motor skills. Wide Range
                    Achievement Test indicated reading, spelling, and math below grade level.

Figure 2   Evaluation request form for case example.

• Does he demonstrate deficits in focusing, maintaining, and/or shifting attention to verbal and nonverbal tasks? and,

• Does he display any verbal or motor deficits that suggest delays in brain development or brain damage?

BEHAVIORAL ASSESSMENT

There are a variety of measures that can provide valuable information on the behavioral characteristics of children. Their standardized format reduces the subjectivity of informant judgments and increases the reliability. This information can have direct relevance to specific evaluation questions or provide important associated information that will help in understanding the evaluation data (e.g., attention problems, internalizing problems such as depression and anxiety, level of defiance and oppositionality). Instruments for behavioral assessment fall into three classes: ratings, completed by respondents who know the child well (parents, other caregivers, teachers); self-report by the patient; and observation by the examiner during the evaluation or in a naturalistic setting (e.g., classroom, home). Table 1 provides a summary of the uses, strengths, and limitations of well-developed ratings and self-report measures.

Ratings

Ratings provide a convenient, efficient, and easily quantifiable method to collect behavioral data. They call for opinions across time and situations, minimizing day-to-day variability which might color ratings. However, they are subject to a variety of factors that may affect their validity, such as social desirability (the desire to present the child in a positive or negative light), halo effects (general negative or positive ratings of one type of behavior carrying over to ratings of another), and variations in views of deviance (a certain numerical rating applied to a level of behavior may reflect different intensities to different people). Also, children's behavior varies from site to site and time to time; thus, one can expect a fair amount of variation between different raters (e.g., home and school). Finally, the correlation between different respondents may vary considerably, depending on the type of behavior assessed (e.g., there is more consistency in the ratings of externalizing behaviors). It is particularly important for the informant to have extensive contact with the child.

Rating scales can be divided into broad and specific, with the former covering a wide range of behavioral, emotional, and social problems and the latter tapping certain areas in more depth (e.g., ADHD, depression, anxiety, parenting stress). The most useful and widely used of the general scales are the Child Behavior Checklists (CBCL) developed by Achenbach and colleagues (1991 a, b, c). These rating scales involve parallel parent and teacher forms which help to improve cross-situational consistency. Parents rate behavior problems as well as completing items covering competency in activities as well as social and academic areas. Responses generate total, internalizing, and externalizing scores as well as eight or nine scale or factor scores, empirically derived, that make up the Child Behavior Profile, separately normed for boys and girls at different age ranges (4–5, 6–11, 12–16) and for 2- to 3-year-olds. Howie's profile, resulting from his father's ratings, is presented in Figure 3. Scores more than two standard deviations above the mean of the general population (98th percentile) are considered clinically significant.

In Howie's case the Hyperactive and Aggressive scales are elevated, reflecting significant ADHD, oppositional, and angry behaviors. In addition, though, the profile indicates that Howie may also possess significant worries, minor physical problems, obsessive-compulsive behaviors, and mood fluctuations which result in elevations of the Somatic Complaints, Immature, and Obsessive-Compulsive scales. Finally, his social problems are reflected by the high Hostile-Withdrawal score.

The broad assessment of adaptive behavior—the ability to meet the natural and social demands of the environment—although a requirement for a diagnosis of mental retardation, is frequently a valuable component of any evaluation. Cognitive and academic skills should be examined in relation to age-appropriate standards for the use of these skills in the environment. The Vineland Adaptive Behavior Scales are most frequently used for this purpose and provide versions for use in the classroom and for major caretakers. The com-

Table 1   Selected Behavioral Assessment Measures
a. Ratings

Title & author	Description	Age range	Strengths and weaknesses
Child Behavior Checklist (Achenbach, 1991a)	Parent ratings providing profiles of social competence and behavior problems. Version for children 4–18 consists of 138 items which take approximately 30 minutes to complete. Separate form for 2–3 year-olds with 100 behavior items.	2–18 years	Widely used in clinical work and research. Behavior checklist information most useful. Computer scoring available including comparison of informants. Standard T-scores for factor-analytically derived scales as well as normative cutoffs.
Teacher's Report Form (Achenbach, 1991b)	Modeled on the Child Behavior Checklist; obtains ratings of behavior problems and academic performance and derives profiles comprised of scale scores for behavior problems.	6–16 years	Provides broader view of child's behavior than other teacher checklists; therefore, more burden on the teacher. Widely used. Standard T-scores for factor-analytically derived behavior scales obtained. Provides opportunity for teacher's written opinions of strengths and weaknesses. Computer scoring.
Conners' Parent Rating Scales (Conners, 1989)	Original (93 items) and revised (48 items) form used extensively in studies of hyperactivity but also contains scales for conduct problems, anxiety, somatic problems, and learning problems.	3–17 years	Adequate validity and reliability for the longer version. Good outcome measure in studies of ADHD. Strong practice effect evident in some studies (scores decrease from first to second administration). Spanish-language version and computer scoring available.
Conners' Teacher Rating Scale (Conners, 1989)	Original (39 items) resulting in 6 factors (hyperactivity, conduct disorder, emotional-over-indulgent, anxious-passive, asocial, daydreams /attendance problems), and revised form (28 items) with 3 externalizing factors only.	3–17 years (suggested norms for original version cover ages 4–16 years)	Good sensitivity to treatment effects. More validity studies for original version. Many versions of scales-need to be careful in use and interpretation.

Table 1   (Continued)

Title & author	Description	Age range	Strengths and weaknesses
Revised Behavior Problem Checklist (Quay & Peterson, 1987)	89 items resulting in 6 broad band dimensions (Conduct Disorder, Anxiety-Withdrawal, Attention Problems-Immaturity, Socialization-Aggression, Psychotic Behavior, Motor Excess)	6–18 years	Limited norms and few, though promising, reliability studies. Excellent discriminant and concurrent validity. Items well based in current conceptions of child maladaptive behavior.
Vineland Adaptive Behavior Scales (Sparrow, Balla, & Cichetti, 1984)	Rating scale that uses interview format with major caretaker or teacher report to tap four domains of adaptive behavior: Communication (receptive, expressive, and written), Daily Living Skills (personal, domestic, and community); Socialization (play, leisure time, responsibility and sensitivity); and Motor Skills (fine and gross) for children under the age of 6 years. Commonly used Survey Form (297 items) requires 20–60 minutes to administer.	birth - 18 years, 3–12 years for Classroom Edition.	Strong normative group although differences in means and standard deviations across age groups makes longitudinal and interdomain comparisons less reliable.

b. Self-Report

Title & author	Description	Age range	Strengths and weaknesses
Youth Self-Report (Achenbach, 1991c)	2 competence and 7 behavior problems scales resulting from 112 items overlapping with other versions of the Child Behavior Checklist. Approximately 30 minute administration time.	11–18 years	One of few instruments gathering a broad assessment of behavior problems. Useful to refer to in initial interviews. Adequate short-term test-retest reliability. Minimal validity data.
Revised Children's Manifest Anxiety Scale (Reynolds & Richmond, 1985)	28 content and 9 social desirability items which use a yes/no format all keyed in the yes direction. Provides an overall anxiety T-score and scaled scores for 3 types of anxiety (worry & oversensitivity, physiological, concentration difficulties)	6–19 years	The most widely used, researched, and employed self-report instrument for anxiety in children and adolescents. Adequate reliability and validity. May relate more to generalized anxiety disorder than other anxiety problems (e.g., separation anxiety).

Table 1   (Continued)

Title & author	Description	Age range	Strengths and weaknesses
Children's Depression Inventory (Kovacs, 1992)	Downward extension of Beck Depression Inventory. 27-item three alternative forced choice measure in which children select the symptom level (minimal, moderate, severe) that best characterizes how they are feeling for the last two weeks. Requires only a 3rd grade reading level.	3–18 years	The most widely used self-report measure of childhood depression with excellent normative data, good reliability, and reasonable correlations with various measures of depression. Mixed results for discriminant validity which may reflect age and defensiveness of children.
Reynolds' Child Depression Scale (Reynolds, 1989)	30 item, 4-point Likert-type response format measure of depressive symptomology	8–12 years	Detailed manual with procedures for administration, scoring, and interpretation. Good evidence of clinical utility.
Reynolds' Adolescent Depression Scale (Reynolds, 1987)	30 item, 4-point response format with items worded at a 3rd grade reading level and covering somatic, motivational, cognitive, mood, and vegetative components of depression.	13–19 years	Cutoff scores validated to determine clinically significant levels of severity. Excellent validity studies showing strong relationships with other self-report depression scales and other related constructs.
Pictorial Scale of Perceived Competence and Social Acceptance for Young Children (Harter & Pike, 1984)	Measures 4 domains of perceived competence (cognitive and physical) and acceptance (maternal and peer) with one form for preschool and kindergarten children and one for 1st and 2nd graders. Uses pictorial format.	4–7 years	One of the few well developed, self-report scales of self-concept and social competence for preschoolers.
Self-Perception Profile for Children (Harter, 1985) and for Adolescents (Harter, 1988)	A 36-item, 4-point, format in which children respond ("really true" or "sort of true") to one of two alternative sentences. Assesses global self worth and 5 domains for children (scholastic, athletic, and work competence, social acceptance, physical appearance, behavioral conduct) with 3 more domains for adolescents (close friendship, romantic appeal, and job competence.	8–13 years for children, 14–18 for adolescents	This excellent measure of perceived competence in different domains provides a richer picture than other measures providing only a single self-concept score. Global self-worth directly tapped, independently of domain-specific scores. Format avoids pulling for socially-desirable responses. Parallel teacher rating scale (15 items) available.

BEHAVIOR RATING DATA

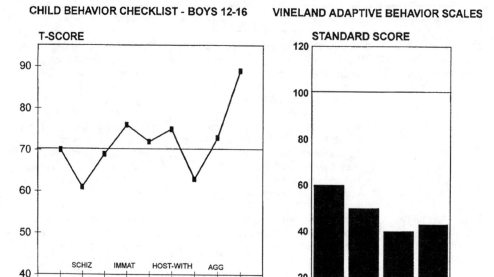

Figure 3 Child Behavior Checklist (CBCL) factor T-scores and Vineland Adaptive Behavior Scales (VABS) domain standard scores for case example. Horizontal line indicates 98th pecentile for CBCL and average score for VABS.

monly used Survey form provides a composite Adaptive Behavior standard score as well as scores for four domains: Communication, Daily Living Skills, Socialization, and Motor Skills for children under the age of 6 years. The Vineland was administered to Howie's father, and the resulting scores presented a serious picture of Howie's current adaptive skills, with extremely low scores across the board (see Figure 3).

We always find it valuable to obtain a general behavior rating instrument during an evaluation, even if the problems appear somewhat circumscribed. However, we employ more narrow-band rating instruments to provide a detailed picture of specific problem areas. Ratings of internalizing disorders have been only rarely implemented because of the belief that parents and teachers are less sensitive to the internal states of children. A large number of rating scales are available for externalizing disorders (see chapters 13 and 14 on ADHD and Conduct and Oppositional-Defiant Disorder, respectively).

Self Report

As defined here, self-report refers to instruments designed to tap a child's view of his or her own feelings and behaviors. It is important to remember various issues in using such reports. First, although less important than in adults, responses may be influenced by social desirability. Some self-report inventories include a "lie" scale which involves items that, if answered in a certain way, suggest a tendency to present oneself in a positive light ("I am never angry."). Second, children and particularly adolescents may sometimes be reluctant to self-disclose information about themselves for fear of the consequences. For instance, hospitalized children may deny suicidal thoughts for fear of delaying discharge. Finally, the usefulness of self-report varies with developmental level. Very few measures are used with children under 7 years of age because of language factors, self-awareness, the ability to differentiate among emotions, and accurate self-monitoring.

Table 1 presents a list of often-used self-report inventories. The best broad behavior inventory for adolescents is the Youth Self Report (YSR) developed by Achenbach (1991c) as an adjunct to the parent and teacher forms of the CBCL. As with other versions of the CBCL, the YSR results in a Behavior Profile comprised of different scales. We have found it useful to go back over the YSR with an adolescent patient to clarify responses and to delve more deeply into certain areas. Unlike rating scales, most of the specific, self-report instruments available for children and adolescents focus on internalizing symptoms. These measures are critical pieces in the assessment of such problems because children have been shown to be reliable reporters, more so than other informants. In this realm, the Revised Children's Manifest Anxiety Scale (RCMAS) is a well-developed, useful instrument that taps different aspects of anxiety and also contains a lie scale to assess social desirability. For depressive symptomology, the Child Depression Inventory is the most extensively used self-report measure and has been employed frequently as a measure of treatment outcome clinically and in research studies. Recently, Reynolds has developed complementary depression scales for children and adolescents with excellent normative data and strong reliability and validity (Reynolds' Depression Scales [Reynolds, 1987]). Self-concept and, more specifically, self-esteem are often important qualities to assess in children and adolescents. This domain has virtually been defined by self-report measures. Harter, nicely integrating developmental theory and careful test construction, has developed Self-Perception Profiles for children and adolescents (Harter, 1985, 1988).

Direct Observation

Within the context of psychological assessment, observational data can be divided into that collected during testing-related activities and in more naturalistic settings. Detailed observations of the patient's appearance, reactions to testing, activity level, language, and other behavioral features contribute to estimates of the validity of the administration, indicating whether test-related, situation-related, or intra-individual factors influenced the results, and inform recommendations for intervention in other structured situations (e.g., the classroom). In Howie's case, it seemed that his attentive difficulties may have lowered his overall scores to some extent.

Direct observation of a patient in more naturalistic settings can provide a window on a child's spontaneous behavior patterns, interpersonal behavior, learning style, and response to daily challenges. Moreover, such observation will help to evaluate the concerns of teachers, parents, and other referral sources and help provide more informed suggestions for behavioral change. It must be kept in mind, however, that the act of observation can influence the child's performance. Observation varies from informal, narrative accounts of a child's behavior in a setting to formalized methods using sophisticated coding systems. The more complex systems tend to require extensive training and lengthy observational periods which may not be viable for most clinicians. For the practitioner, formalized, direct observation systems tend to be most useful when a limited set of behaviors are of interest. Sattler (1990) and Barrios (1993) provided guidelines for developing such systems.

Table 2   Selected Measures of Cognitive Abilities

Test Title & author	Description	Age range	Strengths & weaknesses
Bayley Scales of Infant Development Second Edition (BSID-II; Bayley, 1993)	Standardized measure of infant mental and motor development. Takes about 45 to 75 minutes to administer. Includes standardized scale to operationalize behavior observation.	2 months to 2 years 6 months	The most well conceived and normed measure of infant development available Requires significant training to properly administer.
Kaufman Assessment Battery for Children (K-ABC; Kaufman & Kaufman, 1983)	Standardized test of intelligence for children based on distinction between sequential and simultaneous processing. Relies less on verbal and crystalized abilities that traditional intelligence tests. Takes about 45 to 75 minutes to administer.	2 years 6 months to 12 years 5 months	Useful for children with specific language problems and as a comprehensive test of problem-solving abilities. Not as well developed or clinically useful as Wechsler scales.
McCarthy Scales of Children's Abilities (McCarthy, 1972)	Very useful test of intelligence with young children, and children with known learning problems. Separate scales assessing verbal, perceptual-performance, quantitative, memory, and motor skills. Takes about 1 hour to administer.	2 years 6 months to 8 years 6 months	Well standardized, with good reliability and validity for index scores. Restricted age range; cumbersome scoring procedures to calculate index scores. Lack reliability scores for individual subtests.
Stanford-Binet Intelligence Scale - Fourth Edition (SB: FE; Thorndike, Hagen, & Sattler, 1986)	Standardized test of intelligence comprised of 15 subtests which are divided into 4 areas of cognitive abilities (verbal, abstract/visual reasoning, and quantitative reasoning and short term memory). Complete battery can take about 2 hours to administer.	2 years to 23 years	Large normative sample; can be used for an extensive age range; demonstrated reliability and validity. Long administration time can be difficult for younger children or children with attention problems.
Wechsler Adult Intelligence Scale - Revised (WAIS-R; Wechsler, 1981)	Standardized test of cognitive abilities consisting of 11 subtests divided into 2 scales: Verbal and Performance. Takes about 60 to 90 minutes to administer.	16 years 11 months to 74 years 11 months	Well standardized, with demonstrated reliability and validity. Normative sample is about 15 years old, could use revisions to some items that seem outdated.

Table 2 (Continued)

Test title & author	Description	Age range	Strengths & weaknesses
Wechsler Intelligence Scale for Children - Third Edition (WISC-III; Wechsler, 1991)	Standardized test of cognitive abilities consisting of 13 subtests divided into 2 scales: Verbal and Performance; and 4 Index Scores. Takes about 60 to 90 minutes to administer	6 years to 16 years 11 months	This updated version of the WISC-R is well standardized with demonstrated reliability and validity. Utility with language impaired children is questionable due to high reliance on verbal tasks and responses.
Wechsler Preschool and Primary Scale of Intelligence - Revised (WPPSI-R; Wechsler, 1989)	Standardized test of cognitive abilities for young children consisting of 12 subtests divided into 2 scales: Verbal and Performance. Takes about 60 to 90 minutes to administer.	3 years to 7 years 3 months	Updated version of the original WPPSI has a greater age range, larger standardization sample and demonstrated reliability and validity. Long administration time may be problematic for the youngest children.

Cognitive Assessment

The goal of cognitive assessment is to identify specific strengths and weaknesses in a range of mental processes including verbal processing, visual perception, abstract thinking, problem-solving, and memory. Assessment of cognitive abilities is typically used by school systems to determine a student's need of special education services. Table 2 provides a summary of the uses, strengths, and limitations of selected instruments for cognitive assessment.

The tests of cognitive functioning most frequently used in clinical practice with children and adolescents are the Wechsler Scales, which are highly reliable, have demonstrated validity, and utilize large standardization samples for comparison of individual scores to groups of same-age children and adolescents. The Wechsler Intelligence Scale for Children-Third Edition (WISC-III; Wechsler, 1991) is used for children ages 6 to 16 years 11 months, and consists of 13 subtests, each measuring different skills. The subtests are divided into Verbal and Performance subscales. The WISC-III yields standard IQ scores for the Full Scale and two subscales. Additionally, factor analysis of the subtests has identified four indexes, describing more circumscribed cognitive skills: Verbal Comprehension, Perceptual Organization, Freedom from Distractibility (Arithmetic, Digit Span), and Processing Speed.

Tests similar in structure and presentation to the WISC-III are employed with adolescents age 17 and older—the Wechsler Adult Intelligence Scale-Revised (WAIS-R; Wechsler, 1981)—and for children between the ages of 3 and 6—the Wechsler Preschool and Primary Scale of Intelligence Revised (WPPSI-R; Wechsler, 1989). Brief batteries, like the Kaufman Brief Intelligence Test (K-BIT; Kaufman & Kaufman, 1991), are available to provide estimates of cognitive abilities as well as short forms of the Wechsler scales. Sattler (1990) provided information on the pro-rating procedures that produce summary score estimates of the abbreviated Wechsler scales.

Table 3   Cognitive (WISC-III) Results for Case Example and Interpretation Information
a. WISC-III Subtest and Scaled Scores (mean = 10, standard deviation = 3)

Verbal test	Abilities assessed	Scaled score	Performance test	Abilities assessed	Scaled score
Information (I)	General knowledge acquired through average experiences	8	Picture Completion (PC)	Discriminate essential from non-essential details; recognition of common objects	8
Similarities (S)	Verbal concept formation; abstract reasoning	12	Coding (CO)	Visual-motor speed; focused attention; learning novel tasks	6
Arithmetic (A)	Basic mathematical operations; attention-requiring memory skills	3	Picture Arrangement (PA)	Non-verbal, causal reasoning; planning; social problem solving	4
Vocabulary (V)	Word knowledge; expressive language skills	8	Block Design (BD)	Visual-spatial organization; part-whole relationships; visual motor coordination	7
Comprehension (C)	Use of past experience to problem-solve; reasoning; knowledge of cultural norms	3	Object Assembly (OA)	Use of visual-motor skills to construct familiar object without a model.	7
Digit Span (DS)	Short term verbal memory; attention-requiring memory skills.	3	Symbol Search (SS)	Visual search and discrimination; focused visual attention	4
			Mazes (M)	Non-verbal planning; perceptual organization	9

Table 3 (Continued)
b. WISC-III Summary Scores (mean = 100, standard deviation = 15)

Summary scale/Index	Abilities assessed	IQ/Index score	Percentile rank
Verbal Scale (I, S, A,V, C)	Verbal reasoning, comprehension, receptive and expressive language skills; verbal short-term memory and attention; crystal-ized intelligence; accumulated experience	82	12th
Performance Scale (PC, CO, PA, BD, OA)	Non-verbal reasoning; visual organization; visual-motor coordination; spatial skill; visual-focused attention; visual short-term memory; fluid intelligence; immediate problem-solving with novel stimuli	78	7th
Full Scale Score	Global estimate of cognitive ability	78	7th
Verbal Comprehension Index (I, S, V, C)	Verbal comprehension and reasoning; general knowledge base	88	21st
Perceptual Organization Index (PC, PA, BD, OA)	Visual organization; part-whole understanding; non-verbal reasoning	80	9th
Freedom from Distractibility Index (A, DS)	Attention; concentration; problem solving; numerical facility; short term memory	61	0.5th
Processing Speed Index (CO, SS)	Visual disrimination; visual focused attention; psycho-motor speed	75	5th

The WISC-III results for Howie are presented in Table 3, along with a listing of the skills assumed to be tapped by the different scales, indexes, and subtests. Interpretation is usually carried out in a hierarchical fashion. First, the summary scores are examined and qualitative labels for the level of performance applied. Often, summary scores mask variation among subtests and therefore do not adequately represent the patient's functioning. Examination of the pattern of index and subtest scores provides the most useful information on specific strengths and weaknesses. See Kaufman (1994) for greater detail regarding the full interpretation of the WISC-III.

Howie's IQ scores place him on the boundary between the "Borderline" and Low Average ranges of intellectual functioning. However, the Freedom from Distractibility Index Score is significantly below the other index scores, indicating particular difficulties with verbal tasks that require the ability to focus and maintain attention. He showed his strongest performance on the Verbal Comprehension Index, demonstrating low average ability for word and general knowledge, and a relative strength in abstract reasoning. His scores on the Performance Scale subtests suggest general problems with nonverbal processing, showing weak scores on Perceptual Organization Index tasks involving reproduction and manipulation of visual stimuli. Howie demonstrated a relative strength for attention to detail, but showed below average visual-motor speed on the timed tasks making up the Processing Speed Index.

Neuropsychological Assessment

Neuropsychological investigation differs somewhat in pediatric and psychiatric settings. In the former, goals often center around the behavioral consequences of an identified disease process or injury. In psychiatric settings, questions involve determination of specific impairments related to psychiatric disorders (e.g., attentive problems in ADHD), distinguishing significant cognitive deficits from behavioral interference (e.g., oppositionality), and elucidating cognitive factors underlying learning and behavioral problems. The rate of neuropsychological problems in children and adolescents referred for outpatient psychiatric treatment is quite high (e.g., Tramontana, Sherrets, & Golden, 1980), reaching as high as 60 percent, with difficulties concentrated in the areas of complex, cognitive-perceptual skills.

Assessment can employ either a standardized, fixed battery or an individualized selection of tests. In either case measures usually evaluate sensory-perceptual capabilities, motor and psychomotor skills, attention and memory capabilities, psycholinguistic skills, and higher order conceptual and problem-solving capabilities. The choice of approach tends to reflect both an examiner's training and time available for evaluation as well as the referral questions. In each case, however, the evaluation almost always follows a standard intelligence test which covers basic language and visual-perceptual functions.

Standardized Batteries   Two well-established batteries, the Halstead-Reitan Neuropsychological Test Battery (HRNB; Reitan & Wolfson, 1985) and the Luria-Nebraska Neuropsychological Battery-Children's Revision (LNNB-CR; Golden, 1987), are available for use with children and adolescents. Both were developed through modifications of adult versions. The two batteries discriminate brain dysfunction equally well, at least for general classification purposes; however, the LNNB-CR takes about half the time to administer.

The HRNB has versions for older (9 to 14 years) and younger (5 to 8 years) children and represents the most widely used approach to neuropsychological evaluation in children. However, research suggests that its discriminatory power is limited to broad diagnostic groups (learning disabled, brain damaged, and normal children), and it is quite redundant with standard IQ tests except for basic motor and sensory-perceptual abilities. Moreover, it does not permit a detailed analysis of a child's functional capacities because tests are either too crude (language tests in particular) or too complex to determine the processes underlying poor performance, or important functions are not addressed adequately (e.g., memory, attention). In sum, these drawbacks do not justify the extensive time needed to administer this battery.

Scores on the 149-items LNNB-CR are summarized in 11 major scales, with item composition based on Luria's areas of function rather than for statistical reasons, as well as second-order scales made up of items that best discriminate brain damage (Pathognomonic Scale) and contralateral hand performance (Left and Right Sensorimotor Scale). Criterion rules for each scale determine impairment. Items on the LNNB-CR are simpler than those on the HRNB tests and are assumed to tap component skills more clearly, permitting qualitative analysis of functional strengths and weaknesses. However, the small number of items assessing each skill reduces the reliability of the analysis. Moreover, like the HRNB, it excludes measures of critical skills such as executive functions, learning, and attention.

Flexible Batteries Pure qualitative approaches to neuropsychological evaluation rely less on standardized tests to assess an individual against a normative group and more on a micro-analysis of how and where an individual's performance on tasks succeeds or fails. The emphasis is on determining the cognitive strategies available to an individual that have direct relationship to treatment options. However, this approach is very dependent on the orientation and skills of the examiner. Moreover, the approach does not lend itself to studies of reliability or validity. Process-oriented approaches combine quantitative and qualitative methods and represent the usual practice of neuropsychologists, particularly those who work with children and adolescents. Usually, there is a brief, fixed battery of tasks that provide a reasonable comprehensive assessment of functioning. The rest of the evaluation involves a more flexible assortment of tests, tailored on the basis of the results of the initial battery and particular referral questions. Comprehensive accounts of myriad neuropsychological tests can be found in edited books on child neuropsychology (Hynd & Willis, 1988; Reynolds & Gletcher-Janzen, 1989).

For Howie, the WISC-III and the background data suggested problems with attention. Therefore, a battery of tasks (Mirsky, Anthony, Duncan, Ahearn, & Kellam, 1991) was administered, tapping the abilities to focus attention in the face of distraction, sustain that focus over time, shift focus adaptively, and allocate attentive effort to the encoding of information in short-term memory. Across the different tasks, Howie showed much more difficulty with tasks involving visual as opposed to auditory input. Similarly, on the Wide Range Assessment of Memory and Learning (WRAML; Adams & Sheslow, 1990), Howie showed average to above average performance when asked to remember a list of spoken words or a paragraph of prose. In contrast, his visual memory for details of a picture or the sequence of finger movements was much worse.

Academic Achievement

Tests of academic achievement are comprised of graded items, usually derived from school textbooks and curriculum experts, linked to expected knowledge of basic areas for different ages or grade levels. Within the context of psychological assessment, examination of academic achievement is most often conducted in conjunction with intelligence testing. This comparison provides important data for the assessment of learning disorders; significantly lower academic skills in a particular area compared to measured cognitive abilities are suggestive of a learning disorder. Assessments of academic achievement also are used in decisions regarding school placement and giftedness. Individually administered tests of academic achievement can be divided into screening measures and full batteries. The depth of the assessment depends on whether the goal is to obtain a general sense of academic skills or to identify specific areas or skills in need of remediation.

The most commonly used academic screening tool is the Wide Range Achievement Test-Revision 3 (WRAT3; Jastak & Wilkinson, 1993) which can guide more extensive educational assessments if problem areas are identified. However, it is important to remember the limitations of the WRAT3. It measures word recognition not reading comprehension, knowledge of mathematical operations not more complex problem solving, and spelling not writing skills. The Brief Form of the Kaufman Test of Educational Achievement (K-TEA; Kaufman & Kaufman, 1985a) provides a somewhat broader sampling of skills.

As part of the assessment battery, Howie was administered the WRAT3. Each of his scores fell below the 2nd percentile and were markedly below average based on his age and grade level. Comparing Howie's WRAT3 standard scores to his Full Scale IQ score on the WISC-III indicates a level of achievement only slightly lower than the expected range given his overall level of cognitive abilities. However, limiting analysis to this comparison, as is sometimes done, can hamper understanding and the development of appropriate intervention. The gap between Howie's Verbal Comprehension Index score and the WRAT3 results is much more substantial and suggests that he could be achieving at a higher level (see Table 3). From the previous data, we suspect that his difficulties with visual processing and attention may be factors in his stalled academic progress. Given the poor achievement scores, further academic assessment is warranted to gain a more complete picture of his academic strengths and weaknesses.

The most widely used full academic battery is the Woodcock-Johnson Psycho-Educational Battery-Revised (WJ-R; Woodcock & Johnson, 1991). The Tests of Educational Achievement of the WJ-R include 14 different subtests, allowing for precise assessment of different aspects of reading (phonetics, comprehension, vocabulary), mathematics (calculation, applied concepts), written language (spelling, capitalization, punctuation, sentence construction) and knowledge (science, social studies, humanities). The WJ-R provides an in-depth assessment of academic skills, and is an excellent tool for the identification of specific academic strengths and weaknesses that is crucial for customization of a student's educational plan.

Other comprehensive batteries include the Kaufman Test of Educational Achievement (Kaufman & Kaufman, 1985b) and the recently developed Wechsler Individual Achievement Test (WIAT; Wechsler, 1992). The latter test possesses the additional advantage of direct comparisons between its scores and the WISC-III indices to determine the significance of achievement-IQ discrepancies. Besides the full academic batteries, a number of achievement tests have been developed to test, in a more detailed manner, skills in focal areas.

Personality Assessment

There are two major methods to measure personality in children and adolescents: projective techniques and objective inventories. Opinions concerning the validity and efficacy of these techniques among practitioners vary widely (Goldstein & Hersen, 1984).

Personality Inventories The majority of personality inventories are paper-and-pencil tests that present informants with a specific set of questions or statements concerning their own or their child's attitudes or mental state. Items are clustered into clinical scales by their ability to distinguish diagnosed groups. Although a number of personality inventories exist for use with adults, difficulty in reliably reporting thoughts, feelings, and attitudes has reduced their development in children. One of the few and best developed instruments, the Personality Inventory for Children (Wirt, Lachar, Klinedinst, & Seat, 1977), is administered to long-term caregivers, not to the child. It consists of a total of 600 items (although completion of fewer items can still be meaningfully interpreted) that yield scores on 20 different scales, as well as numerous other experimental scales.

The most frequently used adolescent self-report personality inventory is the Minnesota Multiphasic Personality Inventory-Adolescent (MMPI-A; Butcher et al., 1992). It consists of 478 item statements that provide scores on 10 basic scales, as well as numerous other experimental and supplemental scales. Interpretation involves analyzing the pattern and interrelationships among the scale scores. It is a well-developed measure with solid normative data, reliability, and validity. The MMPI-A and PIC results can be compared to assess the consistency of self and caregiver perspectives on the adolescent's personality functioning.

Projective Tests Most clinical child psychologists use projective techniques in their evaluations even though they acknowledge problems with reliability, validity, and scientific basis (Tuma & Pratt, 1982). Interpretation of these measures ranges from structured to more qualitative approaches. The development of projective techniques was based on theories about the unconscious and internal processes; thus, a more individualistic, qualitative approach to interpretation has been dominant, based on the examiner's experience and notions of personality. This approach has made it difficult to carry out meaningful studies of reliability and validity. More recently, attempts have been made to take a more structured approach, emphasizing the reliability of scoring responses to allow for the assessment of validity. Practitioners generally favor an integration of these approaches, using as reliable a scoring system as possible and then integrating these data with other clinical information to generate hypotheses about an individual's personality and emotional functioning.

The Rorschach remains the most widely used of the projective techniques. It is comprised of a series of 10 cards which are printed with bilaterally symmetrical inkblots, 5 black and white only, and 5 others that contain color. The patient is given each card and asked to state first what the inkblot could be and, in a second exposure, where the percept is located on the card and what characteristics (e.g., color, form, shading) determined their response. Responses are recorded verbatim and scored by one of several systems available. However, most scoring is carried out with Exner's structural or psychometric Comprehensive System (Exner, 1993) which has incorporated empirically supported features of existing systems, advocated procedures allowing for good interrater reliability, and developed a normative database for ages 5 years through adult. However, most practitioners feel that the Rorschach is only useful for children above the age of 7 years.

Various measures are then grouped into related clusters and decision rules allow for interpretation of the scores. Important constructs resulting from the Exner approach include response tendencies (ideational or emotional), stress resistance, emotional control and lability, self-concept, ideational flexibility, and organization of the environment, as well as indices of thought disorder, suicidality, and depression. An important feature of analysis to remember is that measures must be viewed in the context of the whole profile to be accurately interpreted.

Apperception instruments represent a large and commonly used class of projective measures. In these tasks, the individual is presented with a picture and is required to construct a "story" about it. Interpretation is based on the assumption that responses will reflect the individual's needs, desires, and conflicts. The original Thematic Apperception Test (TAT; Murray, 1943), although heavily used, lacks a consistent scoring system, reliability, and validity. For children and adolescents, the TAT is inappropriate because of the outdated and developmentally inappropriate nature of the cards. In addition, the cards tend to pull for negative emotional themes and the content tends to determine responses more than personality characteristics of the child.

The Children's Apperception Test (CAT; Bellak, 1975) provides parallel sets of cards involving young animals and children. Although more age-appropriate than the TAT, the CAT also lacks a reliable scoring system and clinicians tend to use it in a subjective manner. The Robert's Apperception Test for Children (McArthur & Roberts, 1982) has sets of cards with African-American as well as Caucasian children, depicting common conflicts and peer and family stressful and positive situations. The well-developed scoring system measures both adaptive and maladaptive functioning in multiple scales which are converted into normalized T-scores. Interpretation is carried out through both qualitative analysis of themes as well as quantitative analysis of the scale scores. The small normative base and few validity studies temper enthusiasm for this measure. Also, the scoring system is complicated and may reduce its usage by busy clinicians.

Although projective drawing tasks enjoy wide clinical appeal, there are limited data supporting their use in assessments of personality functioning. The three most frequently used forms of projective drawings are the Draw-a-Person Test, the House-Tree-Person Test, and the Kinetic Family Drawing. Apparently face-valid relations between various features of drawings and internal processes (e.g., size of human figures related to self-concept; gender of the figure related to sexual identification) are often espoused but have largely proved to be illusory. Reliable scoring systems have been developed for drawings (Koppitz, 1983); however, the lack of validity data (Cummings, 1986) argues forcefully against the use of drawings by themselves to infer aspects of a child's personality. Drawings provide a good "ice-breaker" at the beginning of an evaluation, allowing a non-threatening entry to testing and limited clinical information through purely qualitative analysis.

The Written Report   The written report of the psychological assessment determines the success of the process because it conveys, in an understandable form, to the referral source and to parents the results, the implications of the results for different aspects of the patient's functioning, and useful educational and treatment recommendations. Thus, the report begins with the questions that prompted the referral. Since a good report does not merely list test scores but also interprets them in the context of other important clinical information, relevant developmental, health, educational, and psychiatric history is usually provided next. As noted earlier, behavioral observations during the evaluation are a crucial factor in interpreting results and determining the validity of the administration. A detailed section of such observations is an important feature of good reports. Results are most usefully organized by function (e.g., intellectual, memory, achievement), integrating information from different assessment procedures. Parallel findings from different sources strengthen hypotheses. Isolated or inconsistent findings should be treated with great caution. A concise summary of findings and their implications should be followed by a recommendation section. The latter is often too general and is most often criticized by consumers. Realistic and concrete interventions should clearly derive from the pattern of data and they should be individualized with specific suggestions regarding the involvement of parents, teachers, and professionals as well as the child in the planning.

CONCLUSION

The process of psychological assessment of children and adolescents in the outpatient setting begins with deriving initial questions from referral and background information. These questions determine the composition of the battery, although, as the process unfolds, modifications are made to follow up on leads stemming from initial results. There is an ever-increasing list of instruments available for use; however, care must be taken in the interpretation of those that do not have solid psychometric qualities (e.g., adequate norms, reliability, validity) or which may not be age-appropriate. Hypotheses are strengthened by supporting data from different sources (e.g., ratings, self-report, clinical material) and must be considered in light of the overall pattern of results. This latter caution is even more important for children and adolescents than for adults because of variations in the developmental course of different mental functions.

REFERENCES

Achenbach, T. M. (1991a). *Manual for the Child Behavior Checklist/4-18 and 1991 Profile.* Burlington, VT: University of Vermont, Department of Psychiatry.

Achenbach, T. M. (1991b). *Manual for the Teacher's Report Form and 1991 Profile.* Burlington, VT: University of Vermont, Department of Psychiatry.

Achenbach, T. M. (1991c). *Manual for the Youth Self-Report and 1991 Profile.* Burlington, VT: University of Vermont, Department of Psychiatry.

Adams, W., & Sheslow, D. (1990). *The Wide Range Assessment of Memory and Learning.* Wilmington, DE: Jastak Associates.

American Educational Research Association, American Psychological Association, & National Council on Measurement in Education (1985). *Standards for educational and psychological testing.* Washington, DC: American Psychological Association.

Barrios, B. A. (1993). Direct observation. In T. H. Ollendick & M. Hersen (Eds.), *Handbook of child and adolescent assessment* (pp. 140–164).

Bayley, N. (1993). *Manual for the Bayley Scales of Infant Development-Second edition.* San Antonio, TX: Psychological Corporation.

Bellak, L. (1975). *The TAT, CAT, and SAT in clinical use* (3rd ed.). New York: Grune & Stratton.

Butcher, J. N., Williams, C. L., Graham, J. R., Archer, R. P., Tellegen, A., Ben-Porath, Y. S., & Kaemmer, B. (1992). *Manual for the Minnesota Multiphasic Personality Inventory-Adolescent.* Minneapolis: University of Minnesota Press.

Conners, C. K. (1989). *Conners rating scales manual.* North Tonawanda, NY: Multi-Health Systems, Inc..

Cummings, J. (1986). Projective drawings. In H. Knoff (Ed.), *The assessment of child and adolescent personality.* New York: Guilford Press.

Exner, J. E. (1993). *The Rorschach: A comprehensive system. Vol. 1. Basic foundations* (3rd ed.). New York: John Wiley & Sons.

Golden, C. J. (1987). *Luria-Nebraska Neuropsychological Battery: Children's Revision.* Los Angeles: Western Psychological Services.

Goldstein, G., & Hersen, M. (1984). Historical perspectives. In G. Goldstein & M. Hersen (Eds.). *Handbook of psychological assessment* (pp. 3–15). New York: Elsevier Science.

Harter, S. (1985). *Manual for the Self-Perception Profile for Children.* Denver: University of Denver.

Harter, S. (1988). *Manual for the Self-Perception Profile for Adolescents.* Denver: University of Denver.

Harter, S., & Pike, R. G. (1984). *The Pictorial Scale of Perceived Competence and Social Acceptance for Young Children.* Denver: University of Denver.

Hynd, G. W., & Willis, W. G. (1988). *Pediatric neuropsychology*. New York: Grune & Stratton.

Jastak, S., & Wilkinson, G. S. (1993). *Wide Range Achievement Test* (3rd ed.). Wilmington, DE: Jastak Associates.

Kaufman, A. S. (1994). *Intelligent testing with the WISC-III*. New York: John Wiley & Sons.

Kaufman, A. S., & Kaufman, N. L. (1983). *K-ABC administration and scoring manual*. Circle Pines, MN: American Guidance Service.

Kaufman, A. S., & Kaufman, N. L. (1985a). *Manual for the Kaufman Test of Educational Achievement (K-TEA) Comprehensive Form*. Circle Pines, MN: American Guidance Service.

Kaufman, A. S., & Kaufman, N. L. (1985b). *Manual for the Kaufman Test of Educational Achievement (K-TEA) Brief Form*. Circle Pines, MN: American Guidance Service.

Kaufman, A. S., & Kaufman, N. L. (1991). *Manual for the Kaufman Brief Intelligence Test (K-BIT)*. Circle Pines, MN: American Guidance Service.

Koppitz, E. M. (1983). Projective drawings with children and adolescents. *School Psychology Review, 12*, 421.

Kovacs, M. (1992). *Children's Depression Inventory*. San Antonio, TX: Psychological Corporation.

McArthur, D., & Roberts, G. (1982). *Roberts Apperception Test for Children: Manual*. Los Angeles: Western Psychological Services.

McCarthy, D. A. (1972). *The McCarthy Scales of Children's Abilities*. San Antonio, TX: The Psychological Corporation.

Mirsky, A. F., Anthony, B. J., Duncan, C. C., Ahearn, M. B., & Kellam, S. G. (1991). Analysis of the elements of attention: A neuropsychological approach. *Neuropsychology Review, 2*, 109–145.

Murray, H. A. (1943). *Manual of the Thematic Apperception Test*. Cambridge, MA: Harvard University Press.

P.L. 94-142, The Education of All Handicapped Children's Act, Federal Register, November 29, 1975.

Quay, H. C., & Peterson, D. R. (1987). *Manual for the Revised Behavior Problem Checklist*. Coral Gables, FL: Author.

Reitan, R. M., & Wolfson, D. (1985). *The Halstead-Reitan Neuropsychological Test Battery*. Tucson, AZ: Neuropsychology Press.

Reynolds, C. R., & Gletcher-Janzen, E. (1989). *Handbook of clinical child neuropsychology*. New York: Plenum Press.

Reynolds, C. R., & Richmond, B. O. (1985). *Revised Children's Manifest Anxiety Scale manual*. Los Angeles: Western Psychological Services.

Reynolds, W. M. (1987). *Reynolds Adolescent Depression Scale: Professional manual*. Odessa, FL: Psychological Assessment Resources.

Reynolds, W. M. (1989). *Reynolds Child Depression Scale: Professional manual*. Odessa, FL: Psychological Assessment Resources.

Sattler, J. M. (1990). *Assessment of children* (3rd ed.). San Diego, CA: Jerome M. Sattler.

Sparrow, S., Balla, D. A., & Cicchetti, D. V. (1984). *Vineland Adaptive Behavior Scales*. Circle Pines, MN: American Guidance Service.

Thorndike, R. L., Hagen, E. P., & Sattler, J. M. (1986). *Guide for administering and scoring the Stanford-Binet Intelligence Scale: Fourth edition*. Chicago: Riverside.

Tramontana, M. G., Sherrets, S. D., & Golden, C. J. (1980). Brain dysfunction in youngsters with psychiatric disorders: Application of the Selz-Reitan rules for neuropsychological diagnosis. *Clinical Neuropsychology, 2*, 118–123.

Tuma, J., & Pratt, J. (1982). Clinical child psychology practice and training: A survey. *Journal of Clinical Child Psychology, 11*, 27–34.

Wechsler, D. (1981). *Manual for the Wechsler Adult Intelligence Scale-Revised*. San Antonio, TX: The Psychological Corporation.

Wechsler, D. (1989). *Manual for the Wechsler Preschool and Primary Scale of Intelligence-Revised (WPPSI-R)*. San Antonio, TX: The Psychological Corporation

Wechsler, D. (1991). *Manual for the Wechsler Intelligence Scale for Children-Third Edition (WISC-III)*. San Antonio, TX: The Psychological Corporation.

Wechsler, D. (1992). *Manual for the Wechsler Individual Achievement Test*. San Antonio, TX: The Psychological Corporation.

Wirt, R. D., Lachar, D., Klinedinst, J. K., & Seat, P. D. (1977). *Multidimensional description of child personality: A manual for the Personality Inventory for Children*. Los Angeles: Western Psychological Services.

Woodcock, R. W., & Johnson, M. B. (1991). *The Woodcock-Johnson Psychoeducational Battery-Revised*. Chicago: Riverside Publishing Co.

Chapter 9

Speech and Language Evaluation

Regina Cicci, Ph.D.

Language characterizes us as human and is the primary mode of communication in all cultures. We understand the language of others, we think with words, and we produce speech that will be understood. For most of us, language enters the human communication system through hearing, is processed through various cognitive mechanisms, and is expressed by speech. Mastery of language comprehension and production is important for developing self-image, as social interaction, as a base to acquire reading, writing, and some math, and relates to ultimate dependence or independence in adulthood.

Speech and language disorders have various etiologies. For example, children and adolescents with cognitive limitations, or cognitive deficits because of neurological insult, will understand and produce language at the general level of their intelligence, and individuals with neuromotor problems may have restrictions on their speech production. Hearing-impaired persons have characteristic speech and language patterns related to the type and extent of their hearing loss. Children within the spectrum of autism are classified by how competent they are in using language and speech. Children born into poverty often lack exposure to a language environment involving varied linguistic structures and verbal interactions with resulting language deficits. Bilingual children can encounter problems with language learning, and it is important to determine if a problem exists in the first language as well as with English. Children and adolescents with any speech and language problem, including those who deviate from expectation for age and ability in language comprehension and/or production, must receive appropriate diagnostic and remedial attention.

Individuals with speech and language difficulties have increased incidence of psychiatric problems including attention disorders. Conversely, children with psychiatric disorders are at higher risk for communicative disorders (Cantwell & Baker, 1987; Beitchman, Hood, Rochon, & Peterson, 1989). Thus, many toddlers or teens, referred for psychiatric evaluation, may benefit from speech and language assessment.

THE LANGUAGE TO BE LEARNED

Language is a rule-governed system, and as children grow they master the rules of the language that is spoken by those around them. The components of a language system include phonology, morphology, syntax, semantics, and pragmatics, and most languages are represented in print by an orthography.

Phonology refers to the sound structure of a language, with a phoneme being a speech sound, a small unit that changes one word to another word. We hear words like tap or top and bit or bat as whole words. A change in a phoneme, in this case the vowel, changes meaning. Syntax refers to the grammar of language, the way words are arranged to form sentences. Grammar is a universal of the world's languages since all languages have a permissible way of placing words in sentences. Word order is different in English when we make a statement or ask a question. We say "The bike is blue" and to ask a question about color, "Is the bike blue?" Adjectives precede nouns in English, but in other languages may be positioned differently. Words that tell about words' relation to other words, such as prepositions, are placed in sentences in particular ways in a language.

Morphology is another part of a language system. A morpheme is the smallest unit of meaning. Morphemes can stand alone or are bound to other morphemes. A word such as caps is made up of two morphemes. One is cap and the other is the s at the end of the word that marks the word caps as being more than one, or plural. Such plurals may be pronounced as /s/, /z/, or /uz/ (as in caps, dogs, and matches) depending on which sound precedes the ending. These morphological changes are referred to as inflectional, and they are formed in a fairly regular way.

Other morphemes are derivational and are not as consistent. In English, for example, how we change verbs to nouns varies. When we change the verb amuse to a noun, the result is amusement, but the resulting noun for prefer is preference.

Semantics refers to meaning—meaning of vocabulary, but also sentences, and extended discourse. A linguistic community's shared meanings of words allow for communication as well as for appreciation of figurative language in metaphor and humor. Pragmatics is the use of language in a social context—how language is used for interaction with others. Language and behavior are modified depending on a situation. How one uses language formally or casually, how politeness is understood and expressed, how we offer a question, request, or demand, expand a point or seek clarification depends on effective use of pragmatics.

SPEECH DISORDERS

Speech disorders are classified as disorders of articulation, voice, or fluency.

Articulation Disorders or Phonological Disorders

Articulation disorders can occur because of dysarthria as in children with cerebral palsy or other neuromotor conditions; because of apraxia for speech which means that the individual has difficulty in voluntarily executing the coordinated motor patterns for speech even though function is adequate at a vegetative level; or because of motor patterning difficulties and/or lack of efficient velo-pharyngeal closure. Such problems are motor expressive output disorders. Causes of articulation disorders are often unclear, but generally relate to some difficulty in matching speech sounds with the motor patterns necessary to produce them.

An articulation problem (a Phonological Disorder in the *Diagnostic and Statistical Manual of Mental Disorders [DSM-IV]* [American Psychiatric Association, 1994]) is identified when a child does not pronounce sounds appropriately for his or her age. A child may distort sounds such as a lisp for production of /s/, saying "thee-thaw" or "shee-shaw" for see-saw. He or she may substitute a sound such as using /w/ for /r/ resulting in "wabbit" for rabbit and "cawit" for carrot or omit a sound as saying "up" for cup or "boon" for balloon.

Some children, with or without deviations in articulation, have difficulty with phonological awareness as they reach school age. They may have trouble perceiving how words can be segmented into sounds; therefore, they cannot relate printed letters with the sounds of speech. A reading and spelling disorder—dyslexia—results.

Voice Disorders

Voice disorders are present when there is deviation from normal expectation for age and sex in areas of pitch, loudness, resonance, tone, and general quality. Voice quality can be affected by fatigue and emotional states. Vocal abuse that includes behaviors such as shouting on the playground or at sporting events or speaking loudly to be heard above noise or music can result in hoarseness, and if such behaviors continue can cause lesions on the vocal folds. Apart from results of such vocal abuse, voice problems are rare in children and adolescents.

Children and adolescents may also show deviations with the prosody of speech. Prosody refers to the melody and rhythm of speech including the patterns of stress and emphasis as kinds of verbal highlighting of words used. Prosodic features inform a listener whether the speaker is making a statement or asking a question. Prosody gives speech its emotional tone. Individuals with some emotional difficulties and others with neurological disorders may show problems with prosody. They may speak in a monotone or show an explosive quality to speech patterns. Their speech lacks typical melodic qualities.

Stuttering   During the preschool years many normal and advanced language users show dysfluent speech with repetitions of words or beginnings of words or prolonging sounds within words. With calm management and with adults refraining from calling attention to the repetitious patterns, most pass through this phase easily. Others persist with the pattern of repetition and come to be referred to as stutterers. Stuttering is a condition that has fascinated and mystified for thousands of years, and continues to be unresolved as to cause. Current thinking classifies three kinds of stuttering: developmental, neurogenic, and psychogenic. Developmental stuttering has been studied the most and is regarded as the most prevalent. The speaker displays hard blocks on words, and may have secondary symptoms such as finger snapping or facial grimacing. Neurogenic stuttering results from disease process such as stroke or head injury. Psychogenic stuttering develops following a period of strain or trauma and generally occurs after the stage at which developmental stuttering occurs.

A condition that mimics stuttering is cluttering. The individual shows dysfluent speech, problems with word retrieval and organization, and may show similar patterns when writing. He or she may lift a pencil from paper several times before beginning a sentence, write a word or two, erase, write a phrase, erase again, and so on, until a single written sentence is completed.

Language Disorders

Each of the language components (phonology, morphology, syntax, semantics, and pragmatics) passes through certain cognitive processes. Information is received via the ear to the brain where it is interpreted, put into storage by way of working memory, and is available to be retrieved, organized, and expressed by speech. A disruption anywhere in these processes results in a language disorder. Such language disorders in children were previously referred to as receptive and or expressive aphasia or dysphasia (McGinnis, 1963; Myklebust, 1971; Eisenson, 1972), but are now classified with the more general term of language disorder.

Expressive Language Disorder   Expressive language disorders are characterized by difficulty in expressing thoughts and feelings using speech. One kind of expressive language problem is difficulty with retrieval of words, which may be referred to as a wordfinding problem or dysnomia. The person knows a word but cannot recall it quickly for use. Individuals may use circumlocutions, such as "that what you cook eggs in" for frying pan or skillet. They may say a word with a similar sound pattern, as "violent" for violin, or confuse word parts as "no tails" for toe-nails or "varicose" for bellicose, or give a semantically related response, as "clock" for watch or "teepee" for igloo. A wordfinding problem can affect conversation, answering questions that must have a single specific-word response, recalling numerals or letter names or sounds, and completing fill-in-the-blank tests.

Children and adolescents with expressive language disorders may also show problems with formulation of ideas. They may confuse word order as in a 4-year-old child saying "What for this is?" for What is this for? or a 14-year-old asking "What do want from me else?" for What else do you want from me? They may omit words saying "I go store" from a 5-year-old boy or "I went Annapolis friends" from a teenager.

Problems with expressive language may be persistent. A youngster followed over many years said at age 3, "Where other train there down a floor?." At 6, he queried, "How many more time?" for How much more time [must I stay here]? and said "fallton" (a possible combination of water falls and fountain) for waterfall. At 9 years, trying to retrieve the title, Robin Hood, he said "Don't tell me. I forget! I know it! Christopher Robin. No, not Christopher Robin. It's Robin Hood!" When he was 11, he defined peninsula as "water surrounding land on three sides" and said, "You take 2,000 into 12" when he meant 2,000 divided by 12. At age 17, he said "reeked" for reaped, commented that "I always get that word right—I mean—wrong," and wrote of "oppressment of women" and "feminitely labeled jobs."

Expressive language disorders can interfere with social communication at home, at school, with peers, and with adults. These problems may cause later difficulties with written expressive language and can affect verbal interaction in a therapy session (Cicci, 1991).

Receptive Language Disorder   Children and adolescents may also have receptive language disorders that result in problems understanding language and that may interfere significantly with daily activities. Those with such problems may not follow oral directions and rules of discipline. They struggle learning new vocabulary and verbal concepts, confuse words used at play and for games, and often fail to appreciate verbal humor. Making inferences from known or given facts is hard. They may have difficulty with written instructions on worksheets or with reading comprehension in general.

Individuals with receptive language problems tend to be literal in their interpretation of language and show rigidity of meaning. They may learn one definition of a word but fail to learn additional ones.

Responding to the question, Is anything hard for you in school? an 8-year-old boy said "A chair is hard in my school." A teenage girl was confused by a question on a test that requested comments on the social climate of the times; she thought of climate as related only to weather. A middle-school boy did not know how a person would feel following events in a story when feelings were not explicitly stated "because it didn't tell me how she feels." A 10-year-old boy was scolded and told to stand in a certain place away from the other children while they were waiting for a bus. The next day, he did not wait with the children for his bus, but again stood in the space he was moved to on the previous day. He told the teacher on bus duty that day that was where he was supposed to stand. She became angry with him for disobeying; he was frustrated at being misunderstood.

Some children and adolescents will show mixed receptive-expressive language disorders—exhibiting difficulty with both understanding language and producing it. However, some youngsters with receptive language disorders may be deceptive. They have good articulation, produce sentences, and use a fair vocabulary. It is not until specifically tested that the receptive part of the receptive-expressive language is exposed.

Who Needs a Speech and Language Evaluation?

Preschool children who:

- show deviations or inconsistencies in response to sound
- use limited vocal play (cooing, babbling) in early months of life
- have recurrent middle ear disease
- do not seem to understand speech (Wave bye-bye, Give the ball to Mommy, Where's Daddy?) when unaccompanied by gesture at 15 months of age
- use no real words, in addition to Mommy and Daddy, at age 2
- do not combine words by age 3
- use speech that cannot be understood most of the time by strangers when they are 4 years old
- repeat, or echo, everything they hear but with little understanding
- have errors in speech production at age 7 years
- never want to be read to.

Children or teenagers who:

- "do not listen" or have trouble following directions
- use vocabulary that is deficient compared with peers
- have trouble retrieving specific words they wish to use
- have difficulty in formulating sentences
- talk spontaneously but fail to engage in give-and-take conversational speech or respond to questions
- do not use language to question, comment, and clarify
- are reluctant to use verbal communication
- do not differentiate use of language with peers and adults
- do not acquire reading and spelling skills as expected

- cannot put thoughts and ideas on paper either by pencil or computer
- at any age, are concerned or have parents who are concerned about development in the areas of language, speech, or learning.

Speech and Language Assessment

For speech and language assessment, the clinician, usually a speech-language pathologist, needs to have a sample of speech and language. A comfortable relationship must be established between a child or adolescent and a clinician so they are willing to talk.

Speech Testing   Questions about speech include:

- Is articulation normal for the individual's age?
- Is speech intelligible?
- Is voice quality appropriate in areas of pitch, loudness, resonance, and quality?
- Is prosody normal?
- Is fluency typical for age and developmental status?
- Is the oral mechanism adequate to support speech development?
- What approaches should be used for management if there are deviations in any of these areas?

Language Testing   Language testing requires sampling how the individual understands and produces language. To measure comprehension in a child with limited language output, it is necessary to select a standardized test or devise tasks that do not require speech as a response. The child can point to a stimulus, manipulate materials, or carry out a motor act, as well as speak, to demonstrate comprehension of vocabulary and syntax.

Obviously, for measuring expressive language the individual must talk. The clinician evaluates the level of vocabulary use and how well the child or adolescent can retrieve words and formulate sentences using correct and varied syntax. Tasks are selected that will elicit information about a child's or adolescent's language through the consistent application of rules (even if the rule cannot be explicitly stated). There must be a recognition that contrived tests and tasks do not necessarily reflect how the person uses language in naturalistic situations with familiar and unfamiliar persons and activities. The verbal give-and-take of conversation is different from more formal language required to respond to questions, to share complex information, and to form the base for later writing.

In the area of language assessment, clinical questions include:

- Is vocabulary understood in a way appropriate for age and ability?
- Is syntax understood?
- Is auditory memory adequate to support verbal learning?
- Are individual words retrieved as needed for communication?
- Can messages be formulated in a way compatible with what the child or adolescent wishes to say?
- What remedial approaches are likely to be successful in management if there are problems?

It is always helpful to observe young children in as natural a setting as possible. Seeing them with a parent is invaluable because it is possible to learn about parent-child interaction and the extent and kind of verbal stimulation typically provided.

Older children and adolescents need to participate actively for good test results; they have to use speech to have speech evaluated. Occasionally, they may refuse to talk or provide only limited verbal output. Such refusal may indicate elective mutism, emotional difficulties, cognitive limitations, or reluctance to communicate for any number of reasons. In nearly all such cases, it is possible to learn how much language individuals understand, even if they provide limited speech. In my experience, children and adolescents who resist using speech often have spoken language disorders.

TREATMENT TECHNIQUES

Problems with language and speech are not benign (Cicci, 1995) and demand attention and appropriate intervention. Speech and language disorders are generally managed by speech-language pathologists, and most disorders are responsive to intervention. Disorders of articulation and voice are often completely remedied. Problems with fluency vary in response to intervention, but many make very good progress and are symptom-free. Children and adolescents with language disorders can make progress in language understanding and use; however, spoken language disorders can endure and influence an individual's lifelong approach to learning and interacting with others (Johnson & Blalock, 1987).

In treating a child or adolescent with a language disorder, the clinician asks these questions:

- Does the individual have the skill? If not, how can we teach it?
- Does he or she have the skill, but need additional practice? If so, we provide practice.
- Does the individual have the skill most of the time in a one-to-one session, but does not generalize to daily use? If this is the case, we provide support to use the skill in various structured situations and then in less structured ones. It is with application and generalization that the individual achieves mastery.

With receptive-expressive problems we need to time the presentation of the language with the experience, whether teaching words for playing with a ball (roll, throw, bounce) to a 3-year-old child or supervising a biology lab for high school sophomores. Experiences are provided to teach what the concept or word is, and what it is not. Much more direct teaching is required because new words are seldom learned in an incidental way for those with receptive difficulties. Since it is hard to observe a problem with language understanding, we must help families and teachers understand the impact of failing to comprehend language that is used every day.

When children and adolescents have expressive disorders, we teach strategies for recalling words and help them feel comfortable with alternative word choices. We teach various kinds of sentence structure and provide practice in using sentences. We help them develop plans for extended discourse so they have a kind of frame on which to hang their thoughts and feelings. We help them understand the nature of their language disorder and provide direct teaching, but also support, until they are comfortable with themselves and the level of their communicative competence.

Proficiency in communication forms an important part of social-emotional development. Inadequate communication interferes with effectiveness at home, in the community, at school, and in the therapy session. Identifying and treating speech and language disorders forms a part of successful treatment of some psychiatric disorders.

CONCLUSION

Research continues to focus on the interactions between spoken language and reading and written expressive language. Translating research findings for general use in educating children is always slow, but as the significance of language problems' effects on long-term growth and development are made clear, efforts should improve. As technology improves, more precise measures of speech and language can be made, and delivery of services will be more efficient and cost-effective. We continue to need more studies of language in naturalistic settings, greater understanding of brain-behavior relationships, better knowledge of genetic transmission, and expanded data sharing across institutions and agencies. Increased interdisciplinary work among physicians and other mental health providers, speech-language pathologists, and educators will allow better diagnosis and management of the language and speech disorders in children and adolescents.

REFERENCES

American Psychiatric Association (APA). (1994). *Diagnostic and statistical manual of mental disorders* (4th ed.). Washington, DC: Author.

Beitchman, J. H., Hood, J., Rochon, J., & Peterson, M. (1989). Empirical classification of speech/language impairment in children. *Journal of the American Academy of Child and Adolescent Psychiatry, 28,* 1, 118–123).

Cantwell, C., & Baker, L. (1987). *Developmental speech and language disorders.* New York: Guilford Press.

Cicci, R. (1991). Teaching language handicapped children. In J. F. Kavanagh (Ed.), *The language continuum: From infancy to literacy.* (pp. 167–194). Parkton, MD: York Press.

Cicci, R. (1995). *What's wrong with me: Learning disabilities at home and school.* Baltimore: York Press.

Eisenson, J. (1972). *Aphasia in children.* New York: Harper & Row.

Johnson, D. J., & Blalock, J. W. (1987). *Learning disabilities: Clinical studies.* Orlando FL: Grune & Stratton.

McGinnis, M. A. (1963). *Aphasic children: Identification and education by the association method.* Washington, DC: Alexander Graham Bell Association for the Deaf.

Myklebust, H. R. (1971). Childhood aphasia: An evolving concept. In L. Travis (Ed.), *Handbook of speech pathology and audiology.* New York: Appleton-Century-Crofts.

Chapter 10

Forensic Community Child and Adolescent Psychiatry

Andre P. Derdeyn, M.D. and Mark Jennings, M.D.

Forensic child and adolescent psychiatry can be considered to have three major realms:

- legal "rules" of the practice of child and adolescent psychiatry (e.g., confidentiality and requirements for commitment)
- testifying as to cause and extent of damage in personal injury or tort claims (e.g., a day care center is sued because a child is alleged to have been sexually molested by a staff member; a physician is sued for admitting a child to an inpatient facility on insufficient grounds), and
- clinical assessments of two rather distinctly different types.

Clinical assessment for the juvenile court involves work with neglected and abused children and those who have been adjudicated delinquent. The goal of such work is to shed light upon which types of facilities and modes of psychiatric intervention might best serve the adjudicated youth, and for the neglected and abused the questions before the court revolve around termination of parental rights, foster placement, return from foster care to biological parent(s), and adoption. The focus of clinical assessment in family or domestic relations court revolves largely around divorce and its aberrations. In recent years allegations of sexual abuse have become quite frequent in domestic relations court. These latter clinical areas comprise most of the work engaged in by psychiatrists in community settings; torts and the law of psychiatric practice will not be treated in this chapter. First, the development of the juvenile court will be discussed, followed by a discussion of custody issues.

THE JUVENILE COURT

Origins and Development

In colonial times the systems for societal care for dependent and for delinquent children were quite indistinguishable. These included outdoor relief (income maintenance), indentured apprenticeship, and almshouses which took in all manner of impaired, destitute, and dependent persons. Children found guilty of significant crimes were sentenced and imprisoned as adults.

In the 19th century, the belief arose that institutions could socialize the child separated from the deleterious influence of their parents' class and culture. Philanthropists and religious charities objected to placing children in adult prisons and advocated special facilities for children emphasizing education, vocational skills, and moral training. Institutions developed which accepted children convicted of crimes as well as those in need of care and supervision. The first state institution specifically for convicted juveniles, the State Reform School in Westborough, Massachusetts, was built in 1847.

In the latter half of the 19th century institutional care was replaced largely by placing-out programs. Sharing a prevalent view, the Children's Aid Society of New York considered the chaotic urban environment to be the major cause of delinquency. The society and many similar organizations collected destitute and delinquent children and provided one-way tickets to farmers' homes in the midwest United States. Several hundred thousand children were so transported.

Many court clinics opened in the early 20th century, beginning with Dr. William Healy's in Chicago in 1909. From the first and continuing to the present there has always been a tension between two quite different views of the juvenile court. One is that the court's purpose is social welfare, with the task of education-treatment-rehabilitation of delinquent youth. The other view is that it is a court of law, and should provide the procedural safeguards that courts for adults do. Both views have always had adherents: some of the activity leading to separate juvenile courts was related to the belief that courts and juries were not finding juveniles guilty because of concern about sending children into the deplorable conditions of the prisons for adults. Generally, over the last several decades there has prevailed diminishing belief in the rehabilitation potential of our institutions for delinquent youth, increasing concerns about crime, and concerns about the legal rights of juveniles before the court. The informality of the court, which originated because of the court's rehabilitative purpose, was sometimes leading to conviction with insufficient proof and generally lacking in basic legal safeguards for the juvenile.

The first U.S. Supreme Court intervention involving juvenile courts related to the policy of transferring or waiving jurisdiction for the juvenile to the adult criminal court. The juvenile courts' informality was not found to be consistent with the potential seriousness of this action for the juvenile. Therefore the Court in *Kent v. United States* in 1966 indicated that more process was due for such transfers.

The Gault case in 1967 vastly increased the due process requirements of the juvenile court. In this instance, a juvenile who did not have the opportunity to confront a witness had been effectively sentenced for five years for a crime (lewd telephone calls) which would have required an adult to serve two months in jail. In 1970 the standard of proof required for adjudication as a delinquent was raised in *In re Winship* to "beyond a reasonable doubt."

The insanity defense is rarely made in juvenile court (and is not common in adult criminal court either). Similarly, competence to stand trial is not often questioned. It should be remembered that the presence of even a major mental illness does not signify that a youth is incompetent to stand trial. For a youth to be incompetent to stand trial he or she must fail to have a factual and rational understanding of the charges against him or her, and must be unable to cooperate in his or her own defense.

Although the juvenile court is currently continuing its process of becoming more of a juvenile criminal court, the psychiatrist's role in disposition, and sometimes in diversion, is in English common law's *parens patriae* tradition of the juvenile court's rehabilitative mission. The *parens patriae* concept refers to the king's guardianship over people who had no other protector. The juvenile and domestic relations courts continue this role with regard to abused and neglected children, and when parents come under court jurisdiction as in paternity, custody, and visitation conflicts.

Procedures

Intake: Diversion or Adjudication   The *parens patriae* concept is also in the fore at intake. When a case is referred to the court, intake staff decide whether to proceed informally or schedule the case for arraignment before the judge, in which case all the due process requirements apply. If the alleged act is not serious or violent, intake staff may conduct an informal hearing, and diversion—a non-judicial resolution of the issue—may be instituted. For example, the youth may agree to perform community service and charges for underage purchase of alcohol may be dropped. For diversion to be considered the youth must admit to and take responsibility for the act. If the youth denies the charges, then the adjudicatory hearing (trial) is held. If the charges are serious and the youth admits guilt, then the need for trial is obviated and a dispositional hearing is held.

There is continuing controversy regarding whether the court should retain jurisdiction over status offenses—acts which are against the law because one is a child—with some courts maintaining jurisdiction, some not, but almost all trying to divert them to non-legal channels. Status offenses include most typically incorrigibility, truancy, and running away.

Transfer or Waiver to Adult Court   Courts obtain psychiatric evaluations as part of the process of transferring adolescents to adult court because of the seriousness of the crime the youth is accused of having committed. The psychiatrist contributes to the question of the adolescent's potential for rehabilitation. The court is attempting to deduce what the offender's future behavior is likely to be, prior to the offender's being convicted of the crime with which he or she has been charged. This question tends to be associated with crimes about which there is considerable public knowledge and emotion. Only the most intrepid of community child and adolescent psychiatrists will want to venture into these cases.

Disposition   It is at this stage, after adjudication, that the court decides what is to be done with the juvenile. Dispositions available to the court include hospitalization, incarceration in a correctional institution, residential treatment, group home placement, custody to the department of social services, and return home, probably with probation and possibly with outpatient services. Recommendation of dispositions may also entail a dilemma for the psychiatrist: is the recommendation for what the child actually needs or is the recommendation altered to what the state can readily provide?

Psychiatric Evaluation in the Forensic Setting   Psychiatric evaluation and care of incarcerated youth and evaluation in relation to the disposition phase of court proceedings are the major reasons psychiatric evaluation is sought in relation to the juvenile justice/corrections system. An adolescent's mental state bears importantly upon the appropriateness of a disposition. A psychotic adolescent will require hospitalization and possibly medication instead of incarceration.

Incarcerated juveniles who voice suicidal ideation are referred to psychiatrists to determine the degree of intent and recommend the level of observation to keep the youth safe. Likewise, homicidal youth may be referred. Although it is impossible to predict accurately who will be dangerous, correctional facility staff need to know which individuals are dangerous as a result of delusions or other aberrant thinking.

Adolescents in the juvenile justice system frequently suffer from mental illness ranging from psychosis and depression to anxiety and eating disorders. The psychiatrist will be asked to evaluate these young people and make recommendations for treatment. Often, these adolescents remain in the juvenile justice system and require ongoing therapy and medication management.

The evaluation of incarcerated adolescents is similar to that done in any other setting. The necessary information includes current problems and functioning, past problems, medical, educational and family history, as well as social background, with particular attention to any legal problems or history of conduct-disordered behavior. This information often may be unavailable, because these young people come from chaotic homes and have limited ability to recall the past. Past records may be unavailable as well. Occasionally, an adolescent will lie, but this abates when he or she realizes that the psychiatrist is uninterested in getting involved in the intrigues at work within the system. Clear communication with the correctional facility staff diminishes the splitting and secondary gain.

It is essential to inform the adolescent of the purpose of the interview and that it is not confidential. By remaining free of any judgmental tone and asking questions calmly and in a straightforward manner, the psychiatrist reassures the youth that nothing will be seen as evil, corrupt, or shocking. The question, "How old were you when you started smoking (drinking, using cocaine, having sex)?" acknowledges the near-universal practice of these behaviors in their peer group, making denial less likely.

A subspecialty within the forensic setting is the evaluation of the juvenile sex offender. The format is essentially the same, with emphasis on sexual practices, paraphilias, fantasies, and any history of abuse. Treatment options range from outpatient to intensive outpatient to foster-care supervision to inpatient to no specific treatment aimed at the sexual offense for those whose perpetration is part of a conduct disorder, which requires treatment aimed at the underlying conduct/personality problems.

Any report to the court should differentiate clearly what the psychiatrist learned firsthand, and what was read in reports and told him or her by persons other than the youth (hearsay). Similarly, it is important to separate clearly the facts (and hearsay) on which the psychiatrist's opinion is based, and the opinion itself. Brevity is key, with headings and a clear, brief summary and recommendations.

It is possible for the psychiatrist to "identify with the aggressor," taking a somewhat callous attitude with this population. Any child (and his or her family) before the court is in a crisis situation, no matter how some may cover their feelings with nonchalance or anger. It is possible for the psychiatrist to slip into an identification with a somewhat hostile and dehumanized view of the juvenile. This is sometimes discernable as an "us and them" attitude, which seems to be present among adults to some degree in all institutions connected with adolescents. If the psychiatrist begins to notice that he or she fails to empathize regarding the child's crisis, the psychiatrist should realize that he or she is losing touch with the qualities for which he or she is useful to the court.

Occasionally, a juvenile will be seen as a "victim" by the correctional facility staff. While it is not the purpose of this chapter to discuss the parataxic distortions at work in either extreme, the psychiatrist should be alert to the prevailing attitude within the setting to any individual juvenile. Adopting the role of "Devil's Advocate" often gives a balanced perspective to the entire evaluative process.

Custody Disputes

Abuse and neglect, foster care placement, return from foster care, termination of parental rights, and adoption usually are handled in the juvenile court. The juvenile court's jurisdiction may also include divorce custody and visitation, but usually that is the business of family or domestic relations court.

Psychiatrists are called upon to act as consultants in two general types of child custody disputes. The first is a private dispute, usually between the parents in the context of divorce but sometimes between a parent and a grandparent or other long-term caretaker. In these cases, the parties become involved in the legal system because they are not able to decide the issues themselves. If they could come to some agreement, the court would typically not intervene but would simply ratify the decision made by the parties. The other type of custody issue is one in which there has been an allegation of parental abuse or neglect, and the child is usually in foster care. In these cases, the state (usually in the form of a welfare department) is intervening in the family. Because this kind of case represents an intrusion by the state in the privacy and integrity of the family, the applicable law differs quite markedly from that governing private disputes, in recognition of the imbalance of power between an individual and the state.

In community settings the psychiatrist is most likely to be working in a contractual arrangement, with the parties ordered by the court to participate in the evaluation. This arrangement avoids the powerful conflicts of interest inherent in being in the employ of one of the parties.

Divorce Custody Disputes   In recent years, the law throughout the states has evolved from the previous "tender years presumption" favoring mothers toward a sex-neutral standard. It has become much more possible for fathers to gain custody or primary physical residence, although the number of fathers doing so remains quite low. The judge may consider a wide range of issues in assessing which parent's custody will be in the best interests of the child. The parent's lifestyle and behavior, especially sexual orientation, may strongly influence the outcome of a custody dispute. An important function a psychiatric consultant may have is to focus the court's attention on factors which relate to the child's psychological well-being and to help the court consider the lifestyle of a parent only as it affects the child. The psychiatric consultant, by taking the child's view and by being well-informed on child development and relevant empirical research, can address the question of whether or not the parental behavior is likely to be harmful to the child. In this way, psychiatric consultants may defuse inflammatory, distracting issues and help maintain the focus of the inquiry on the child's well-being.

Grandparent and Stepparent Visitation Disputes   Under the English common law from which our domestic relations law is derived, a grandparent did not have a legal right to petition a court to consider whether that grandparent should be allowed to visit a grandchild. In the interval from 1977, when six states had laws permitting grandparents to petition a court for visitation upon the death or divorce of their adult child, to the late 1980s, every state passed legislation allowing grandparent visitation rights.

As the question of visitation revolves entirely around the court's determination of what is in the best interests of the child involved, these cases constitute an important area for psychiatric consultation. In addition to the new rights accorded grandparents, legislatures and courts are extending visitation rights to include siblings, former stepparents, and others.

Custody Disputes in Which the State Is a Party

Child Abuse and Neglect and Foster Care   Cases in which the state (i.e., a welfare department) intervenes in a family and gains custody of a child raise policy considerations which are different from those of divorce custody and other private disputes. In private disputes, the parents have, in effect, asked for the court's involvement, having been unable to resolve the dispute themselves. This is not the case in abuse or neglect cases, where the family's involvement with the court is usually involuntary and its adversary is the state. A number of U.S. Supreme Court cases have established a constitutional right of family privacy that includes the right of parents to raise their children free from state intrusion. This right is not absolute, and the state has a responsibility to intervene under the *parens patriae* doctrine when a child is abused or neglected.

The major question to be answered in these cases is whether or not the child should be returned to the parent(s). Issues to be considered in making such a decision are ability to provide reasonable consistency; capacity for empathy; and capacity to use available parent training activities. In cases where return to parents or termination of parental rights is an issue, assessment should include observation and interaction of the child with the family. Observation of attachment behaviors is particularly important.

In recent years various systems of foster care review have been instituted to keep track of children so that they do not slip into the interminable foster care that has occurred so much in the past. This review has provided a stimulus both in returning children to their homes and in effecting termination of parental rights and adoption.

Termination of Parental Rights   Termination of the right of a parent to the custody of his or her child is considered a grave step that courts are extremely reluctant to take. Termination of parental rights frees the child for adoption and traditionally severs the relationship of the parent and the child. For older children coming from foster care who have maintained contact with their parents, there is widespread acceptance of having them continue such contact after adoption.

Most states have statutes which spell out in detail the criteria for termination of parental rights. These criteria include such items as abandonment; neglect; perpetration of, or failure to protect a child from, physical or sexual abuse; commitment of a crime such as murdering a child's sibling or other parent; failure to maintain contact with a child in foster care; or failure to remedy with reasonable assistance the conditions which led to removal of a child. All states require a plan for the rehabilitation and reunification of families whenever a child is placed in foster care. Such a plan is an integral part of the state's foster care review system mentioned previously.

In 1982 the U.S. Supreme Court, in *Santosky v. Kramer,* struck down the prevailing standard that required proof by "fair preponderance" of the evidence that the child was permanently neglected. The court found that due process requires that allegations supporting termination of parental rights be proven by at least "clear and convincing evidence," a high standard to achieve in cases like these.

Because of the strong emphasis on parental rights, the child's interests in a termination case are often not the focus of the proceeding. The courts are largely concerned with the question of whether the parents' right to their child is abrogated by the extent of the parents' failure to take remedial steps. The judge's decision is usually based upon relatively concrete evidence: the frequency and extent of injury, neglect, or abandonment, and the state's diligence in carrying out rehabilitative activities.

The Evaluation   Divorce custody contests between two capable parents generally require the most comprehensive evaluation and are the most common type of child placement case for which psychiatric consultation is sought. The guidelines that follow are geared to this type of evaluation. Not all facets of the evaluation may be required in other types of contested custody. The psychiatric consultant may draw upon two categories of data in carrying out child custody evaluations. The first is observations made in interviewing the child and parents and in observing interactions between the child and family members. The second may include indirect sources such as social service records, school reports, psychological test results, and medical and psychiatric records.

Confidentiality   While there are many similarities between custody evaluations and other types of clinical work, the practice regarding confidentiality is not one of them. The psychiatric consultant must actively dispel the expectation that confidences will be kept. Some clinicians require adults to sign a release even when the court has ordered the evaluation. The psychiatric consultant generally presents himself or herself to the child as a person who is helping the judge think about with whom the child should live.

The Major Issues   The psychiatric consultant can contribute to resolution of the custodial question by providing information to the court regarding at least four major areas:

- the child's preference
- the reciprocal attachment between a parent and a child
- the child's needs and the adult's capacity as a parent, and
- the relevant family dynamics.

The Child's Preference   The child's wishes or preference regarding custody and visitation are considered an important determinant in custody determinations. However, the child's wishes are often difficult to ascertain, are of uncertain validity, and are subject to change. Central to any discussion of the child's preference is a consideration of the loyalty conflict. The child's wishes or preference are concise terms, and suggest ready availability to a child of a reliable, constant body of established information or opinion. In many instances, nothing could be further from the truth. The loyalty conflict children feel when between warring or even cooperative, friendly parents is powerful and subjects the child to very different feeling states and opinions at different times.

The child's loyalty conflict can play a role in a child's holding strong opposing opinions about parental preference which can be powerfully felt in favor of one parent at one time and the other parent at another. A curious example is provided repeatedly in cases in which sexual abuse of a young child is alleged. The child whose statements are interpreted as alleging sexual abuse in the home of father and stepmother will often later, while in the father's home, indicate that the sexual abuse took place at the hands of the stepfather or someone else in the mother's home. Whatever home and parent the child is with, the abuse (if any indeed occurred) took place in the "other" home.

Direct questions regarding preference are likely to be experienced by the child as threatening and confusing, and often children refuse to answer. Most children will be firmly attached to both parents. Sometimes a child will express a preference for the parent not "chosen" by a sibling, or for the parent with whom a degree of role reversal has occurred, with the child choosing the parent who appears to be the most in need of the child's care and attention. Should the child express a preference, it is important for the clinician to seek to engage the child in a discussion, so that motivations can be identified such as keeping the mother from being lonely or staying with the father to take care of the meals and the house because the child views him as incompetent to do so.

Some consultants approach the issue of who is the more suitable parent in indirect ways such as asking the child whom would he take on vacation with him if only one person could come, whom would he save first from a burning building, and things of that sort. Most children, however, are not fooled by this approach and refuse to answer, change the question, or reply "both." Not only do they see through this approach, but they probably resent its disingenuousness and respond in an oppositional fashion, explaining the frequent failure of this method.

A clinical approach which sometimes elicits useful material is to inquire about the good parts and the not-so-good parts about living with mom and with dad. This method is direct, not tricky, and not nearly as threatening as being asked for a preference. The child may be willing to join the consultant in an analysis of this sort. Surely the majority of qualified consultants approach the preference issue through even more indirect means, talking with the child at length about activities, problems, and relationships with both parents. With older children, especially those above age 14, the child's preference dominates other issues. The court in most instances will go along with the wishes of an older child.

The Reciprocal Attachment between Parent and Child   The meaning of a child to a parent provides useful information about the nature of the parent's attachment to the child. For example, a parent may regard the child as a personal possession or as an extension of the parent. A parent may have unrealistic, unconscious expectations that the child should fulfill the parent's fantasies or conflicted needs. Alternatively, a parent may realistically view the child as a separate and temporarily dependent being who needs support and guidance toward achieving autonomy. A parent's description of the child can provide an indication of the parent's awareness of the child's existence separate from that of the parent and may offer some indication of the parent's knowledge of and respect for the child's strengths, weaknesses, fears, and other attributes.

The importance of the child to the parents can be determined by assessing the extent of the parent's constructive involvement in the child's life, attentiveness to the child's needs, and consideration of the child in activities and in planning for the future. A technique which can provide useful information is for the psychiatric consultant to ask a parent to discuss a living plan for the child in the event he or she gains custody. A thoughtful and realistic plan may give some indication of the extent of the parent's caring for the child and capability as a parent.

Observation of the nature of the interaction between a child and a parent can provide an indication of parental empathy and ability to communicate with the child. Physical interaction with young children and verbal exchange with older children provide clues about the quality of the relationship between child and parent. Many consultants spend some time observing the child and parent playing together.

Family drawings by the child may provide indications of how the child views a parent. Family drawings are an excellent means of exploring the child's feelings; they may indicate the child's view of who is close to whom and can lead to extended discussions of a variety of family issues. Similarly, a kinetic family drawing, a drawing of the family doing something together, can add further to the consultant's understanding of the child's world.

Typically, the child is unsure of whether to include the non-custodial parent, or includes that parent in the background, to the side, or makes him or her smaller than the custodial parent. That in itself is a good reflection of a child's symbolic thinking: however, it indicates nothing reliable regarding how that person is viewed as a parent and the nature of the child's relationship with that parent. The drawings in themselves are generally of little consequence. The contribution of drawings rests primarily in what the child has to say about them. Otherwise, conclusions based on family drawings might depend on what the child saw on television the night before, or on some other spurious issue.

Another technique routinely used in psychiatric work with children is also useful in child custody evaluations. The child is asked to make three magic wishes. Usually first is the wish the family were still together. Such a response can lead into a useful discussion of how the child perceives and is affected by the current emotional climate generated by the parents, and can provide the child with an opportunity to share the pain.

The Child's Needs and the Adult's Parenting Capacities   Parental affection, protection, and guidance are necessary to promote the child's development of social and learning skills, self-control, socially oriented values, positive self-esteem, and a coherent sense of self—all part of the process of development toward autonomous adulthood. An understanding of a child's developmental needs is necessary to determine which of the potential custodians may be more helpful to the child in accomplishing these goals.

The ability to relate adequately to people depends upon having been valued and cared for early in life. Young children need parents who can accept and respond to their bodily functions as well as communicate with them to facilitate the acquisition of language. Children also need parents who can set limits and model coping techniques: the abilities to tolerate frustration and postpone gratification permit the development of the self-control needed for social cooperation and task performance. A range of learning skills is required to gain information about oneself, other people, and the world. Parental help in channeling curiosity and supporting education is important. A value system which accommodates self-interest to social realities must be modeled and taught by caring parents. Children benefit from learning recreational, creative, and pleasure-affording skills.

Parental awareness and acceptance of the child as a unique person is essential to the development of positive self-esteem and a sense of autonomy. The presence of physical, educational, or emotional disorders in a child poses special challenges for a parent in working toward these child-raising goals. The clinician may be able to shed some light on the ability of each parent to assist the child to achieve these goals.

The psychiatric consultant sees the parents and child for individual interviews, the child and each parent together, and perhaps other persons of importance such as grandparents, stepparents, and child care persons. In addition to general observations in the interview situation, the psychiatric consultant may obtain further data about the parent-child relationship by assigning a task. For example, the psychiatric consultant may provide blocks and request that the parent and child build something together. Important observations may include the pair's ability to cooperate, the child's degree of initiative in the presence of each parent, the parent's ability to allow the child some autonomy, and the parent's ability to help or make suggestions without belittling the child.

Often, the clinician will find that each parent has different strengths in the relationship with the child and may meet different needs in the child. One parent may be consistent and set appropriate limits for the child, while the other is more erratic but also more nurturing. In some cases the clinician's role may be to describe to the court the strengths and weaknesses of each parent, leaving the court to make what is ultimately a value judgment in deciding which parent should have custody. Particularly when the case is not clear-cut, courts in determining custody are often inclined to seize upon a parent's personal characteristics, lifestyle, and any other qualities that may serve to differentiate the contesting persons.

The psychiatric consultant may serve a useful role in directing the court's attention to those parental qualities that have a known positive or negative effect upon the child while minimizing the importance given to other issues. For example, in a situation where a capable custodial parent who is homosexual or who has been psychotic in the past is challenged for custody, the psychiatrist can address the specific implications of the parent's sexual preference or psychiatric condition on the child.

Family Dynamics   A parent seeking custody may have important motivations in addition to affection and concern for the child. The parent's behavior often is complicated by emotional reactions to the disruption of the spousal relationship. Custody may be sought as a way to maintain a sense of identity when one's sense of self and continuity is threatened by the separation or divorce. A parent may seek custody and may seek to disrupt visitation out of anger at the former spouse.

A parent's anger at the former spouse may come to involve a child as stand-in for the other parent. With the diminution of generation boundaries between parent and child that characterizes the new one-parent family, there may develop in the mind of the parent a blurring of the boundary between the former spouse and the child, often, but not necessarily, with a child of the same sex as the other parent. This can result in a partial re-creation of the former spousal relationship by the custodial parent and child. Often this relationship contains many elements reminiscent of the struggle with the former spouse. Parents who are caught in this type of problem typically drift from talking about their daughter or son to talking angrily about the former spouse.

An important consideration in divorce is the custodial parent's ability to promote and protect the child's relationship with the non-custodial parent who maintains an interest in the child. Studies indicate that children benefit when they have regular access to both parents after divorce. Awarding custody or primary physical residence to a parent who supports the child's relationship with the other parent may help to mitigate post-divorce problems and loyalty conflicts for the child.

A phenomenon that has come to prominence is the allegation by one parent, typically the mother, that the father is physically or sexually abusing the child. The children involved are generally of preschool age and the allegations are brought by the parent. In many instances, the allegations are probably not brought maliciously, but are rooted in rage and in a variety of complex overreactions on the part of the mother to the father's affectionate involvement in the physical and emotional care of the child. The mother's anxiety regarding sexual abuse may then fuel the child's anxiety and foster regressive behavior that the mother then interprets as proof of sexual abuse. Because of the response of public agencies and the inherent difficulty in establishing that an event such as sexual abuse did not occur, such allegations can effectively interrupt the child's contact with the father.

Possibilities for Useful Interventions   Parents can sometimes begin to think more flexibly about their children's situations and needs as they engage in the consultation process. Sometimes a constructive resolution is possible if the psychiatric consultant sees his or her task as more than simply to help the judge decide who wins and who loses. The psychiatric consultant should arrange for ample time for a custody evaluation. It cannot be predicted how many interviews will be required, although most divorce custody evaluations require between five and fifteen interviews.

In the course of many types of consultations, it is possible for the psychiatric consultant to be directly helpful to the children and adults involved. The psychiatrist can usually share with the caretaking adults ways of understanding and helping children with the various changes and losses occurring in their lives. In a divorce custody consultation, the evaluation process may include help to parents and children in dealing with the divorce and perhaps even assisting the parents in learning to deal with each other.

Testimony

While the juvenile courts tend to readily accept reports regarding many matters, termination of parental rights and custody/visitation issues usually require the psychiatrist to testify. It is not sufficient to conduct an evaluation and write a good report; one must also be able to communicate clearly and explain convincingly one's findings and recommendations. The psychiatric consultant must be able to document carefully the process of opinion formation, including a description of the sources of information relied upon. A report should be written in all cases as part of the process of organizing the consultant's thinking and delivery of the information.

Clinical findings should be stated in objective and descriptive terms. The consultant often can convey greater clarity by sharing observations or quoting persons interviewed rather than expressing conclusions. Direct quotations from subjects involved in the evaluation tend to be clearer and to stand up better under cross-examination than do subjective judgments. For example, a father's statement, "I must get my child away from my former wife's evil ways, and I've looked into a boys' home since I can't care for him myself," speaks for itself more clearly than any conclusion drawn from such statements. Similarly, if a mother is attempting to interrupt visitation by the father on the basis of his alcoholism, quoting her statement that the children look forward to his visits and that she had never observed him to be inebriated on those visits can be very helpful to the court's understanding of the situation.

The importance of a psychiatric diagnosis regarding parent or child can vary greatly from case to case. When a child is disturbed, a parent's understanding of the disturbance and attitude about therapeutic intervention may be of relevance to the custodial question. If a parent carries a psychiatric diagnosis, it is the psychiatric consultant's task to address the implications for parenting ability. A psychiatric diagnosis by no means disqualifies a person from adequately carrying out parental functions, and this needs to be made clear to the court. In addition, if the condition is readily remediable and the person is willing to engage in therapy, this should be included in the report. In the case of a parent with manic-depressive illness, for example, it would be important to state that this has been well controlled with medication and therefore does not importantly interfere with the parent's ability to care for the child. On the other hand, where a parent's psychiatric condition significantly impairs that person's response to or ability to care for the child, then that should be stated by the psychiatric consultant.

The psychiatric consultant may be tempted to cite professional literature, but in so doing will open the door to creative and confusing cross-examination. The best preparation for cross-examination is a tightly constructed statement that does not contain unclear or extraneous material. For the psychiatric consultant, the evaluation and recommendations are generally of central importance; for the judge, the psychiatrist's findings are one of many factors to be weighed. The psychiatric consultant should be aware that his or her opinion may not be a central issue in the decision and he or she should not feel insulted if the recommendations are not followed. The weight accorded to the testimony in a given instance, however, will generally be related to the psychiatrist's credibility and conduct in court.

CONCLUSION

Child psychiatry in this country originated as a partner to the developing juvenile courts. From that beginning there have been many paths, and child psychiatry continues its growth in the community. Although some of the challenges related to health care and financing changes are not particularly welcomed by the profession, some of the current adaptations made by community-oriented child and adolescents psychiatrists and training programs are taking us to some of the places where we can do the most good, such as the juvenile and domestic relations courts. The better one understands the territory, the less anxiety the psychiatrist will have, and the better the psychiatrist can function.

Expertise in psychodynamic issues continues to be sought. The courts are a crossroad for many systems of thought, of care, and of orientation. There is challenge and reward in the exercise of psychiatric skill and clinical judgment in this real-world environment.

SUGGESTED READINGS

American Academy of Child and Adolescent Psychiatry. In press (Herman et al.). *A report by the work group on quality issues. Practice parameters for custody disputes.* Washington, DC: American Academy of Child and Adolescent Psychiatry.

American Psychiatric Association (1988). *A report by the Task Force on Clinical Assessment in Child Custody. Child custody consultation.* Washington, DC: American Psychiatric Association.

Benedek, E. P. (1996). Testifying in court: A psychiatrist's viewpoint. In M. Lewis (Ed.), *Child and adolescent psychiatry: A comprehensive textbook* (pp. 1150–1154). Baltimore: Williams & Wilkins.

Derdeyn, A. P. (1996). Adoption. In M. Lewis (Ed.), *Child and adolescent psychiatry: A comprehensive textbook* (pp. 1110–1118). Baltimore: Williams & Wilkins.

Fritz, G. K., Mattison, R. E., Nurcombe, B., & Spirito, A. (1993). *Child and adolescent mental health consultation in hospitals, schools, and courts.* Washington, DC: American Psychiatric Press.

Nordhaus, B., & Solnit, A. J. (1996). The role of the child expert in court-requested evaluations. In M. Lewis (Ed.), *Child and adolescent psychiatry: A comprehensive textbook* (pp. 1160–1166). Baltimore: Williams & Wilkins.

Nurcombe, B., & Partlett, D. F. (1994). *Child mental health and the law.* New York: The Free Press.

Rosen, D. N. (1996). Testifying in court: A trial lawyer's perspective. In M. Lewis (Ed.), *Child and adolescent psychiatry: A comprehensive textbook* (pp. 1154–1160). Baltimore: Williams & Wilkins.

Rosenfeld, A. A., Pilowsky, D. J., Fine, P., Thorpe, M., Fein, E., Simms, M. D., Halfon, N., Irwin, M., Alfaro, J., Saletsky, R., & Nickman, S. (in press). Foster care: An update. *Journal of the American Academy of Child and Adolescent Psychiatry.*

Schetky, D. H., & Benedek, E. P. (1992). *Clinical handbook of child psychiatry and the law.* Baltimore: Williams & Wilkins

Wallerstein, J. S., & Corbin, S. B. (1996). The child and the vicissitudes of divorce. In M. Lewis (Ed.), *Child and adolescent psychiatry: A comprehensive textbook* (pp. 1118–1127). Baltimore: Williams & Wilkins.

Wizner, S. (1996). The mental health professional in the juvenile justice system. In M. Lewis (Ed.), *Child and adolescent psychiatry: A comprehensive textbook* (pp. 1131–1134). Baltimore: Williams & Wilkins.

Workgroup on Psychiatric Practice in the Juvenile Court, Kalogerakis, M. G., Chair (1992). *Handbook of psychiatric practice in the juvenile court.* Washington, DC: American Psychiatric Association.

Part 3

Common Disorders of Childhood and Adolescence

Chapter 11

Affective Disorders in Children and Adolescents

Paramjit T. Joshi, M.D.

INTRODUCTION

In the last decade there has been an explosion in the number of articles written about depressive disorders in children and adolescents. Major depression and dysthymic disorder are known to contribute significantly to serious psychiatric disturbance in childhood and adolescence. Studies have in fact indicated that the incidence of depressive disorders in children and adolescents may be increasing. Until about two decades ago several investigators felt that the occurrence of major depression in very young prepubertal children was rare or even nonexistent (Kovacs & Beck, 1977). However, since then, several investigators have reported depression in young children and concluded that major depression exists in preschoolers and that stressful life events are associated with depressive symptoms. The incidence of major depression in clinical populations is widely varied ranging from 3 percent to 33 percent (Robins, 1979).

The increase in the prevalence of depression as children get older has been reported by several investigators who found a tripling of the rate of depression in 1–0 to 14-year-olds. In two different age groups the prevalence of major depression has been reported to be 4.7 percent in younger children and 20.8 percent in junior and high school students.

Epidemiological studies in adults have clearly demonstrated a preponderance of depressive illness in females versus males. This finding has not been borne out in children and adolescents and studies to date do not report a preponderance of depressive disorders in young girls Although prevalence studies in depressed adults have found increased rates in African Americans compared to Caucasians, there are no studies to describe this same finding in young children. There are reports of increased depressive symptoms in junior high school students of African-American descent, but this finding may have been confounded by the marked disparity in the socioeconomic status of the two populations studied. Socially and economically disadvantaged youngsters, based on paternal education, maternal occupation and family income have been found to be at increased risk for depression.

The natural history of depressive disorders has been examined extensively in adults since Kraepelin (1921) first described the phenomenology of "Manic-Depressive Insanity and Paranoia." However, there is a paucity of literature studying the natural course of mood disorders in children and adolescents. Youngsters who have dysthymia and/or major depression have protracted episodes, are at high risk for further episodes of depression, may spend 50 percent of their young lives being depressed, and many of them exhibit suicidal behaviors (Kovacs, 1984, 1985, 1992). These characteristics, including the fact that 30 percent to 50 percent of young patients with major depression also have underlying dysthymia, are very similar to findings reported in adults suggesting continuity of these disabling conditions across the life span. Adding to this concern is evidence that childhood depression significantly disrupts normal emotional development and academic progress. Therefore, it is imperative to recognize and identify depressive disorders in youngsters and institute appropriate treatments to minimize the morbidity that can result.

CLASSIFICATION OF MOOD DISORDERS

There are three depressive disorders described in the *Diagnostic and Statistical Manual of Mental Disorders* (4th edition) (*DSM-IV*) (American Psychiatric Association [APA], 1994). There are no separate criteria for any of the following disorders in children and adolescents, and therefore they are subsumed under the adult criteria:

- Depressive Disorders: Major depressive disorder (MDD), Dysthymic disorder (DD), and Depressive disorders not otherwise specified
- Bipolar disorders: Bipolar I disorder, Bipolar II disorder, Cyclothymic disorder, and Bipolar disorder not otherwise specified
- Mood disorder as a result of a medical condition and substance-induced mood disorder.

The focus of this chapter is on major depressive disorder in children and adolescents (MDD).

Major Depressive Disorder

The diagnostic criteria of major depressive disorder in children and adolescents is based on distinct clinical phenomena which are similar to those applied to adult affective disorders. Mood disorders are seen on a continuum during the life span and the core phenomenology and symptoms described is similar for children, adolescents, and adults (APA, 1994). However, there is data to suggest that the prominence of characteristic symptoms may change with age. Therefore, certain symptoms such as somatic complaints, irritability, and social withdrawal are particularly common in depressed children and adolescents, whereas psychomotor retardation, hypersomnia, and delusions are less common, especially in prepubertal children. Despite limitations posed by the criteria published in *DSM-IV*, the description of the criteria allow uniformity in identifying affective disorders in prepubertal children and adolescents. This further allows for rigorous criteria applied to youngsters to be included in research studies, thereby decreasing the obstacles and difficulties encountered in some of the earlier studies where the criteria used were much more general and sometimes vague.

To validate psychiatric diagnoses, follow-up studies along with family and treatment studies have been used over the years. In this way, recurrent episodes of a mood disorder in children and adolescents lend validity to and support the original diagnosis as it continues into adulthood.

The *DSM-IV* diagnostic criteria for a major depressive episode are the following:

- depressed mood, irritability, and/or pervasive anhedonia of at least two weeks duration, either by subjective report or objective observation by others. These changes should represent a change from previous level of functioning.
- five out of the following nine symptoms also of at least two weeks duration either by subjective report or objective observation:
  - Depressed mood and/or irritability; the irritability being the most common affective state seen in children and adolescents almost every day or nearly every day.
  - Appetite disturbance, usually a decrease in appetite with or without weight loss. Failure to make expected weight gains in children and adolescents is considered significant. Infrequently there is an increase in appetite resulting in weight gain.
  - Sleep disturbances seen in children and adolescents are similar to those reported in adults—that is, initial insomnia, middle of the night awakening, and terminal insomnia or early morning awakening occurring nearly every day. Parents are often not as aware of sleep changes in their adolescents as they are if they occur in the younger children, because parents are much more involved in bedtime rituals with younger children.
  - Motor restlessness, fidgetiness, and trouble sitting still is suggestive of motor agitation; conversely moving and talking slowly is reflective of motor retardation. The symptoms of motor agitation are often misdiagnosed to be symptoms of an attention deficit hyperactivity disorder and in the latter the symptoms of motor retardation considered to be a sign of laziness and oppositional behavior.
  - Loss of interest in activities that the youngsters usually engage and participate in is readily observed by parents and teachers. Youngsters tend to become withdrawn, isolated, and retreat into themselves. These changes are often of great concern to parents, teachers, and friends.
  - Loss of energy and lethargy almost daily is often evident in children and adolescents suffering from major depression. Youngsters complain of feeling tired, resist getting up to go to school, tend to nap during the day, lie around, and complain of feeling exhausted. This feeling of tiredness and low energy is often puzzling to the youngster and the parents. It often leads to trying to find a medical etiology for the low energy: often the child is seen by the pediatrician.
  - Feelings of guilt and self-reproach, often seen in depressed adults, can also be a symptom of depression in children and adolescents as well. However, the concept of guilt is an abstract one and therefore developmentally is often not readily elicited in very young children.
  - Academic impairment secondary to a decrease in the ability to concentrate is a symptom that is readily noticed by teachers, parents, and the youngster. Grades tend to drop or the student may have to work much harder to keep up. Often, youngsters describe their mind as blank and empty or find themselves daydreaming excessively.
  - Recurring thoughts of death and suicide often occur even in young children. It is important to ask about such painful thoughts. Most children despite their age and cognitive abilities have some concept of death, even if at a very simple, concrete psychological level. These thoughts are of three types: passive death

wishes such as "I wish I was never born" or "'I wish I was dead"; active death wishes where the youngster actually thinks of a method to put an end to his or her life such as taking an overdose, and, proceeding with a suicidal attempt or gesture.

- The *DSM-IV* has exclusionary criteria for the diagnosis of a major depressive episode. These include schizophrenia, direct physiological effects of a substance (e.g., a drug of abuse, a medication), or a general medical condition (e.g., hypothyroidism) and uncomplicated bereavement.
- Functioning in social, occupational, school, or other areas is significantly impaired and causes serious distress as a result of the depressive disorder.
- The symptoms do not meet criteria for a mixed episode which is characterized by a period of time lasting at least one week in which the patient meets criteria for both a manic episode and a major depressive episode.

It is important to keep in mind that children very often will have one or more of the above symptoms during their childhoods. One should be suspicious of the development of a mood disorder when there is clustering of these symptoms over a given period of time

Bipolar Disorders

There remains controversy about the occurrence and presentation of mania, especially in prepubertal children. Though much less common than major depression, mania has now been well documented by several researchers and clinicians in children and adolescents. Just as with the diagnostic criteria for major depression, there are no separate criteria for bipolar disorders in children and adolescents. Therefore one is left adopting the adult criteria to apply to youngsters.

There are six separate criteria sets for Bipolar I disorder. According to the *DSM-IV*, these are as follows:

- single manic episode
- most recent episode hypomanic
- most recent episode manic
- most recent episode mixed
- most recent episode depressed, and,
- most recent episode unspecified.

This chapter's focus is Bipolar I disorder, a single manic episode which is used to describe individuals who have had a first episode of mania. The other criteria are used to describe the nature of the current or most recent episode in those patients who have had recurrent mood episodes—Bipolar II disorder, Cyclothymic disorder, and Bipolar disorder not otherwise specified.

The *DSM-IV* diagnostic criteria for a manic episode are:

- a distinct period of abnormally and persistently elevated, expansive, and/or irritable mood, lasting at least one week (or of any duration if hospitalization becomes necessary).
- the presence and persistence to a significant degree of at least three (or more) of the following symptoms (four if the mood is only irritable, which is often the case with youngsters):

- Inflated self-esteem, grandiosity, and in children often a heightened sense of being superior to their peers.
- Decreased need for sleep (not sleeping all night or feeling rested after only a few hours of sleep).
- being much more talkative than is usual, feeling the pressure to keep talking and at a greater speed than is normal.
- Flight of ideas or a subjective feeling that thoughts are racing and being unable to keep up with them.
- Distractibility, which is often difficult to assess in those with a preexisting attention deficit hyperactivity disorder.
- Increase in goal-directed activity socially, in school/work, sexually in older children, and/or psychomotor agitation (which can be mistaken for hyperactivity).
- Excessive involvement in pleasurable activities leading to negative consequences or indulging in unusual risk-taking behaviors (i.e., "daring behaviors").

- the symptoms do not meet criteria for a Mixed Episode.
- the disturbance in mood is sufficiently severe to cause marked impairment in school/occupational functioning or in usual social activities or relationships with others, or necessitating hospitalization to prevent harm to self or others, or has the presence of psychotic symptoms.
- the symptoms are not a result of the direct physiological effects of a substance (e.g., drugs, medications, or other treatments) or a result of a general medical condition (e.g., hyperthyroidism).
- the *DSM-IV* makes a note of not including manic-like symptoms or an episode that may result from somatic antidepressant treatment such as medications, electroconvulsive therapy, and light therapy toward a diagnosis of Bipolar I Disorder.

Several patients in recent years with symptoms of impulsiveness, distractibility, behavioral problems, and irritability are being diagnosed to have bipolar disorder. It is important to remember that patients with ADHD usually develop the symptoms of impulsiveness, distractibility, and hyperactivity before the age of seven years. When these symptoms appear for the first time at a later age in a child, they are usually not a result of ADHD. A family history of bipolar illness also helps in identifying those patients who may be at risk for developing bipolar disorder. Another diagnosis that is gaining popularity is Impulse Control Disorder, which has all the features of a behavior disorder, but without the consistent affective changes that are seen in patients with a bipolar disorder.

ETIOLOGICAL CONSIDERATIONS

The argument about nature versus nurture continues to be an important one in the etiology of depression in humans. The issue may not be so much of one or the other, but, rather, the lack of nurture and presence of environmental stress and learned helplessness as precipitating or potentiating depressive symptoms in a patient who has the substrate for developing major depression, based on the genetic etiology of major depressive disorder. The type and distribution of psychiatric disorders in the child and adolescent members of extended pedigrees identified through bipolar probands showed that it is 5.1-fold higher than in the offspring of healthy parents.

In writing about the etiological aspects of child and adolescent mood disorders, McCracken (1992) described an interactional approach to understanding depression. The three-factor approach consists of provoking agents, vulnerability factors, and symptom formation factors. The provocative factors are bereavement, impairment of relationship with parents, physical illness, and use of certain medications. These provocative factors may interact with vulnerability factors such as positive family history of major depressive disorder, maladaptive cognitive-behavioral patterns, and maternal dysfunction such as depression in the mother or poor parenting skills and emotional unavailability. Therefore, the provoking agents and the vulnerability factors then interact with symptom formation influences which may include the presence of vulnerabilities to develop phobias and anxiety symptoms, especially separation anxiety. Epidemiological studies in addition have shown a higher risk of suicidality in children and adolescents who experience high levels of perceived family stress. However, at present it remains unclear how these various forces interact with each other to precipitate a depressive episode in children and adolescents and if there is change in these interactions and their impact as the child gets older.

There is a growing body of knowledge suggesting that genetic factors play an important role in affective disorders. The lifetime risk in first-degree relatives is 25 percent and 20 percent, respectively for bipolar and unipolar affective disorder. Concordance studies also show an increase of monozygotic over dizygotic twins in bipolar and unipolar affective disorder with a ratio of 4:2.8 (Weissman, Fendrich, Wasner, & Wichramaratne, 1992). There remains a scarcity of genetic studies in children and adolescents but there are reports of increased history of depression in parents of depressed children.

The most systematic longitudinal studies examining the natural course of mood disorders (Kovacs, 1992) suggested the average length of an untreated major depressive episode to be 32 weeks in duration, with a recovery rate from the depressive episode to be within 18 months in 92 percent of the patients from the start of the episode. Kovacs also reported that the younger the child at the time of the onset of the episode the longer it would take for recovery. Therefore, there is an inverse relationship between the length of the depressive episode and the age of the child. A pessimistic finding reported by Kovacs was a recurrence rate of major depression in 70 percent of the children within five years from the onset of the first episode and 40 percent experience a second episode within two years from the time the child recovers from the first episode. The only predictors and risk factors for a second episode that could be identified in children with major depression in Kovacs' study were the concurrence of a diagnosed dysthymic disorder, referred to as a "double depression." Others have concluded that there is continued risk for recurrences of major depressive disorder into adulthood with a recurrence rate of up to 69 percent over a period of seven years.

DIAGNOSIS

Diagnosis must always be based on clinical information obtained from the family and the patient along with a thorough mental status examination. Diagnosis can be aided by the use of checklists and questionnaires designed to measure depressive symptomatology in children and adolescents including the Beck Depression Scale-BDI (Beck, Ward, & Mendelson, 1961), the Children's Depression Inventory-CDI (Kovacs, 1985a), and the Johns Hopkins Depression checklist for children-HDCL (Joshi, Capozzoli, & Coyle, 1990). Unlike the latter, the first two are subjective rating scales relying on self-report from the patients with no input from the parents. Furthermore, children's self-ratings may be much more sensitive to, and affected by, immediate life circumstances than adults, and therefore, more variable over time. The Johns Hopkins Depression Checklist-HDCL, a 38-item checklist, has been normalized on a large normal population, ages 5 to 13 years. Unlike the subjective scales, the HDCL is an objective measure, completed by the parents. It has been shown to be sensitive when used in depressed inpatients, showing change over time. Structured and semi-structured interviews, such as the Kiddie Schedule for Affective Disorders and Schizophrenia-K-SADS (Chambers et al., 1985), Diagnostic Interview for Children and Adolescents-DICA-R (Herjanic & Reich, 1982), and the Diagnostic Interview Schedule for Children-DISC (Costello, Edelbrock, Kalas, Dulcan, & Klaric, 1984) are also being used for clinical and research purposes to identify children and adolescents who may suffer from major depression and/or bipolar disorder.

In addition to the various diagnostic instruments, clinicians often rely on other methods to help support clinical impressions. Some of these include cognitive and projective testing—for example, responses on the Rorschach cards or the Thematic Apperception Test (TAT) stories. Themes indicative of depression, self-blame, undue guilt, hopelessness/helplessness, abandonment, and self-harm or suicide are often prevalent. Scores on the cognitive tasks related to memory and concentration are often negatively effected, usually abating after the child gets well. Children's artwork is somewhat reflective of their mental state. In our experience, depressed children typically draw ill-defined, sad-appearing figures, with decreased intensity of lines, with pictures that are disorganized and that lack color. Because drawing is an activity that most young children engage in, it could be helpful to follow a child's artwork, reflecting the clinical changes we see as clinicians (see chapter 8, The Process of Psychological Assessment for a thorough discussion of the use and misuse of testing).

Biological Markers

Several biological markers such as cortisol secretion and sleep EEG changes have been associated with depression in adults. In children, the one that has been studied fairly extensively has been cortisol secretion (Dexamethasone Secretion Test-DST). As with most of the adult studies with DST, the results in children and adolescents are inconclusive. Growth hormone secretion tests have also been conducted showing a blunting of the growth hormone secretion after administration of 5 units of insulin in patients with major depression, compared to normal controls. However, none of these tests have proven to be specific or conclusive, therefore they are not currently being routinely administered in children and adolescents with major depression.

Case Examples

Three case studies are presented to highlight two important points: the importance of obtaining a family history, and the description of clinical symptoms as seen in different age groups from the very young child to adolescence.

Case 1: Kristin   Kristin was a six-and-one-half-year-old girl when first referred by her pediatrician secondary to severe temper tantrums and increasing behavior problems of six month's duration. Family history was strongly positive for major depression in the patient's father, paternal aunt, and paternal grandmother, who had all been treated with antidepressants. There was no family history of psychiatric illness on the mother's side of the family.

Early development was unremarkable, with the patient achieving developmental milestones well within the normal time frame for her age. However, the patient experienced more than the usual amount of separation anxiety when left with caretakers and at nursery school. She was described as a perfectionist by nature, getting easily upset and distraught if she did not do her schoolwork just right. Academically Kristin did exceedingly well in first grade and had several friends at the parochial school she attended.

Medical history was negative except for some lactose intolerance. The patient was seen in therapy at age five for the symptoms of separation anxiety, which would always reemerge at the start of the school year, subsiding within a few weeks. However, more recently the symptoms had worsened, with increased tearfulness, irritability, trouble settling for bed, an increase in tantrums, waking up in the middle of the night, looking unhappy, and making self-deprecatory statements— for example "I am stupid and ugly," "No one loves me," "I wish I was dead." She was diagnosed to have a major depression when first evaluated in the clinic at age six-and-a-half and was started on Prozac 5 mg. a day with her symptoms of depression and anxiety completely resolving in about four to five weeks. Six years later, now almost 13 years of age the patient remains on Prozac at 10 mg. a day and doing well. She has not needed any other psychotherapeutic interventions besides pharmacotherapy.

Case 2: James   James was a 16-year-old high school student in a competitive private school who had not experienced any difficulties until a few months before being seen in the clinic. He was referred by his school for suddenly having marked deterioration in academic functioning, increased absenteeism, and looking unhappy and feeling alone. James' family history was positive for major depression in only one paternal uncle who had been treated for it with medications. There were several members in the extended family who were described as low-key, quiet, and socially withdrawn.

Early development and childhood was unremarkable. However, James had always been described as somewhat of an introvert, with few friends, and somewhat shy. When James became depressed it was unclear at first both to the family and the school whether this was just a shy, reserved James or if in fact he was becoming much more withdrawn and quiet secondary to the onset of major depression. At the time of the first clinic visit the patient was sad, felt more lonesome than ever, and described a sense of emptiness and boredom. In addition, he had the neurovegetative symptoms of low energy, low appetite, and hypersomnia. He had come to believe that life was not worth living and felt hopeless, helpless, and completely demoralized about his future.

James was diagnosed to be suffering from major depression and was started on 10 mg. of Prozac, which was increased over the next few weeks to 20 mg. a day. There was no improvement in the depressive symptoms after a total of six weeks of Prozac treatment. It was therefore discontinued. After a two-week wash out period James was started on Nortriptyline which was gradually titrated into a therapeutic range; achieving and main-taining blood levels between 75 and 90 ng/ml (Range 50–140ng/ml) on 75 mg/day. Two years later James is looking forward to graduating from high school and starting college. James needed supportive psychotherapy for a few weeks at the start of treatment, as he became more despondent when he did not respond to Prozac and his depression worsened. At present he is seen every three months for management of pharmacotherapy.

Case 3: John   John was a nine-year-old boy who was referred to the clinic by his pediatrician secondary to looking unhappy and being restless and fidgety. He had been diagnosed to have an attention deficit hyperactivity disorder since kindergarten and had a positive response with Ritalin. His family history was positive for depression in both parents who were being treated with two different SSRIs with a good response. Family history was also positive for major depression in two maternal aunts, maternal grandmother, and several other extended family members with a history of alcoholism. On the father's side of the family there was major depression in both paternal aunts, as well as major depression in the paternal grandfather and the paternal grandmother's mother.

Early childhood was significant for John, always having trouble with peers, not knowing how to make friends, socially awkward, and being learning-disabled. During the clinic evaluation John described feeling "blah," gloomy all day long, and feeling that no one could help him out of his misery. He also was much more irritable and cranky with difficulties at bedtime. In addition, he had several somatic complaints— headaches, stomachaches, and his legs hurting. He also felt that he was having a much harder time paying attention and completing his schoolwork. He had contemplated dying but never actually attempted suicide.

Given the positive response of several family members to SSRIs John was started on 5 mg. of Prozac. Three weeks later he was much improved but still complained of feeling easily annoyed, and not wanting to participate much in activities. The dose of Prozac was increased to 10 mg. After another 10 days his mother called to say that John was acting "weird," being much more restless, acting funny and somewhat disinhibited. The dose of Prozac was decreased to 8 mg/day with return to baseline mood state. However, after becoming euthymic he continued to have problems with social awkwardness, restlessness, and short attention span. Ritalin was reintroduced at 5 mg at a.m. and noon with positive results. In addition, the patient benefited greatly from individual therapy to help him with improving his social awkwardness and teaching him social skills. (See chapter 17, Pharmacotherapy in Children and Adolescents, for further discussion on the use of SSRIs and stimulant medications).

The following case is an example of the presentation of bipolar disorder in a latency-age child.

Case 4: Ila   Ila was an 11- year-old Caucasian female who was first seen in the clinic after discharge from an inpatient unit where she was admitted secondary to symptoms of agitation, irritability, increased energy, irrational behaviors (jumping out of a moving car), and the inability to sleep. She was diagnosed to have a behavior disorder which was not specified. Treatment included individual therapy, behavioral work with the family, and pharmacological treatment with a neuroleptic to get her behavior under control. On obtaining further history from the parents it was learned that the father was being treated for bipolar disorder with Lithium and a paternal aunt also suffered from a similar disorder.

Ila had been a model student prior to the onset of these symptoms. A few weeks before the presenting symptomatology she had experienced excessive tearfulness, tiredness, and an inability to concentrate. This was explained by the family to be a result of her getting into a fight with her best friend who was no longer talking to her. Since her discharge from the hospital she had continued to experience difficulties both behaviorally and affectively. She cut her hair with scissors, stated that she was an excellent pianist when she had just started piano lessons, and was extremely disruptive in school.

She was diagnosed in our clinic with bipolar disorder and was started on Lithium. The neuroleptic was gradually tapered and discontinued over a period of several weeks. Lithium was titrated into a therapeutic range. Four years later Ila has continued to do well on Lithium except for a very mild depressive episode one winter which did not require hospitalization. She reached menarche at age 12 with no change in the course of her illness. She has a good understanding of bipolar illness and is doing well in school, at home, continues to play the piano, and now also the violin for the school orchestra.

These four cases point out the importance of obtaining thorough family histories to make correct diagnoses and institute appropriate treatment. It is seldom that a prepubertal child with an affective disorder will have a negative family history of a mood disorder in my experience. These clinical vignettes also point out the differences between children and their individual treatment needs. The biopsychosocial model was applied in different "dosages" to the four patients.

DIFFERENTIAL DIAGNOSIS

The issue of major depression occurring in a "pure"' form has been examined by several investigators. Studies suggest that at least one-half of prepubertal children who meet DSM criteria for major depression have a co-morbid psychiatric diagnosis, particularly anxiety disorders and conduct disorders. It is unclear if there is a difference in the clinical presentation, treatment response, and longitudinal outcome in those patients with a "pure depressive illness" versus those with additional psychiatric co-morbidity.

The differential diagnosis should include the following disorders:

• Anxiety disorders, which can often be a co-morbid diagnosis. Often, children can have symptoms of separation anxiety disorder presenting clinically with school refusal. It is important to identify children with school refusal secondary to a mood disorder and those without a mood disorder. The differentiation is important in order to make appropriate treatment interventions.

• Mood disorder secondary to a medical condition such as hypothyroidism. The symptoms of hypothyroidism are almost identical to those found with a mood disorder—low energy, tiredness, sleep, appetite and weight change, and a decrease in concentration. It is therefore important to obtain thyroid function tests. Another medical condition which can simulate a mood disorder is chronic fatigue syndrome, which may or may not be a result of infectious mononucleosis. The most salient feature of this is the very low energy level and the inability to function. Infectious mononucleosis can be diagnosed by obtaining a mono screen which is positive if there is presence of the Epstein-Barr virus. A third medical condition which can have some of the symptoms of a major depression is neurally mediated hypotension. This usually causes lethargy, with somatic symptoms such as headaches and a decrease in concentration. This condition can be readily diagnosed by obtaining a "tilt test." The treatment of this condition often relieves the symptoms.

• Affective changes can also be caused by various medications. The most notorious medication to cause such mood changes are steroids. It is amazing how often parents fail to mention at the original interview that their child is taking steroids.

TREATMENT

Treatment of children and adolescents with major depressive disorder is often more complicated than in adults because of the variables that are often encountered such as developmental issues, cognitive immaturity, dependence on the adults in their lives, resistance from the adolescent patient, and lack of clarity of the diagnosis. As mentioned previously the biopsychosocial approach to treatment perhaps encompasses the three aspects of treatment that should be emphasized: a) education and "illness teaching" once the patient has been diagnosed to have major depression, b) pharmacotherapy, and c) supportive therapy, depending on the individual needs of a particular child. As described with the examples of Kristin, James, John, and Ila, some need more emphasis on the biological aspects of treatment, others the psychosocial, and others all three.

Education

Education involves an open discussion with the child and his or her parents about the general nature of the disorder; its clinical presentation and prognosis, and specific aspects as it applies to the child in question. Since major depressive illness is episodic, the patient and family should be taught to be able to better recognize recurrences and seek treatment in a timely fashion. The child/adolescent and the parents can often be referred to important readings on the subject, seminars, and other materials available from their child's treating psychiatrist and also from local and national organizations like the Depression and Related Affective Disorders Association (DRADA) and the National Association of the Mentally Ill (NAMI) and the National Institute of Mental Health (NIMH)..

Pharmacotherapy

Pharmacotherapy in the treatment of childhood depression includes the use of antidepressants, mood stabilizers, and anticonvulsants. With the advent of clearer diagnostic criteria came studies examining the efficacy of the use of antidepressants. Though most of the open studies have shown antidepressants to be effective in the treatment of major depression in the young, most of the rigorous, double-blind, placebo-controlled studies have repeatedly been unable to demonstrate any superiority of antidepressants to placebo in children and adolescents. Most of the patients in these studies had a chronic, unremitting course of depressive illness, with a very high degree of co-morbidity. In adults the same drugs have been shown to be efficacious in the treatment of depression, though not to the same degree in those who have a high degree of co-morbidity However, compared to the number of adult studies including thousands of subjects, there have only been eight randomized placebo-controlled TCA studies published involving approximately two hundred youngsters. More recently, the use of fluoxetine in children and adolescents has been demonstrated to be efficacious in a double-blind control trial using an "intent to treat" model, where the goal was to treat the patients.

The use of antidepressants and mood stabilizers is described in much more detail in chapter 17, "Pharmacotherapy in Children and Adolescents," therefore discussion of the use of these medications in this section is brief.

The three groups of antidepressants that have been used in the treatment of depression in children and adolescents have been the tricyclic antidepressants (TCAs), the monoamine oxidase inhibitors (MAOIs), and the selective serotonin reuptake inhibitors (SSRIs). Lithium, a mood stabilizer, is a naturally occurring salt which has been used in children and adolescents for a variety of disorders and symptoms, including bipolar disorders, organic mood disorders, the management of aggression, and as an adjunct to tricyclic antidepressants and SARIS in the treatment of major depression. Several anticonvulsants have also been shown to be effective in the treatment of major depression and manic depressive illness in children and adolescents. The most commonly used anticonvulsant is carbamazepine (Tegretol). In adults, it has been shown to be prophylactic in mania and depression in patients who are resistant to lithium. Several reports have shown carbamazepine to decrease impulsiveness, agitation, and affective lability in children and adolescents. The author has had experience also using Valproic Acid either alone or synergistically with Tegretol or Lithium (Joshi, Coyle, & Walkup, 1994).

SUPPORTIVE TREATMENT

Supportive treatment includes illness teaching to families and patients, especially adolescents. Denial of the depressive illness is common, not only with the young patient but also with the family. Many times the patient and family feel stigmatized and need supportive counseling to help with their feelings of inadequacy, anger, and despair. This can be done in supportive individual therapy, family therapy, or by referral to local support groups formed especially for those suffering from a major depressive disorder. Several groups have been formed for all ages and their families to discuss the effect of having a depressive disorder on themselves or their loved ones, as mentioned previously. Supportive treatment in the young may also include talking with school counselors and the child's teacher to acquaint them better with the signs and symptoms of the disorder, and to get them involved in helping the child or adolescent in the context of the school setting.

Other interventions may include referring the young patient's ill parent for treatment of a condition which may not have been identified earlier. Since there is often evidence of very strong family histories in children and adolescents with depressive disorders, there are usually other family members who get identified, who may need psychiatric interventions and appropriate treatment. Treatment with the young also includes helping the child sees himself or herself in context with his or her friends, school, and future goals and aspirations. In the adolescent it is important to help him or her gradually take responsibility for his or her own care as he or she gets ready to move into the adult world and away from the confines of the immediate family.

CONCLUSION

Millions of children and adolescents suffer needlessly from undiagnosed depression, bipolar disorder, and other mood disorders. It is imperative that educators, parents, and health care providers recognize these disorders in the young and become more skilled in identifying those children and adolescents who are at risk. It is equally important to identify the disorders correctly and initiate treatment.

Research efforts in the areas of understanding mental illness in children and adolescents hold exciting possibilities. The inseparable roles of genes and the environment are being further clarified. Well-designed prospective, longitudinal studies and genetic family studies hold the key to answer many questions related to the risk and protective factors of child and adolescent mental illness and the outcome of disorders such as major depression and bipolar disorder.

REFERENCES

American Psychiatric Association (APA). (1994). *Diagnostic and Statistical manual of mental disorders* (4th ed.) *(DSM-IV)*. Washington, DC: the Association.

Beck A. T., Ward, C. H., & Mendelson, M. (1961). An inventory for measuring depression. *Archives of General Psychiatry, 4,* 561–571..

Chambers W. J., Puig-Antich J., Hirsh, M., Paez P., Ambrosini, P. J., Tabrizi, M. A., & Davies, M. (1985). The assessment of affective disorders in children and adolescents by semi-structured interview: Test-retest reliability of the schedule for affective disorder and schizophrenia for school age children, present-episode version. *Archives of General Psychiatry, 42,* 696–702.

Costello, A. J., Edelbrock, C. S., Kalas, R., Dulcan, M. D., & Klaric, S. H. (1984). Development and testing of the NIMH diagnostic interview schedule for children in a clinical population (Contract No. RSP-DB-81/0027), Rockville, MD: Center for Epidemiologic Studies, NIMH.

Herjanic, B., & Reich, W. (1982). Development of a structured psychiatric interview for children: Agreement between child and parent on individual symptoms. *Journal of Abnormal Child Psychology, 10,* 307–324.

Joshi, P. T., Capozzoli, J. A., & Coyle, J. T. (1990). The Johns Hopkins Depression Scale: Normative data and validation in child psychiatry patients. *Journal of the American Academy of Child and Adolescent Psychiatry, 29*(2): 283–288.

Joshi, P. T., Coyle, J. T., & Walkup, J. T. (1994). Pharmacotherapy in children and adolescents. In H. S. Ghuman & R. M. Sarles (Eds.), *Handbook of adolescent inpatient psychiatric treatment* (pp. 104–131). New York, Brunner/Mazel.

Kovacs, M., & Beck, A. T. (1977). An empirical-clinical approach toward a definition of childhood depression. In J. G. Schulterbrandt & A. Rasken (Eds.), *Depression and childhood: Diagnosis, treatment and conceptual models.* New York, Raven Press,

Kovacs, M. (1985a). The Children's Depression Inventory (CDI). *Psychopharmacology Bulletin, 21,* 995–998.

Kovacs, M. (1985b). The natural history and course of depressive disorders in children. *Psychiatric Annals, 15* (6), 387–389.

Kovacs, M. (1992). A prospective study of DSM-III adjustment disorders in childhood. Paper presented at the Institute on Long-Term Outcome of Childhood Disorders at the Annual Meeting of the American Academy of Child and Adolescent Psychiatry, Washington, DC. Kovacs, M., Feinberg, T. L., Crouse-Novak, M. A., Paulauskas, S. L., & Finkelstein, R. (1984a). Depressive disorders in childhood I: A longitudinal prospective study of characteristics and recovery. *Archives of General Psychiatry, 41,* 229–237.

Kovacs, M. & Beck, A. T. (1977). An empirical-clinical approach toward a definition of childhood depression. In: Schulterbrandt, J. G. & Rasken, A. (Eds.) *Depression and childhood diagnosis: Treatment and conceptual models.* New York: Raven Press.

Kovacs, M., Feinberg, T. L., Crouse-Novak, M.A., Paulauskas, S.L., Pollack, M., & Finkelstein, R. (1984b). Depressive disorders in childhood: II. A longitudinal study of the risk for a subsequent major depression. *Archives of General Psychiatry, 41,* 643–649.

Kraepelin, I. (1921). *Manic-Depressive insanity and paranoia.* Edinburgh: E & S Livingston.

McCracken, J. T. (1992). The epidemiology of child and adolescent mood disorders. *Child & Adolescent Clinics of North America, 1*(1), 53–72.

Robins, L. N. (1979). Longitudinal methods in the study of normal and pathological development. In K. P. Kisker, J. E. Meyer, C. Meyer, & C. (Eds.), *Psychiatric der gegenwart, band I, forscchung und praxis, grundlagen und methoden der psychiatrie teil I* (p. 627). Heidelberg, Springer-Verlag.

Weissman, M. M., Fendrich, M., Warner, V., Wichramaratne, P. (1992). Incidence of psychiatric disorder in offspring at high and low risk for depression. *J. Am. Acad. Child Adolesc. Psychiatry. 31*(4): 640–648.

Chapter 12

Obsessive-Compulsive Disorder, Tics and Tourette's Syndrome, and Separation Anxiety Disorder

Jacqueline Haimes, M.D., Harinder S. Ghuman, M.D., and Richard M. Sarles, M.D.

OBSESSIVE-COMPULSIVE DISORDER

Once a rare illness in childhood and adolescence, obsessive-compulsive disorder (OCD) is now recognized much more frequently. According to the *Diagnostic and Statistical Manual of Mental Disorders* (4th edition) (*DSM-IV*) (American Psychiatric Association [APA], 1994), which classifies OCD as an anxiety disorder, patients with this illness experience obsessions and/or compulsions of a distressing, time-consuming, and excessive nature. However, unlike adults with OCD, children and adolescent OCD patients are not required by *DSM-IV* criteria to possess insight into the fact that their obsessions and compulsions are unreasonable.

Obsessions are defined as "recurrent and persistent thoughts, impulses, or images that are experienced as intrusive and inappropriate and that cause marked anxiety or distress" (APA, 1994). In a major National Institute of Mental Health (NIMH) study of child and adolescent OCD patients, obsessions involving dirt or germs, danger to self or loved ones, symmetry, and religiosity were most frequently reported (Swedo, Rapoport, Leonard, Lenoine, & Cheslow, 1989). In the Yale Child Study Center study, fears of contamination were also observed as a commonly occurring obsession but images of an aggressive and violent nature as well as somatic obsessions were each additionally described in 38 percent of patients (Riddle, Hardin, Towbin, Ort, Lackman, & Cohen, 1990).

Compulsions are "repetitive behaviors or mental acts that the person feels driven to perform in response to an obsession or according to rules that must be applied rigidly" (APA, 1994). The intention of these compulsions is to stave off an anticipated disaster or feared event. In the NIMH study mentioned previously, 85 percent of the patients displayed washing rituals; repeating and checking compulsions were also often observed. Riddle et al. (1990) noted that repeating rituals were seen most frequently in their study followed by washing, ordering and arranging, and checking.

Epidemiology

In 1984, the Epidemiology Catchment Area survey estimated that 2.5 percent of the population studied (about 10,000 probands) had a history of symptoms that met *DSM-III* criteria for OCD (Regier, Myers, Kramer, Robins, Blazer, Hough, Eaton, & Locke 1984). Prior to that study, the prevalence of OCD in the general population was considered much lower largely because these patients often failed to seek treatment because of embarrassment and secrecy (Towbin & Riddle, 1996). Zohar, Ratzoni, Pauls, Apter, Bleich, Kron, Rapoport, Weizman, & Cohen (1992) reported a prevalence of 3.56 +-.72% among Israeli adolescent army inductees although half of those had obsessions only.

In an epidemiological study of a community sample of young adolescents, Valleni-Basile and colleagues (1994) reported the prevalence of OCD to be 3 percent. They noted no significant difference between black and white adolescents or among socioeconomic classes. Regarding gender differences in OCD, the 1989 NIMH study observed that boys diagnosed with OCD outnumbered girls with this disorder by a 2 to 1 ratio. They noted that boys tended to have earlier age of onset (9 years, 6 months) as compared with girls (11 years). It does appear, however, that by adolescence, the ratio between males and females becomes about equal (Zohar et al., 1992; Flament, Davis, Berg, Kalikow, Sceery, & Shaffer, 1988; Valleni-Basile, Garrison, Jackson, Waller, McKeown, Addy, & Cuffe, 1994).

Etiology

At one time OCD was thought to develop secondary to unresolved, unconscious internal conflicts, often of an aggressive and sexual nature. Although there is a rich anecdotal psychoanalytic literature regarding treatment of obsessive and compulsive symptomatology, these theories have never been formally tested by scientific studies. Over the past 20 years, there has been increasing evidence to substantiate OCD as a primarily neurobehavioral disorder whose course can be exacerbated by social and psychological stressors. The exact etiology of OCD is uncertain at present.

It does appear that a vulnerability for OCD is genetic which is supported by the high prevalence of OCD among a patient's family members. In addition, there is some evidence that OCD and Tourette's syndrome may represent varying expressions of the same gene and that these disorders are transmitted via autosomal dominant inheritance with variable penetrance (Pauls & Leckman, 1986). Between 25 percent to 30 percent of adolescents with OCD have at least one first-degree relative with the disorder (Lenane, Pauls, Sceery, & Rapoport, 1990; Swedo et al., 1989a). In Swedo's 1989 study, 25 percent of probands had a family history of OCD, with father-son pairs predominating. Symptom clusters among affected family members were noted to differ suggesting that a simple modeling hypothesis is not enough to explain family transmission (Lenane et al., 1990; Swedo et al., 1989a).

It is also likely that neurotransmitter dysregulation is involved in the etiology of OCD. In particular, the important role of serotonin has been suspected because of the efficacy of serotonin reuptake inhibitors on OCD symptoms. Dopamine abnormalities are also considered another feasible cause given the worsening of OCD symptoms with psychostimulants and the augmenting effects of dopamine receptor antagonists (Goodman, McDougle, & Price, 1992).

Another possible source of OCD involves abnormal information processing in the corticostriatothalamocortical circuitry. It has been observed by positron emission tomography (PET) that patients with OCD demonstrate increased metabolic activity in the right and left prefrontal., left orbital frontal, left premotor, and right sensorimotor regions as well as the bilateral anterior cingulate gyri (Swedo, Schapiro, Grady, Cheslow, Leonard, Kumar, Friedland, Rapoport, & Rapoport, 1989b). Involvement of the basal ganglia in the etiology of OCD has also been suspected largely because Sydenham's chorea, which involves autoimmune inflammation of the basal ganglia following streptococcal infection, has frequently been correlated with subsequent development of obsessive and compulsive symptoms (Swedo, Rapoport, Cheslow, Leonard, Ayoulo, Hosier, & Wald, 1989c). It remains unclear, however, whether the current theories of the etiology of OCD represent one as yet unintegrated cause or separate sources of this pathology.

Clinical Presentation

OCD in children and adolescents appears to have a remarkably similar presentation to adult-onset OCD (Rappaport, Swedo, & Leonard, 1992). Most pediatric patients with this disorder possess both obsessions and compulsions. Initially, OCD patients often hide and attempt to minimize their highly ritualized compulsions; an example is disguising washing rituals as more frequent voiding. Swedo and colleagues (1989a) observed that the children in their study had performed rituals an average of four to six months before their parents detected a problem. Teachers and peers often have no knowledge of the symptoms. Additionally, except in severe OCD cases, there is partial control so that the child is often able to suppress rituals at school and with friends. However, at home, the earlier suppressed rituals become "unleashed" and the child can spend hours occupied by his or her particular ritual or rituals. Attempts to interrupt these activities by others often lead to tantrums among younger patients. The symptoms usually cause subjective distress in older children and adolescents.

In Hanna's 1995 study of 31 OCD clinic patients, the mean age of onset was 10 years with most cases developing between ages 8 and 12. However, OCD has been reported as early as age 3 (Hollingsworth, Tanguay, & Grossman, 1980). The onset of OCD can develop in a variety of ways, but it seems that most commonly symptoms increase insidiously in their number and severity over the span of years (Hanna, 1995). Less frequently, symptoms can present more rapidly over the course of weeks to months or even in a few days.

Many OCD patients remain functional in certain areas including academic achievement and recreational activities. In fact, it has been observed that having others structure the patient's time and participating in physical activity can temporarily alleviate symptoms (Swedo et al., 1989a). OCD patients usually have more difficulty in areas of social functioning and peer relations (Riddle et al., 1990), and psychosocial stressors dramatically worsen obsessive and compulsive symptoms.

Family History

OCD is often found in more than one family member. Interestingly, other Axis I disorders are quite prevalent among first-degree relatives. In Lenane and colleagues' 1989 study,

45 percent of fathers, 65 percent of mothers, and 36 percent of the siblings of probands received a no-OCD Axis I diagnosis with affective disorders, alcoholism, and other anxiety disorders being the most frequent.

Family dynamics are also considered an integral part of this illness. It is quite anxiety-provoking for families to observe their child's rituals and to acknowledge their own help-lessness in reducing their child's symptoms. It is often the case that one's parents and family become absorbed in aiding the child to perpetuate their particular rituals while be-lieving that they are actually assisting their child (Towbin & Riddle, 1996). For example, family members may help supply patients with various detergents for their cleaning rituals.

Developmental History

There have not been major perinatal or developmental abnormalities that have been asso-ciated with OCD but minor ones have been observed including delayed eye-hand coordi-nation, reading difficulties, and poor speech articulation (Riddle et al., 1990).

Comorbidity

Comorbid Axis I disorders are more the rule than the exception among children and adoles-cents with OCD; the prevalence of comorbid diagnoses ranges from 62 percent to 84 per-cent (Riddle et al., 1990; Hanna, 1995; Swedo et al., 1989). In Hanna's study, 52 percent of probands had two or more additional diagnoses. Affective disorders (29%–35%) and anx-iety disorders (26%–40%) are the most common comorbid conditions (Riddle et al., 1990; Hanna, 1995; Swedo et al., 1989) with major depression and overanxious disorder (now classified as generalized anxiety disorder) the most frequently seen comorbid conditions, respectively (Leonard, Swedo, Lenane, Rettew, Hamburger, Bartko, & Rapoport, 1993). It appears that about half the time affective and anxiety disorders predate the development of OCD (Swedo et al., 1989a).

Several studies also have identified a prevalence of motor tics among 20 percent to 26 percent of OCD patients (Riddle et al., 1990; Hanna, 1995; Swedo et al., 1989a). Dis-ruptive disorders are also frequent comorbid findings. Hanna, who reported a concurrent diagnosis of a disruptive behavior disorder in 29 percent of probands, noted that attention-deficit/hyperactivity disorder tended to develop prior to onset of OCD whereas oppositional defiant disorder and conduct disorder generally developed in conjunction with OCD.

Tourette's disorder has been identified in families in which one or more members have OCD. Additionally, OCD and Tourette's can occur concurrently in about 15 percent of OCD patients (Hanna, 1995). Specific developmental disorder appears in about 25 percent of OCD patients (Hanna, 1995; Swedo et al., 1989a). In a 1993 study by Thomsen and col-leagues, it was observed that personality disorders are not more common in OCD patients as compared to other psychiatric patients. However, among OCD patients there were sig-nificantly more individuals diagnosed with avoidant personality disorder, but not a higher frequency of obsessive-compulsive personality disorder.

EVALUATION

Interview

When assessing a child for a potential OCD diagnosis, it is important to talk to several indi-viduals who interact with the child in different contexts. Parents, siblings, and teachers can be helpful in eliciting a more complete picture of the child's behavior, level of functioning, and areas of difficulty. Keeping in mind that patients with OCD are often secretive and embarrassed about their symptoms, the clinician should take care to be tactful yet thorough in the diagnostic interview and additionally address potential comorbid conditions.

Medical

A thorough history and physical exam are indicated as part of all evaluations. In patients with suspected OCD, special attention should be paid to the neurological exam and the presence of any motor tics. Although there are no pathognomonic laboratory findings in OCD, more routine laboratory studies including CBC with differential, electrolytes, liver, kidney, and thyroid functions, and drug screen are generally indicated (Towbin & Riddle, 1996). If the patient is to be initiated on clomipramine, an ECG is essential. A head CT or MRI is recommended if tics or a focal neurological finding is detected. In cases where a seizure is suspected, an EEG is indicated.

Standardized Instruments

Both the Leyton Obsessional Inventory -Child Version (Berg, Rapoport, & Flament, 1986) and the Yale-Brown Obsessive Compulsive Scale (Goodman, Price, Rasumussen, Mazure, Fieischmann, Hill, Heninger, & Charney, 1989) are objective measures used to assess the severity of one's obsessive and compulsive symptoms and to follow the patient's course over time.

DIFFERENTIAL DIAGNOSIS

There are many psychiatric disorders in which obsessive, compulsive, or similarly appearing symptoms are present and can be potentially confused with OCD. Looking at the particular content of these symptoms is often helpful in differentiating these disorders (Swedo et al., 1989a). Patients with eating disorders often have a specific preoccupation with and rituals involving food. In major depressive disorder, ruminations involving worthlessness and guilt are frequently present. Excessive fears involving a specific situation or object are seen in phobias. Subclinical obsessions and/or compulsions are quite common and must be distinguished from full-blown OCD by the severity of impairment.

Patients with pervasive developmental disorder can have stereotypies but these are simpler in form than compulsions and are not particularly distressing to them. In Tourette's syndrome, compulsions that may be present are less severe and less likely to involve washing if OCD is not present as a comorbid condition (Swedo et al., 1989a). It is sometimes difficult to distinguish a delusion from an obsession. Usually OCD patients can identify the source of their obsession as deriving from their own mind as opposed to an external agent. However, if reality testing and insight are lost, the obsession reaches delusional proportions and a comorbid psychotic disorder must be seriously considered (APA, 1994).

Among children, it is imperative to differentiate OCD from normal developmental issues. Toddlers frequently display ritualistic behavior and a fondness for routines, but by age 3 or 4 they start to become less rigid in this manner (Leonard, Goldberger, Rapoport, Cheslow, & Swedo, 1990). As compared to normal developmental rituals, OCD rituals are initiated at an older age and cause distress and interference in one's life (Swedo et al., 1989a) whereas normal developmental rituals are functional in that they serve to master anxiety and improve one's socialization (Leonard et al., 1990). Childhood superstitions must also be distinguished from OCD. Superstitions, which are often utilized in situations of a dangerous and unpredictable nature, do not involve washing or grooming rituals (Leonard et al., 1990). There has been no documentation that there is a continuum between superstitions or developmental rituals and OCD (Leonard et al., 1990).

Occasionally, OCD is confused with obsessive-compulsive personality disorder (OCPD). OCPD involves a "pervasive pattern of preoccupation with orderliness, perfectionism, and mental and interpersonal control" (APA, 1994) that is ego syntonic; true obsessions or compulsions are not present. Additionally, most OCD patients do not have nor do they develop OCPD (Towbin & Riddle, 1996).

TREATMENT

Pharmacotherapy

Similar to the case with adults, OCD among the pediatric population has generally responded well to medication. Clomipramine, and several of the serotonin specific reuptake inhibitors (SSRIs) have proved to be effective in this group of patients. Clomipramine is best studied among children and adolescents with OCD. a tricyclic, clomipramine possesses greater potency of serotonin reuptake as compared to other tricyclics. Leonard's 1989 double-blind crossover trial comparing clomipramine and desipramine showed that clomipramine was superior and reduced OCD symptoms significantly more than desipramine. In Flament and colleagues' 1985 double-blind controlled trial of clomipramine, 74 percent of probands were at least moderately improved on the medication and generally showed relapse once the medication was discontinued. In an eight-week multicenter double-blind trial of clomipramine versus placebo, DeVeaugh-Geiss, Moroz, Biederman, Cantwell, Fontaine, Greist, Reichler, Katz, & Landau (1992) showed that clomipramine reduced the score on the Yale-Brown Obsessive Compulsive Scale an average of 37 percent as compared to 8 percent in the patients receiving placebo.

The side effects of clomipramine are essentially related to its anticholinergic, antihistaminic, and alpha-blocking activity. Commonly seen side effects include dry mouth, tremor, sedation, dizziness, insomnia, and sweating (March, 1995). Other side effects include headache and constipation. There appears to be a mild tachycardia and slight reduction in systolic blood pressure that can occur with clomipramine therapy (DeVeaugh-Geiss et al., 1992). In several clinical studies involving clomipramine, no malignant electrocardiographic changes occurred; however, slightly increased PR, QRS, and QT intervals were observed, suggesting the development of cardiotoxicity as a possibility. (Flament, Rapoport, Berg, Sceery, Kilts, Mellstrom, & Linnoila, 1985), As a result, obtaining an ECG prior to initiating treatment as well as periodic ECG monitoring is indicated.

The dose of clomipramine generally ranges from 3 mg/kg up to but not exceeding 5 mg/kg or 250 mg (March, Leonard, & Swedo, 1995). Clomipramine levels are not routinely warranted except in situations in which the patient is receiving high doses of medication and has not responded or exhibited side effects. It is usually sufficient to regulate the dose by monitoring target symptoms and side effects. Clinical improvement often does not commence until the third or fourth week of treatment and often shows increasing efficacy until the eighth week on average (DeVeaugh-Geiss et al., 1992).

In recent years, the SSRIs have been observed to be effective in reducing OCD symptoms. In 1992, Riddle, Scahill, King, Hardin, Anderson, Ort, Smith, Leckman, & Cohen found fluoxetine to show clinical improvement of OCD pediatric patients that is comparable to clomipramine, although they were not directly compared. An open fluvoxamine trial by Apter and colleagues (1994) also showed significant clinical improvement but not until the sixth week on medication. Both sertraline and fluvoxamine are being assessed for their efficacy in multicenter trials. Common side effects of these SSRIs include insomnia, fatigue, motoric activation, and gastrointestinal disturbance. Fluvoxamine can also cause dermatitis. Unlike clomipramine, the SSRIs have no cardiovascular side effects.

Children with OCD can respond to doses of fluoxetine as low as 2.5 mg/day (March, Leonard, & Swedo, 1995). Because fluoxetine takes about two to three weeks to reach steady state, it is recommended that dose increases be performed slowly as to minimize side effects. At times a dose of up to 80 mg/day is required to alleviate OCD symptoms.

About one third of patients fail to be helped by monotherapy (DeVeaugh-Geiss et al., 1992). Generally, one should wait at least eight weeks before changing the medication or adding an augmenting agent. Augmentors that have been found to be somewhat helpful include clonazepam (Leonard, Topol, Bukstein, Hindermarsh, Allen, & Swedo, 1994) and haloperidol (March et al., 1995). If a comorbid tic disorder is present, the addition of a neuroleptic can be effective. With coexisting ADHD, psychostimulants may be added but one must use caution in those patients with a family history of Tourette's disorder as psychostimulants may evoke tics (March et al., 1995). Both lithium and buspirone therapy have proven disappointing as augmenting agents.

Psychotherapy

The psychotherapy that has proven most useful in reducing obsessive-compulsive symptoms is cognitive-behavioral therapy (CBT). In March and colleagues' 1994 open trial of CBT, they found that improvement of OCD patients continued even after withdrawal of medication and noted that the average magnitude of improvement in these patients was larger than usually seen with medication therapy alone. CBT in OCD patients usually includes anxiety management training and exposure-based treatments where the goal is to extinguish anxiety by exposing the patient to the feared stimulus. Additionally, the patient is taught response prevention to block rituals.

Although individual case reports have demonstrated improvement of obsessive and compulsive symptoms in the psychoanalytic literature, the general consensus in the psychiatric community is that OCD is resistant to psychodynamic psychotherapy (Hollingsworth, Tanguay, & Grossman, 1980). However, psychodynamic psychotherapy may be useful for improving self-esteem and interpersonal difficulties among children and adolescents with OCD (March et al., 1995). Family therapy is recommended if there is significant family dysfunction, particularly if pathological family dynamics interfere with the treatment regimen.

CLINICAL COURSE

Generally, the symptom cluster of particular obsessions and/or compulsions evolves over the course of the illness leading to different or additional predominant symptoms (Swedo et al., 1989a). For example, a child preoccupied by fears of contamination and washing rituals one year may show a decrease of these particular symptoms while demonstrating increasing perseveration on counting and symmetry the following year. Hanna reported that the mean number of lifetime obsessions and compulsions in his study of OCD probands was 3.5 and 4.8, respectively. It has been observed that an individual's specific obsessions and compulsions often reflect their developmental stage (Riddle et al., 1990). For example, sexual obsessions and rituals are common among adolescents but infrequently observed among latency-age patients in which collecting and ritualized play are hallmarks.

The course of OCD is variable and somewhat unpredictable. Over time, the symptom constellation generally fluctuates in intensity and makeup. In Rettew and co-workers' 1992 chart review of 79 OCD patients at NIMH, a pattern was identified which involved a gradual increase in the number of symptoms followed by a reduction of symptoms in late adolescence and early adulthood. However, no specific pattern regarding particular symptoms or age was observed. Most commonly, the course involves fluctuation of severity of symptoms without a complete remission (Flament, Koby, Rapoport, Berg, Zahn, Cox, Denckla, & Lenane, 1990). Less commonly, remissions lasting from six months to nine years occur; rarely, there is only one circumscribed episode of OCD. In less than 10 percent of pediatric cases, the course involves a deterioration over many years (Leonard et al., 1993).

Despite continued advances in psychopharmacotherapy and cognitive-behavioral therapy, OCD remains for many a chronic and impairing illness. In medium- and long-term follow-up studies, between 43 percent and 68 percent of patients continued to meet the criteria for OCD (Flament et al., 1990; Leonard et al., 1993; Bolton, Luckie, & Steinberg, 1995). A large number of patients continue to require psychoactive medication although for many the severity of the symptoms is significantly reduced. A substantial number of patients remain impaired in their overall functioning.

TICS AND TOURETTE'S SYNDROME

Tics are defined as a "sudden, rapid, recurrent, nonrhythmic, stereotyped motor movement or vocalization" (APA, 1994). Frequently involved are muscles of the head, neck, and respiratory tract. Tics range in severity and form and have been grouped into transient tic disorder, chronic motor or vocal tic disorder, and Tourette's syndrome (chronic motor and vocal tic disorder). Simple tics involve a single muscle group; examples include eye blinking or throat clearing. Complex tics involve several muscle groups and are more elaborate in nature. These tics, such as grooming behavior and facial gestures, often appear intentional. Tourette's syndrome includes multiple motor and vocal tics that fluctuate in intensity and makeup over time. In its most severe form, Tourette's syndrome may involve coprolalia (obscene words) and self-abusive motor tics.

Unlike the onset of OCD which can occur in childhood or adulthood, tic disorders by definition must begin before age 18 (APA, 1994). Tics frequently begin in early to middle latency (the average age of onset is 7 years) but diagnoses have been made as early as age 2 (Chappell, Leckman, & Riddle, 1995). The incidence of transient tic disorder is 5 percent to 20 percent (Chappell et al., 1995) whereas Tourette's syndrome is much less common, with an incidence of about .04 percent (Apter, Pauls, Bleich, Zohar, Kron, Ratzoni, Dycian, Kotler, Weizman, Gadot, & Cohen, 1993). The ratio of boys to girls in Tourette's syndrome is about 3–4 to 1 (Pauls & Leckman, 1986).

ETIOLOGY

It has been observed that family members of patients with Tourette's syndrome are at relatively high risk of having not only a tic disorder but also obsessive-compulsive disorder

(Pauls & Leckman, 1986). There has been substantial evidence that the various tic disorders actually represent a continuum of symptoms. It is believed that probable autosomal dominant transmission with variable penetrance and expression of a specific gene influences this spectrum which also may include a subset of obsessive-compulsive disorder (Pauls & Leckman, 1986). As of yet no specific chromosomal location has been implicated. Additionally, the basal ganglia possibly has a major role in these disorders; on average Tourette's syndrome patients have decreased volume and abnormal lateralization of their basal ganglia (Peterson, 1995).

CLINICAL PRESENTATION

The differences among the three major tic disorders involve duration and type of tics present. In transient tic disorder, motor and/or vocal tics must be present for at least four weeks but less than one year. Chronic tic disorder lasts at least one year and includes either motor or vocal tics; chronic motor tics are more common than vocal tics. In Tourette's syndrome, multiple motor and at least one vocal tic must occur over the course of at least one year. Additionally, in all three of these disorders, the tics must cause significant distress and interfere in one's functioning for a diagnosis to be made.

Tics in patients with tic disorders are abrupt in onset, often paroxysmal in nature, and frequently occur in bouts. Although tics are mostly preceded by increased tension that is substantially reduced by the tic, generally tic sufferers have some degree of voluntary control over suppression of tics. Tics usually become exacerbated by stress and decrease substantially during sleep. The onset of tics in Tourette's syndrome is usually gradual and often presents with motor tics first (Leckman & Cohen, 1996). In less severe cases, tics can be cleverly masked in normal behaviors so that these disorders may go unnoticed to the undiscerning eye.

COMORBIDITY

Many patients with Tourette's syndrome and other tic disorders have accompanying comorbid conditions. In fact, frequently it is these coexisting disorders that impair one's functioning more than the tics themselves. Attention-deficit hyperactivity disorder is found in about 50 percent of Tourette's sufferers (Chappell et al., 1995). Obsessive and compulsive symptoms are identified in about 60 percent of patients with Tourette's syndrome (Chappell et al., 1995). These patients tend to display rituals that include repetitive touching or rubbing. Other frequently seen co-occurring disorders include depressive and anxiety disorders.

COURSE

In Tourette's syndrome, tics wax and wane frequently into adulthood. These tics are often most severe during the first 10 years of the disorder (Chappell et al., 1995). Occasionally, debilitating Tourette's syndrome continues in adulthood but there is generally a good prognosis with symptoms stable at a reduced severity.

EVALUATION

When evaluating a child with tics, it is important to look at the overall functioning of the patient to identify the extent of impairment in everyday activities and assess any comorbid disorders and behavioral disturbances that may be present. In severely affected Tourette's patients, soft neurological signs may be elicited. There are no specific laboratory findings that are associated with tic disorders; therefore, head imaging and EEG need not be done on a routine basis unless a history of seizures or focal abnormalities on a neurological exam is elicited (Leckman & Cohen, 1996).

DIFFERENTIAL DIAGNOSIS

Tics must be distinguished from abnormal movements seen in certain neurological disorders. Myoclonus, tremors, athetosis, dystonia, and chorea can be confused with tics. Generally, tics can be differentiated by their more consistent nature and location as well as their rapidity (Leckman & Cohen, 1996) and the maintenance of normal muscle tone during the tics.

Complex tics can appear similar to stereotypes found in pervasive developmental disorder (PDD) and compulsive rituals found in obsessive-compulsive disorder (OCD). The presence of vocal tics helps in the diagnosis of Tourette's syndrome. One must also look for accompanying symptoms such as language delay found in PDD to help make the specific diagnosis. Tics can be distinguished from self-stimulating behavior by their involuntary and more restrictive nature. In addition, tics generally have a later onset and do not evoke pleasurable feelings the way self-stimulating behaviors do.

TREATMENT

The treatment of tic disorders varies depending on the specific disorder and severity of dysfunction. Mild tics in transient tic disorder generally require only reassurance, education, and support. If the tics are more severe and impairing, as in Tourette's syndrome, pharmacotherapy is usually indicated. The neuroleptics haloperidol and pimozide and the alpha-2 adrenergic agonist clonidine have been the major pharmacological agents used in the treatment of Tourette's syndrome.

About 70 percent of patients respond favorably to haloperidol or pimozide (Shapiro, Fulop, Hubbard, Mandeli, Nordlie, & Phillips, 1989). The severity of symptoms usually improves by an average of 70 percent to 80 percent in these individuals (Leckman & Cohen, 1996). When using haloperidol, it is recommended to start with a low dose of 0.25 mg/day and gradually titrate the dose to about 0.5–6 mg/day (Chappell et al., 1995). Usually a single dose at bedtime is appropriate. Pimozide therapy should also be begun at a low dose starting with 1 mg/day and slowly increased to a maximum of 10 mg/day. The limiting factor in using these medications is most often the side effects. Both haloperidol and pimozide can cause dystonia, akathisia, pseudoparkinsonian symptomatology, cognitive impairment, weight gain, sedation, and tardive dyskinesia. Additionally, pimozide may cause cardiac conduction abnormalities such as increased QT interval and abnormal T waves. Thus, a baseline ECG is necessary in addition to follow-up ECG's at regular intervals while the patient receives pimozide.

Clonidine, although less effective that haloperidol and pimozide, overall has fewer side effects. About 25 percent of Tourette's syndrome patients show improvement on clonidine with an average of 20 percent to 30 percent reduction in symptoms (Leckman, Hardin, Riddle, Stevenson, Ort, & Cohen, 1991). Dosing should begin at 0.05 mg/day and be increased to a dose greater than 0.25 mg/day (about 5 micrograms/kg/day). Adverse side effects can include sedation, irritability, dizziness, low blood pressure, headache, and dry mouth. Clonidine has been found to be particularly effective in Tourette's patients with comorbid accompanying hyperactivity.

In addition to pharmacotherapy, individual and family therapy can be helpful in reducing the stress and anxiety that may exacerbate the severity of tics. Comorbid disorders should also be treated. In general, the disorder that is most problematic to the patient's functioning should be treated most aggressively.

SEPARATION ANXIETY DISORDER

There have been significant changes in the classification of anxiety disorders with adults, children, and adolescents. In the *Diagnostic and Statistical Manual of Mental Disorders (DSM-I)* published in 1952, all the disorders of psychogenic origin were named "reactions" and anxiety disorders were grouped under psychoneurotic reactions. In *DSM-II*, published in 1968, anxiety was considered as the chief characteristic of the neurosis. Neuroses were further divided into anxiety neurosis, hysterical neurosis, phobic neurosis, obsessive-compulsive neurosis, depressive neurosis, neuroasthenic neurosis, depersonalization neurosis, and hypochondriacal neurosis. Childhood and adolescence disorders were classified separately under the category of behavior disorders of childhood and adolescence, with a subcategory of "overanxious reaction of childhood (or adolescence)" describing children with chronic anxiety, excessive and unrealistic fears, sleeplessness, nightmares, and exaggerated autonomic responses. In *DSM-III* (1980) and *DSM-III-R* (1987), in addition to a broad category of anxiety disorders, there was inclusion of separation anxiety disorder, overanxious disorder, and avoidant disorder under the section of disorders usually first evident in infancy, childhood, or adolescence.

In *DSM-IV* (1994), the anxiety disorder section contains criteria for panic disorder with/without agoraphobia, agoraphobia, specific phobia, obsessive-compulsive disorder, post-traumatic stress disorder, acute stress disorder, generalized anxiety disorder, anxiety disorder due to a general medical condition and anxiety disorder NOS. All of these diagnoses can be applied to children and adolescents. In addition, there is diagnosis of separation anxiety disorder under other disorders of infancy, childhood, or adolescence. The *DSM-III-R* diagnoses of overanxious disorder and avoidant disorder of childhood or adolescence have been deleted.

In *DSM-IV* (1994), separation anxiety disorder has been defined as "excessive anxiety concerning separation from the home or from those to whom the person is attached" and the anxiety is beyond that which is expected for the person's developmental level. The duration of the disturbance must be at least four weeks with the onset before age 18 years.

Epidemiology

The prevalence of separation anxiety disorder is reported to be from 3.5 percent to 5.4 percent (Costello, 1989) with a peak incidence about 11 years of age. In clinical samples, this disorder is equally common among boys and girls but in epidemiological samples the disorder is more frequent in females (APA, 1994). Last and colleagues (1987) reported lower socioeconomic status as a significant factor for having separation anxiety disorder.

Etiology and Risk Factors

Children at risk include those who have recently experienced serious illness or death in the family or disruption in family life, and children with malignant neoplasm, diabetes,

Tourette's syndrome, and the combination of ADD and reading disorder (Livingston, 1990).

Studies of adult patients with anxiety disorder have shown increased prevalence of anxiety disorders in their children (Turner, Beidel, & Costello, 1987). Weissman and colleagues (1984) reported that children of depressed patients with agoraphobia or panic disorder were more likely to display separation anxiety than children of depressed probands without anxiety disorders. Children with family histories of depression and alcoholism also appear to be at increased risk.

Communication or contagion of anxiety within the family often result in a vicious cycle in which anxiety of the child and the parent feed in to each other (Eisenberg, 1958).

Clinical Description

Separation anxiety is a normal developmental phenomenon during late infancy and the toddler stage and is often seen in mild forms during kindergarten, first grade, and under stressful circumstances. This anxiety is considered clinically relevant if the symptoms are severe enough to interfere in daily functioning and in achieving developmental tasks. Separation anxiety symptoms are expressed differently at different ages. Francis, Last, & Strauss (1987) reported that children ages 5 to 8 years were more likely to present with worries about unrealistic harm to attachment figures, nightmares, and school refusal; children ages 9 to 12 years showed excessive distress at times of separation; and adolescents ages 13 to 16 years often presented with school refusal and physical complaints.

The child with separation anxiety often comes to the attention of a physician as a result of school refusal and somatic complaints including recurrent abdominal pain, headache, and palpitations. In addition, the child may have difficulty going to sleep and staying asleep and often ends up sleeping in the parent's bed or in the same room. The child has excessive worries and experiences nightmares with themes of harm befalling major attachment figures or to self and fears of being lost. The child frequently shows clinging and shadowing behavior with the parent and may refuse to go to school, camp, and a friend's house. The child may develop fears of monsters, burglars, car accidents, or the dark, and the younger child may report unusual perceptual experiences—for example, hearing sounds or his or her name being called. The child may become withdrawn, sad, and at times clinically depressed and the relationship between the child and the parent is often strained by the excessive demands of the child.

Case Examples

Casey is a 4-year-old who was brought to the clinic by her foster mother because of her concerns that Casey was "too fragile." Casey followed her foster mother about the house from room to room and if her foster parents like to go somewhere she runs to the door and cries resulting in the foster parents taking Casey with them. Casey insisted on sleeping with her foster mother and experienced frequent nightmares. She was described as timid, crying easily, and having limited peer interaction, talking little to others except her foster mother. She was unable to stay with a babysitter. Casey was born to a 14-year-old and experienced several abandonments by her mother and separations from family members. When placed in the present foster home at age 2 years she was described as extremely withdrawn, unwilling to touch anything, and having to be carried everywhere by her foster mother.

Sam, a 7-year-old boy, was brought to the clinic by his mother. For the previous two to three months, Sam had been refusing to go to school, experienced frequent stomachaches in the morning, and had a frequent nightmare in which he was left in a shopping mall without his mother. At night he had difficulty going to sleep and often awoke in middle of the night coming to his mother's room to sleep in her bed. In addition, Sam started to wet his bed. Sam's parents have serious conflicts and are in the process of divorce and a custody battle.

Differential Diagnosis

Separation anxiety disorder can be distinguished from generalized anxiety disorder by a predominance of the child's concerns being related to separation from major attachment figures. Panic disorder may occur in children with or without separation anxiety disorder. A child with panic disorder without separation anxiety is overwhelmed with anxiety related to anticipation of panic attack rather than separation issues.

Phobic avoidance of school has been becoming more frequent in children because of the increase in violence in schools. Children have been threatened, bullied, physically attacked, or exposed to violent acts in school. This avoidance is a result of fears other than separation from major attachment figures. In some cases school refusal may be caused by social phobia. Truancy in conduct disorder children should be distinguished from school refusal of separation anxiety disorder children by lack of anxiety about separation and the child's staying away from home.

Treatment

Behavioral Interventions   School refusal is a frequent presenting symptom of separation anxiety disorder resulting in the parent seeking professional help. In addition, the parent may be stressed related to the child's refusal to stay with a babysitter, clinging behavior, and sleep difficulties. Behavioral interventions are based on both classical and operant conditioning models. The classical-conditioning-based interventions including systematic desensitization, and exposure and flooding procedures (Croghan, 1981; Miller, 1972). The operant conditioning interventions include rearranging contingencies in home and school to improve school attendance by the child receiving positive and negative reinforcements for school attendance (Doleys & Williams, 1977; Brown, Copeland, & Hall, 1974). In mild cases, the diagnosis and nature of the disorder (including contagion effect) are carefully explained to the parents and child. The child is made to go to school with help by the parents and school staff, and is expected to sleep in his or her room. A reward system including significant praise and reinforcement is initiated.

Pharmacological Interventions   In resistant cases, medication can be tried in addition to the supportive and behavioral measures. Gittelman-Klein and Klein (1971) studied 35 children, ages 6 to 14 years, with separation anxiety disorder who had missed at least two weeks of school. These children were treated with Imipramine, 100 to 200 mg/d or placebo with significant improvement in returning to school in children receiving imipramine (81%) than those receiving placebo (47%) being reported. In addition, fluoxetine (Birmaher, Waterman, Ryan, Cully, Balach, Ingram, & Brodsky, 1994) has been tried with some success in children and adolescents with separation anxiety disorder.

Other Interventions   In addition to interventions described previously, individual psychotherapy for the child and parent counseling may be required depending upon the child's condition and family circumstances. Often, the parent suffers from anxiety symptoms and is conflicted in relating to the child. The parent usually needs significant support from the clinician in implementing a treatment plan. In extreme cases hospitalization may be necessary to force separation. The clinician may seek court assistance when school non-attendance is severe and parents are ineffective in getting the child to school or encourage the child to stay home.

Course and Prognosis   Onset of separation anxiety disorder may be very early in the child's life and related to some stress—for example, illness or death of a family member or moving to a new home or school. Separation anxiety disorder may persist for years marked with periods of exacerbation and remission. More intelligent children, older onset, and greater severity have a worse outcome (Livingston, 1991).

CONCLUSION

In separation anxiety disorder the child/adolescent experiences excessive anxiety related to separation from a primary attachment figure. Anxiety symptoms are manifested through school refusal, somatic complaints, and sleep disturbance. Behavioral interventions, medication, individual therapy and parent counseling are effective in treating this disorder.

REFERENCES

American Psychiatric Association (APA). (1994). *Diagnostic and statistical manual of mental disorders* (4th ed.) *(DSM-IV)*. Washington, DC: the Association.

Apter, A., Pauls, D. L., Bleich, A., Zohar, A. H., Kron, S., Ratzoni, G., Dycian, A., Kotler, M., Weizman, A., Gadot, N., & Cohen, D. J. (1993) An epidemiological study of Gilles de la Tourette's syndrome in Israel. *Archives of General Psychiatry, 50*, 734–738.

Apter, A., Ratzoni, G., King, R., Weizman, A., Iancu, I., Binder, M., Riddle, M. A. (1994). Fluvoxamine open-label treatment of adolescent inpatients with obsessive-compulsive disorder or depression. *Journal of the American Academy of Child and Adolescent Psychiatry, 33*, 342–348.

Berg, C. J., Rapoport, J. L., & Flament, M. (1986). The Leyton Obsessional Inventory-Child Version. *Journal of the American Academy of Child and Adolescent Psychiatry, 1*, 84–91.

Birmaher, B., Waterman, G. S., Ryan, N., Cully, M., Balach, L., Ingram, J., & Brodsky, M. (1994). Fluoxetine for childhood anxiety disorder. *Journal of the American Academy of Child and Adolescent Psychiatry, 33*, 993.

Bolton, D., Luckie, M., & Steinberg, D. (1995). Long-term course of obsessive-compulsive disorder treated in adolescence. *Journal of the American Academy of Child and Adolescent Psychiatry, 34*, 1441–1450.

Brown, R., Copeland, R. E., & Hall, R. V. (1974). School phobia effects of behavior modification treatment applied by an elementary school principal. *Child Study Journal, 4*, 125–133.

Chappell, P. B., Leckman, J. F., & Riddle, M. A. (1995). The pharmacologic treatment of tic disorders. *Child and Adolescent Psychiatric Clinics of North America, 4*, 197–216.

Costello, E. J. (1989). Developments in child psychiatric epidemiology. *Journal of the American Academy of Child and Adolescent Psychiatry, 28*, 836–841.

Croghan, L. M. (1981). Conceptualizing the critical elements in a rapid desensitization to school anxiety: A case study. *Journal of Pediatric Psychology, 6*, 165–170.

DeVeaugh-Geiss, J., Moroz, G., Biederman, J., Cantwell, U. D., Fontaine, R., Greist, J. H., Reichler, R., Katz, R., Landau, P. (1992). Clomipramine hydrochloride in childhood and adolescent obsessive-compulsive disorder-A multicenter trial. *Journal of the American Academy of Child and Adolescent Psychiatry, 31*, 45–49.

Doleys, D. M., & Williams, S. C. (1977). The use of natural consequences and a make-up period to eliminate school phobic behavior: A case study. *Journal of School Psychology, 15*, 44–50.

Eisenberg, L. (1958). School phobia, a study in communication of anxiety. *American Journal of Psychiatry, 114*, 172–178.

Flament, M. F., Rapoport, J. L., Berg, C. J., Sceery, W., Kilts, C., Mellstrom, B., & Linnoila, M. (1985). Clomipramine treatment of childhood obsessive-compulsive disorder. A double-blind controlled study. *Archives of General Psychiatry, 42*, 977–983.

Flament, M. F., Whitaker, A., Rapoport, J. L., Davis, M., Berg, C. Z., Kalikow, K., Sceery, W., & Shaffer, D. (1988). Obsessive compulsive disorder in adolescence: An epidemiological study. *Journal of the American Academy of Child and Adolescent Psychiatry, 27*, 764–771.

Flament, M. F., Koby, E., Rapoport, J. L., Berg, C. J., Zahn, T., Cox, C., Denckla, M., Lenane, M. (1990). Childhood obsessive-compulsive disorder: A prospective follow-up study. *Journal of Child Psychology and Psychiatry, 31*, 363–380.

Francis, G., Last, C. G., & Strauss, C. C. (1987). Expression of separation anxiety disorder: The role of age and gender. *Child Psychiatry and Human Development, 18*, 82–89.

Gittleman-Klein R., & Klein D. F. (1971). Controlled imipramine treatment of school phobia. *Archives of General Psychiatry, 25*, 204–207.

Goodman, W. K., Price, L. H., Rasmussen, S. A., Mazure, C., Fleischmann, R. L., Hill, C. L., Heninger, G. R., & Charney, D. S. (1989). The Yale-Brown Obsessive Compulsive Scale. *Archives of General Psychiatry, 46*, 1006–1011.

Goodman, W. K., McDougle, C. J., & Price, L. H. (1992). The role of serotonin and dopamine in the pathophysiology of obsessive compulsive disorder. *International Clinical Psychopharmacology, 1*, 35–38.

Hanna, G. L. (1995). Demographic and clinical features of obsessive-compulsive disorder in children and adolescents. *Journal of the American Academy of Child and Adolescent Psychiatry, 24*, 19–27.

Hollingsworth, C., Tanguay, P., & Grossman, L. (1980). Long-term outcome of obsessive-compulsive disorder. *Journal of the American Academy of Child Psychiatry, 19*, 134–144.

Last, C. G., Hersen, M., Kazdin, A. E., Finkelstein, R. & Strauss, C. C. (1987). Comparison of DSM-III separation anxiety and overanxious disorders: Demographic characteristics and patterns of comorbidity. *Journal of the American Academy of Child and Adolescent Psychiatry, 26*, 527–531.

Leckman, J. F., & Cohen, D. J. (1996). Tic disorders. In M. Lewis (Ed.), Child and adolescent psychiatry: A comprehensive textbook (2nd ed.) (pp. 622–629). Baltimore: Williams & Wilkins.

Leckman, J. F., Hardin, M. T., Riddle, M. A., Stevenson, J., Ort, S. I., & Cohen, D. J. (1991). Clonidine treatment of Gilles de la Tourette's syndrome. *Archives of General Psychiatry, 48*, 324–328.

Lenane, M. C., Swedo, S. E., Leonard, H., Pauls, D. L., Sceery, W., & Rapoport, J. L. (1990). Psychiatric disorders in first degree relatives of children and adolescents with obsessive compulsive disorder. *Journal of the American Academy of Child and Adolescent Psychiatry, 29*, 407–412.

Leonard, H. L., Topol, D., Bukstein, O., Hindermarsh, D., Allen, A. J., & Swedo, S. E. (1994). Clonazepam as an augmenting agent in the treatment of childhood-onset obsessive-compulsive disorder. *Journal of the American Academy of Child Psychiatry, 33*, 792–794.

Leonard, H. L., Swedo, S. E., Lenane, M. C., Rettew, D. C., Hamburger, M. S., Bartko, J. J., & Rapoport, L. L. (1993). A 2- to 7-year follow-up study of 54 obsessive-compulsive children and adolescents. *Archives of General Psychiatry, 50*, 429–439.

Leonard, H. L., Swedo, S. E., Rapoport, J. L., Koby, E., Lenane, M., Cheslow, D., & Hamburger, M. S. (1989). Treatment of obsessive-compulsive disorder with clomipramine and desipramine in children and adolescents. A double-blind crossover comparison. *Archives of General Psychiatry, 46*, 1088–1092.

Leonard, H. L., Goldberger, E. L., Rapoport, J. L., Cheslow, D. W., & Swedo, S. B. (1990). Childhood rituals: Normal development or obsessive-compulsive symptoms? *Journal of the American Academy of Child and Adolescent Psychiatry, 29*, 17–23.

Livingston, R. (1990). Psychiatric comorbidity with reading disorder. *Advanced Learning Behavior Disabilities, 6*, 143–155.

Livingston, R. (1991). Anxiety disorder. In M. Lewis (Ed.), Child and adolescent psychiatry (pp. 673–684). Baltimore: William & Wilkins.

March, J. (1995). Cognitive-behavioral psychotherapy for children and adolescents with obsessive-compulsive disorder: A review and recommendations for treatment. *Archives of General Psychiatry, 34*, 7–18.

March, J. S., Leonard, H. L., & Swedo, S. E. (1995). Pharmacotherapy of obsessive-compulsive disorder. *Child Adolescent Psychiatric Clinics of North America, 4*, 217–236.

March, J. S., Mulle, K., & Hervel, B. (1994). Behavioral psychotherapy for children and adolescents with obsessive-compulsive disorder: An open trial of a new protocol-driven treatment package. *Archives of General Psychiatry, 33*, 333–341.

Miller, P. M. (1972). The use of visual imagery and muscle relaxation in the counterconditioning of a phobic child: A case study. *Journal of Nervous and Mental Disease, 154*, 457–460.

Pauls, D. L., & Leckman, J. F. (1986). The inheritance of Gilles de la Tourette syndrome and associated behaviors: Evidence for autosomal dominant transmission. *New England Journal of Medicine, 3, 5*, 993–997.

Peterson, B. S. (1995). Neuroimaging in child and adolescent neuropsychiatric disorders. *Archives of General Psychiatry, 34*, 1560–1576.

Rapoport, J. L., Swedo, S. E., & Leonard, H. L. (1992). Childhood obsessive compulsive disorder. *Journal of Clinical Psychiatry, 56*, 11–16.

Regier, D. A., Myers, J. K., Kramer, M., Robins, L. N., Blazer, D. G., Hough, R. L., Eaton, W. W., & Locke, B. Z. (1984). The NIMH epidemiologic catchment area program. *Archives of General Psychiatry, 41*, 934–941.

Rettew, D. C., Swedo, S. E., Leonard, H. L., Lenane, M. C., & Rapoport, J. L. (1992). Obsessions and compulsions across time in 79 children and adolescents with obsessive-compulsive disorder. *Journal of the American Academy of Child and Adolescent Psychiatry, 31*, 1050–1056.

Riddle, M. A., Scahill, L., King, R., Hardin, M. T., Towbin, K., Ort, S. I., Leckman, J. F., Cohen, D. J. (1990). Obsessive compulsive disorder in children and adolescents: Phenomenology and family history. *Journal of the American Academy of Child and Adolescent Psychiatry, 29*, 766–772.

Riddle, M. A., Scahill, L., King, R., Hardin, M. T., Anderson, G. M., Ort, S. I., Smith, J. C., Leckman, J. F., & Cohen, D. J. (1992). Double-blind, crossover trial of fluoxetine and placebo in children and adolescents with obsessive-compulsive disorder. *Journal of the American Academy of Child and Adolescent Psychiatry, 31*, 1062–1069.

Shapiro, E., Shapiro, A. K., Fulop, G., Hubbard, M., Mandeli, J., Nordlic, J., & Phillips, R. A. (1989). Controlled study of haloperidol, pimozide, and placebo in the treatment of Gilles de la Tourette's syndrome. *Archives of General Psychiatry, 46*, 722–730.

Swedo, S. E., Rapoport, J. L., Leonard, H., Lenane, M., & Cheslow, D. (1989a). Obsessive-compulsive disorder in children and adolescents. Clinical phenomenology of 70 consecutive cases. *Archives of General Psychiatry, 46*, 335–341.

Swedo, S. E., Schapiro, M. B., Grady, C. L., Cheslow, D. L., Leonard, H., Kumar, A., Friedland, R., Rapoport, S. I., & Rapoport, J. L. (1989b). Cerebral glucose metabolism in childhood-onset obsessive-compulsive disorder. *Archives of General Psychiatry, 46*, 518–523.

Swedo, S. E., Rapoport, J. L., Cheslow, D. L., Leonard, H. L., Ayoub, E. M., Hosier, D. M., & Wald, E. R. (1989c). High prevalence of obsessive-compulsive symptoms in patients with Sydenham's chorea. *American Journal of Psychiatry, 146*, 246–249.

Thomsen, P. H., & Mikkelsen, H. U. (1993). Development of personality disorders in children and adolescents with obsessive-compulsive disorder. A 6- to 22-year follow-up study. *Psychiatrica Scandinavica, 87*, 456–462.

Towbin, K. E., & Riddle, M. A. (1996). Obsessive-compulsive disorder. In M. Lewis (Ed.), Child and adolescent psychiatry: A comprehensive textbook (2nd ed.) (pp 684–693). Baltimore: Williams & Wilkins.

Turner, S. M., Beidel, D. C., & Costello, A. (1987). Psychopathology in the offspring of anxiety disorder patients. *Journal of Consulting Clinical Psychology, 55*, 229–235.

Valleni-Basile, L. A., Garrison, C. Z., Jackson, K. L., Waller, J. L., McKeown, R. E., Addy, C. L., & Cuffe, S. P. (1994). Frequency of obsessive-compulsive disorder in a community sample of young adolescents. *Archives of General Psychiatry, 33*, 782–791.

Weissman, M. M., Leckman, J. F., Merikangas, K. R., Gammon, G. D., & Prusoff, B. A. (1984). Depression and anxiety disorders in parents and children. *Archives of General Psychiatry, 41*, 845–852.

Zohar, A. H., Ratzoni, G., Pauls, D. L., Apter, A., Bleich, A., Kron, S., Rapoport, M., Weizman, A., & Cohen, D. J. (1992). An epidemiological study of obsessive-compulsive disorder and related disorders in Israeli adolescents. *Archives of General Psychiatry, 31*, 1057–1061.

Chapter 13

Attention Deficit/Hyperactivity Disorder

Bruno J. Anthony, Ph.D.

The most frequent problem encountered in outpatient child and adolescent mental health settings is Attention Deficit/Hyperactivity Disorder (ADHD), representing from one-third to one-half of all referrals (Popper, 1988). Prevalence estimates of ADHD vary between 3 percent and 9 percent, depending on diagnostic criteria. Reports suggest that the prevalence of ADHD has more than doubled in the past few years, resulting in part from increased recognition and awareness but also from changes in diagnostic criteria and their less rigorous application. There has been controversy concerning the relative importance of the core symptoms of inattention, impulsivity, and overactivity, and whether these symptoms represent a distinct syndrome. However, there is no question that these symptoms and their associated emotional, social, and educational problems result in significant impairment in adaptive functioning.

At the same time, ADHD is arguably the most treatable of the childhood disorders. A large corpus of research has demonstrated the short-term efficacy of both pharmacological and psychosocial treatments. Questions still exist about these treatments, however, including their long-term effects and their specificity for different subgroups of ADHD children, prompting a multisite study sponsored by the National Institute of Mental Health (NIMH) (Richters et al., 1995). In particular, evidence pointing to significant differences between subgroups of ADHD children based on comorbid conditions and associated problems adds to the clinical complexity and has significant implications for course and treatment.

CLINICAL FEATURES

Core Symptoms

The conceptualization of ADHD in the fourth edition of *the Diagnostic and Statistical Manual of Mental Disorders (DSM-IV)* (American Psychiatric Association [APA], 1994) represents the most recent attempt to describe a condition that has been formally recognized for almost a century. Roughly synonymous labels that have been applied over the years include minimal brain dysfunction, hyperkinetic reaction (*DSM-II*), attention deficit disorder (*DSM-III*), and attention-deficit hyperactivity disorder (*DSM-III-R*). The criteria for *DSM-IV* include three subtypes based on the division of symptoms into Inattention and Hyperactivity/Impulsivity criteria. Individuals with the Predominantly Inattentive type do not display enough signs of excessive motor activity (e.g., fidgeting, excessive running, climbing, and talking, little quiet activity) or impulsivity (difficulties in delaying speech or action) but do show deficits in sustained attention, listening, following instructions, and completing work in a careful manner, organizational and memory skills, and avoiding distraction. This type appears equivalent to the ADD without hyperactivity subtype of *DSM-III* (Morgan, Hynd, Riccio, & Hall, 1996).

The *DSM-IV* ADHD disorder also contains a Predominantly Hyperactive-Impulsive type that describes individuals who present with inattention symptoms but significant levels of overactivity and impulsivity. There is some controversy as to whether this type exists; however, the lack of recognition may result from the possibility that such individuals would never have met criteria for any ADD or ADHD diagnosis in the past. A third, Combined ADHD type consists of those individuals who meet criteria for both sets of symptoms.

Recent surveys have suggested that the rate of diagnosis of ADHD will increase with the use of *DSM-IV* criteria. In one study using teacher ratings to derive diagnoses (Wolraich, Hannah, Pinnock, Baumgaertel, & Brown, 1996), there was a 57 percent increase in the frequency of ADHD based on *DSM-IV* (11.4%) compared with *DSM-III-R* (7.3%) criteria.

Field trials for *DSM-IV* and more recent work support the multidimensional view of ADHD by showing that, with appropriate multi-method, multi-informant assessment, these subtypes can be reliably distinguished. The Predominantly Inattentive type and the Combined type differ on cognitive and behavioral measures as well as comorbidity. Children meeting criteria for the Combined type tend to have more parent-and teacher-rated aggressive, conduct, and delinquent behavior problems and more peer difficulties. In keeping with these findings, the Combined group also tends to have a greater frequency of comorbid Disruptive Behavior Disorders. Certain internalizing symptoms, particularly withdrawal and somatic complaints, may be more frequent in the Predominantly Inattentive type. The data are conflicting regarding differences in the prevalence of learning disorders in the two ADHD types; when present, the Inattentive type appears to show more math disabilities.

Associated Problems and Comorbidity

The core symptoms of ADHD define the diagnosis but tend not to be the reason that parents seek outpatient treatment for their children and adolescents. The high level of comorbid conditions and associated functional problems increase the complexity of assessment and treatment. Most often, children are referred because of significant academic difficulties, mainly involving incomplete and disorganized work resulting in poor grades. Children with ADHD early on develop poor attitudes toward school because of lack of success and negative feedback from teachers and parents. In addition, the prevalence of learning disabilities is much higher in ADHD children than in those without ADHD. Estimates of learning disabilities vary widely (Biederman, Newcorn, & Sprich, 1991) because of diagnostic differences and populations studied; however, at least 20 percent of ADHD children have a comorbid learning disability compared to a rate of about 3 percent in the general population.

Interpersonal problems, both within the family and with teachers and peers, plague children with ADHD. These problems are so profound that it has led some to conceptualize ADHD as a "transactional disorder, located in the interface between the child and his social worlds" (Henker & Whalen, 1989). Families with ADHD children are characterized by increased levels of conflict and anger and have difficulties defining problems, generating alternatives, and implementing strategies to solve the problems. Parents' views of negative events often contain misattributions both toward their child (e.g., behavior is intentional) and themselves ("I am a poor parent."). Just as disturbing as family conflict for the ADHD child is the rejection by peers, which happens with shocking speed (Pelham & Bender, 1982). High levels of peer rejection and low levels of peer acceptance are correlated with psychiatric problems and antisocial behavior and predictive of early school withdrawal (Asher & Coie, 1990). Children with ADHD tend to be interpersonally awkward, aggressive, intense, and attention-demanding. They lack basic social skills such as how to initiate friendly interactions, how to play a leadership role, and how to act in considerate ways which appear linked to their difficulties with sustained and focused attention (Wilcox, Anthony, Feldstein, Rebok, & Mirsky, 1997). These interpersonal problems are heightened in ADHD children with co-occurring aggression.

Aggressive behavior frequently characterizes children with ADHD. Estimates from this country and others shows that almost half of ADHD children have comorbid Oppositional Defiant Disorder (ODD) or Conduct Disorder (CD). Outcome studies consistently show that the presence of such behaviors leads to greater persistence of ADHD (Biederman et al., 1996) and more problematic outcomes, such as school failure, antisocial behavior, and substance abuse (Barkley, Anastopoulos, Guevremont, & Fletcher, 1991). In fact, negative behavioral outcomes are mainly determined by the presence of aggressive symptoms. Significantly elevated rates of mood and anxiety problems also characterize ADHD children and adolescents. Estimates of comorbidity in clinically referred children range from 15 percent to 75 percent for mood disorders and about 25 percent for anxiety disorders (Biederman, Newcorn, & Sprich, 1991).

DIFFERENTIAL DIAGNOSTIC ISSUES

It is important to recognize several issues which can influence the diagnostic process. First, misdiagnosis can result from an over-reliance on a single source of information. Observation of a child on an outpatient visit is unlikely to provide the type of information necessary to make an accurate diagnosis of ADHD; parental and teacher reports are critical. In the majority of cases, parents seek help from professionals after concerns have been raised at school. Teachers' observations coupled with academic problems have become the major source of data in making diagnostic decisions concerning ADHD; however, relying solely on such reports is problematic. Prevalence estimates based only on teacher ratings are consistently higher than those based on multi-informant sources. Positive parental reports of ADHD are confirmed by teachers' reports in a high percentage of cases; however, negative parental reports tend not be corroborated by teachers to the same degree. Part of the reason for elevated teacher-based identification of ADHD may be what is called a "negative halo" effect—that is, the presence of other disruptive behaviors markedly increases teachers' ratings of ADHD symptoms (Abikoff, Courtney, Pelham, & Koplewicz, 1993).

Diagnostic inaccuracy may also result from misattribution of symptoms. It is always critical to remember that the core symptoms of ADHD are common behaviors that can arise for a variety of reasons. For instance, these symptoms may be transitory, particularly in young children, resulting from normal developmental tasks (e.g., entry into structured formal schooling) or in response to stressors. Recent research has identified a percentage of children who are diagnosed early in childhood but who no longer meet criteria shortly thereafter. For instance, Taylor, Sandberg, Thorley, and Giles (1991) reported that 37 percent of 6- and 7-year-olds showed a lack of significant ADHD symptoms nine months after diagnosis. Biederman and his colleagues (1996) identified a small subset (8%) of a population of ADHD children who showed remission of symptoms prior to age 12 years. These "early remitters" or non-persistent ADHD children were characterized by a lack of familial patterning, reduced family conflict and psychopathology, and lack of comorbidity. It is unclear whether these examples of "transient" ADHD represent mild forms of the disorder or short-lived flare-ups of symptomatology brought on by other factors. In either case, care must be taken to assess other reasons for commonly occurring increases in overactivity and inattention.

Diagnosis is also complicated by the variety of psychiatric and neurological conditions that include the core symptoms of ADHD among their defining criteria or as associated conditions. Of most importance are other disruptive disorders and mood and anxiety problems. In ODD, the pattern of refusal to comply with requests can be mistaken for inattention (e.g., not listening), and the intrusive, annoying behavior may appear as impulsive. In addition, common associated characteristics of ADHD include symptoms of ODD such as temper outbursts (mood lability), low frustration tolerance (easily annoyed), and angry, hostile behavior.

Anxious children may show a pattern of restlessness and an inability to concentrate; however, they tend not to show the pervasive and persistent pattern of disturbance in core symptoms. They rarely show impulsive behavior. Stressful life events can lead to transitory increases in ADHD-like symptoms. Symptoms of depression in children such as psychomotor agitation, lack of concentration, and sleep problems could be viewed as related to ADHD if not investigated thoroughly. Temporal aspects of these symptoms are important in distinguishing their source. Lack of concentration is more pervasive in depressive illness, not a function of the interest value of the activity as it is in ADHD. Conversely, the agitation of depressed children and adolescents is less consistent and does not have the early onset of overactivity seen in ADHD. Sleep problems in ADHD rarely involve insomnia, as they do in depression; rather, ADHD children tend to prolong bedtime to garner more attention and display early-morning rising.

A thorny diagnostic issue involves distinguishing ADHD and Bipolar Disorder. Symptomatic overlap includes distractibility, impulsivity, hyperactivity, and emotional lability, particularly irritability (Carlson, 1984). The relatively chronic presentation of manic symptoms, their mixture with depressive symptoms, and the lack of euphoria creates an "atypical" clinical picture of bipolar disorder in children and makes the discrimination from ADHD more difficult. Several differences emerge, however. First, the overactivity of bipolar children tends to be more goal-directed and the impulsivity in pursuit of pleasurable activities (often with adverse consequences), whereas in ADHD children these symptoms tend to be more pervasive. Feelings of grandiosity tend to be rare in ADHD children and they are less likely to show agitation or belligerence as part of their emotional lability. In a recent study, Wozniak et al. (1995) found that 98 percent of children diagnosed with clinically significant manic episodes also met criteria for ADHD while only 20 percent of a comparison ADHD group also received a mania diagnosis. Of note, the children with mania had significantly more ADHD symptoms than did ADHD children. Thus, mania is not a particularly common correlate of ADHD; however, the presence of both types of problems appears to signal a more severe disorder.

Children with undetected learning problems may respond to their lack of understanding and difficulties in processing by daydreaming and inattention to class activities. They may garner more rewards from interactions with peers and therefore appear disruptive and impulsive.

ASSESSMENT

It is rare to see a "simple" ADHD case in the outpatient child and adolescent psychiatry setting. The high rate of comorbidity, the many other reasons why the common symptoms of ADHD can arise, and the importance of associated problems in the course of the illness call for multiple-informant and wide-ranging assessment of behavior, medical-developmental history, a family assessment, and, when necessary, psychological/neuropsychological testing.

Behavioral Assessment

Behavioral checklists from home and school are mandatory in the assessment of ADHD. Because of the high levels of comorbidity and associated problems, we strongly suggest that, for initial evaluation, broad band instruments, such as the Child Behavior Checklist (CBCL) (Achenbach, 1991a) (see chapter 20, Individual Psychotherapy with Adolescents, for further information) be employed, coupled with more specific ADHD symptom checklists. The latter are listed and evaluated in Table 1.

Interviews

The interview with parents sets the tone for the rest of the evaluation and subsequent treatment. Besides providing symptom information, it can also allow the gathering of data that can focus later assessment activities (differences between parental views of the problems, level of family distress, parental personality and conflict). Barkley (1991) published a useful compendium of instruments for the assessment of ADHD as an addition to his scholarly handbook (1990) which includes a clinical interview form for parents as well as relevant checklists and informational handouts.

Medical/Developmental Evaluation

An adequate review of pre-and perinatal events, developmental progression in motor, sensory, and speech and language areas, and health history are important as in any psychiatric evaluation. However, certain areas should be covered in detail in an ADHD evaluation. First, a thorough understanding of the child's genetic history provides important diagnostic clues given that twin, adoption, and segregation analyses indicate the strong familiarity of the disorder. We have found that asking these questions often elicits feelings from parents that one of them was "just like" the patient when growing up and that they still suffer from ADHD symptomatology. It is important to assess for other mental health problems in the family given the greater incidence of substance abuse, antisocial behavior, and depression in relatives of ADHD probands.

Second, it is important to rule out medical conditions that may contribute to the ADHD symptoms or may affect treatment options. For instance, a high percentage of children with

Table 1   Selected Behavioral Assessment Measures for ADHD
a. Ratings

Title & author	Description	Age range	Strengths and weaknesses
ADD-H Comprehensive Teacher's Rating Scale–2nd Edition (ACTeRS-2; Ullman, Sleator, & Sprague, 1991)	Screening device (5-point scale) comprised of 24 items clustered under 4 dimensions (attention, hyperactivity, social skills, oppositional behavior) and 2 additional 2-item sets tapping peer acceptance and need for teacher's attention. Separate profiles for males and females.	K–6th grade	Adequate internal consistency and test-retest and inter-rater reliability. Helpful in diagnosing attention disorders with and without hyperactivity as well as distinguishing ADHD from LD. Useful in monitoring treatment effects.
Attention Deficit Disorders Evaluation Scale (ADDES; McCarney & Bauer, 1989)	60-item School version and 46-item Home version. Overall percentile ranks can be obtained as well as standard scores for three factor-analytically-derived scales (inattention, impulsiveness, and hyperactivity) based on multiple age-sex standardization groups	4.5–18 years	Excellent assessment tool. High degree of reliability, internally, across raters, and across administrations. Excellent normative data. Strong discriminating power for ADHD versus non-ADHD children particularly with age-sex norms. Useful manuals to assist in development of behavioral goals and interventions linked to problem behaviors.
Children's Attention and Adjustment Survey Lambert, Hartsough, & Sandoval, 1990)	31-item (4-point scale) for each of two versions: Home (parent) and School (teacher). Provides standard scores, percentile ranks, and cutoff scores for 4 scales (inattention, impulsivity, hyperactivity, conduct problems) factor-analytically-derived for each version. Compositive ADD and ADHD scores can also be derived. Administration time: 2–5 minutes	K–5th grade	Thoughtful, research-based item development, allowing for separation of ADHD components, with good reliability and internal consistency for scales. Possibly unrepresentative normative sample, particularly for Home version, and lack of age norms reduces enthusiasm for instrument. No clear rationale for selection of cutoff scores. High false positive rate.

Table 1 (Continued)

Title & author	Description	Age range	Strengths and weaknesses
Conners' Abbreviated Symptom Questionnaire Parent and Teacher (Conners, 1993)	10-item brief versions of Conners' Parent Rating Scales (CPRS-48) and Teacher Rating Scales (CTRS-28) composed of items most frequently marked on the longer forms of hyperactive children. Scores greater than 15 identify children 2 standard deviations above the mean.	3–17 years	Widely used in clinical work and research. These forms are commonly referred to as the "Hyperactivity Index." Very sensitive to drug effects. Because of nature of items, high levels of aggressive behavior could classify a child as hyperactive.
IOWA Conners Teacher Rating Scale (Loney & Milich, 1982)	10-item, 4-point scale derived from the Conners' Abbreviated Symptom Questionnaire-Teacher Version. Consists of two 5-item subscales (inattention/overactivity and aggression). Means, standard deviations, and cutoffs provided.	6–12 years	Allows important discrimination of aggressive and attentive/hyperactive behavior. High test/retest and internal reliability. Strong validity data. Very useful, quickly administered assessment instrument for subtyping ADHD children.

seizure disorders have significant ADHD symptoms which may be worsened by the use of certain anticonvulsants. Also, medications used in the treatment of allergies, which are quite common in ADHD children, can produce impairments of attention and also make ADHD symptoms worse. Thyroid dysfunction can result in ADHD-like symptoms and questions should be asked about such problems. Recently, reports showing a high percentage of children with generalized resistance to thyroid hormone have prompted calls for routine assessment of thyroid functioning in ADHD children. However, only a very small percentage (perhaps 1%) of ADHD children exhibit GRTH and there is no statistically greater prevalence of thyroid abnormalities per se (Spencer et al., 1996). Disturbed sleep patterns are common among ADHD children. Often, because of various circumstances (oppositionality, lack of structure, individual differences) young ADHD children may be sleep-deprived which may exacerbate symptoms.

A variety of environmental influences appear linked with ADHD symptoms and need to be assessed. Maternal use of alcohol and cigarettes during pregnancy is related to the presence of inattention and overactivity in their offspring. It is not established whether this connection is causal. The relationship may merely be a reflection of the genetic ADHD link since those with ADHD use substances more than others. Lead intoxication is correlated with a higher prevalence of inattention and hyperactivity, although the relationship is weak in the general population.

Family Functioning

Children and adolescents place heavy demands on the family unit, imposing greater care-taking demands, increasing stress, producing discord, and reducing feelings of competence in their parents as well as creating maladaptive divisions and alliances. We have found it crucial to explore family structure and functioning in a separate interview, involving both parents and children. Information garnered from these interviews as well as direct obser-vation of parent-child and marital interactions provide important insights into discipline styles, resources within the family, routines, and the extent of cooperation between par-ents. We pay close attention to the levels of parental stress and the communication between and marital satisfaction of parents or caretakers. It is useful to supplement interviews with self-report instruments concerning parent perceptions of family functioning such as the Parenting Stress Index (Abidin, 1986) and the Moos Family Environment Scale (Moos & Moos, 1974).

Educational Evaluation

The high incidence of poor academic progress, learning disabilities, and inappropriate classroom behavior in ADHD children calls for careful investigation of cognitive skills and educational achievement as well as peer relationships. Checklist data from staff at the patient's school is valuable; however, we feel that contact with teachers, principals, and counselors often allows for freer exchange of information. This contact can provide reports of peer interactions, interventions that have been tried to ameliorate behavioral or learn-ing problems, clarification of parent's report of special services, and the school's plans for assessment. These reports often provide a more complete picture of the classroom perfor-mance of the child by allowing further exploration of behavioral difficulties. This more direct contact also begins the development of a relationship that facilitates the implemen-tation of school-based interventions. In gathering information, it sometimes helps to go "off the record" with school staff to allow exchange of information which they would feel uncomfortable imparting to the child's parents.

Psychological and Neuropsychological Testing

The possibility that learning or cognitive difficulties may underlie academic or behavioral problems often calls for assessment involving an intelligence test and a screen of academic achievement. These issues are discussed more completely in the chapters on Psychological Assessment (chapter 8) and Learning Disorders (chapter 16).

Several tests of attentive and executive functioning, on which ADHD children have shown deficits in performance, have become widely used in evaluations. Over the past several years, substantial progress has been made in the standardization, norm develop-ment, and psychometric properties of these instruments. The most useful tasks continue to be based on vigilance or continuous performance tasks (CPT), first developed in the 1950s, which require close monitoring of rapidly presented stimuli for certain targets for several minutes. Several CPT systems are now commercially available such as the Gordon Diagnostic System (GDS; Gordon, 1983) and the Conners' Continuous Performance Test (Conners, 1994). However, it is important to note that no single score on these tests should be the sole determinant of a diagnosis of ADHD. The rate of false negatives (children with ADHD who score within normal limits on these tests) is high. Because the false positive rate (children without ADHD who score over the clinical cutoff score) is low, it is best to view these tests as strong confirmatory evidence for a diagnosis of ADHD, integrating with other clinical information.

We have employed the CPT along with several other neuropsychological tasks to assess different aspects of attentive functioning (Mirsky, Anthony, Duncan, Ahearn, & Kellam, 1991), such as the ability to focus, sustain, and shift attention. Patterns of deficits on the attention performance tasks were linked to different types of behavioral profiles and academic problems, suggesting the usefulness of a comprehensive battery in devising. For instance, while some children might need to be taught to maintain task orientation and inhibit impulsive responding by considering alternatives, others might need help in avoiding distraction or in maintaining and manipulating information in active memory.

TREATMENT

The heterogeneous nature of the group of children who fall under the diagnosis of ADHD and their wide range of associated problems makes it unlikely that a single treatment will produce significant, long-term, generalizable positive outcomes. This will likely be the case for most cases referred to a child and adolescent outpatient setting. A survey of a random sample of pediatricians who treated ADHD children in their practices showed that 98 percent prescribed methylphenidate (Kwasman, Tinsley, & Lepper, 1995). Therefore, it is likely that the 20 percent to 40 percent of children referred to specialists were not responding completely to the medication regimen coupled with brief family counseling. Children with ADHD presenting in an outpatient setting exhibit a wide range of associated, functional deficits, comorbidity, and family backgrounds and characteristics which argues for a multimodal treatment approach specific to their circumstances.

We believe strongly that a family approach is the most effective way to treat ADHD in children and adolescents. First, family problems are often the reason that outpatient treatment is sought, particularly in adolescent patients. The presence of an ADHD child is disruptive to family functioning, presenting serious management problems, sparking interactional conflicts and negative communication patterns, engendering sibling resentment because of their excessive demands on parent time, and leading to increased stress on parents and their relationship. Outcome studies show that chronic family conflicts represent one of the strongest predictors of later maladjustment (Barkley et al,, 1991; Hechtman, Weiss, Perlman, & Amsel, 1984); therefore, these problems need to be approached directly. Second, setting the treatment in the family context reduces the feeling that ADHD children have of being "the problem" and it is our experience that it increases compliance with interventions. Third, the family emphasis reinforces the need for a coordinated effort to attack problems and act as a family, reducing sometimes destructive alliances, and avoids the sense that the therapist, family, and patient have separate roles to play.

Psychopharmacological Interventions

Pharmacotherapy for children and adolescents was first employed for ADHD problems in the 1930s. The various alternative medications to address core symptoms of ADHD are covered in depth in chapter 10, Forensic Community Child and Adolescent Psychiatry. Particular issues concerning the use of medication with ADHD children are briefly mentioned in the following discussion.

Stimulants The widespread use of stimulant drugs stems from numerous demonstrations of their short-term efficacy in reducing the frequency and intensity of core ADHD

symptoms in the classroom, improving peer- and parent-child interactions, and in laboratory tasks of attention, memory, and learning. Stimulants have also been shown to reduce
aggressive behavior and antisocial acts in conduct-disordered adolescents and improve peer
status.

Although large, the corpus of work on stimulant treatments is largely limited to the
effects of methylphenidate in Caucasian, latency-age males (Spencer et al., 1996). At least
in the latter age group, there appear to be few differential effects between methylphenidate
and other stimulants. Anecdotal accounts and clinical lore report that pemoline is not
as effective as methylphenidate; however, as suggested by Pelham, Swanson, Furman,
& Schwindt (1995), this belief may have stemmed from the use of low initial dosages.
Estimates of the number of nonresponders hovers around 25 percent to 30 percent with
some age variation; although robust effects have been observed in adolescents, more variable outcomes have been reported in the few studies of preschoolers (Mayes, Crites, Bixler,
Humphrey, & Mattison, 1994).

Many parents claim good success at school with stimulants but are plagued by angry, defiant, and emotionally labile behavior in the afternoon and evening. The lack of
cross-site effectiveness appears partly the result of dosing effects; the usual twice a day
regimen (morning and noon) results in the effects wearing off at night sometimes resulting
in heightened levels of core symptoms accompanied by emotional lability and oppositionality. Treatment options for these interdose "rebound effects" include manipulating the
time of the administration, adding a third dose in the late afternoon, switching to long-
acting preparations of stimulants, or using alternative medications, such as antidepressants
or beta-blockers. Rebound effects are not easy to ameliorate. It is likely that family issues
can serve to exacerbate symptomatology and reduce the effectiveness of the stimulants.
Modification of evening schedules and demands can often have significant positive effects.

It is important to note that short-term effects on target behaviors (e.g., on-task behavior, aggressive behavior) are often not matched by positive longer-term effects on academic
achievement, peer, teacher, and family relations, school failure, and antisocial behavior.
Limitations of the few outcome studies may account in part for the lack of findings of long-
term effects (Elia, Borcherding, Rapoport, & Keysor, 1991; Schachar & Tannock, 1993).
However, it is our view that the often dramatic decrease in core symptoms may reduce emphasis on important comorbid conditions, attributional issues, educational concerns, and
family issues..

Antidepressants   Tricyclic antidepressants have been shown to be effective in the
treatment of core behavioral symptoms of ADHD for children, adolescents, and adults,
although less positive response has been noted on cognitive symptoms. Direct comparisons between tricyclics and stimulants have produced about equal distribution of findings
showing an advantage for one or the other (Spencer et al., 1996). Responses to other antidepressants, such as monoamine oxidase inhibitors, fluoxetine, and venlafaxine, appear less
robust or produce more significant side effects. Recent evaluation of bupropion has been
encouraging; however, it has been associated with a greater risk for seizures, particularly
when used with high doses.

Other Medications   Clonidine and the more selective α_2-noradrenergic agonist
gaunfacine have shown positive effects on impulsive and hyperactive behaviors of ADHD
children (Hunt, Arnsten, & Asbell, 1995). These compounds, particularly clonidine, are

short-acting and sedating and have uncertain effects on cognitive symptoms. Anti-anxiety drugs have not been shown to have major effects on ADHD symptoms.

Psychosocial Interventions

A great deal of research on ADHD treatment indicates the need for a broad-based, multimodal approach (Satterfield, Satterfield, & Cantwell, 1981). Limiting therapy to one approach (e.g., stimulant treatment, parent training, social skills training, or individual therapy) has simply not proven effective (e.g., Abikoff, 1991). For example, we have found too often that practitioners, patients, and parents concentrate heavily on the minutiae of medication management and ignore larger psychosocial issues. As noted previously, we have found it most helpful to ground multimodal efforts at the family level. Surprisingly, little emphasis has been placed on family-based approaches to address the multiple difficulties of ADHD children and adolescents at school and home.

The family model of treatment has several goals. First, it allows a clearer understanding of the systemic nature of the effects that an ADHD child has on a family and the negative feedback loops that act to maintain defiant and oppositional behavior and conflictual interactions. Second, it reduces the emphasis on the ADHD child as the source of all the problems, which can impede progress. Third, through in vivo demonstration and role-playing, it promotes mutual problem solving and more adaptive communication, areas often lacking in ADHD families. Fourth, it helps to realign hierarchies and alliances within the family. A defiant ADHD child may have gained too much power or one parent may have aligned too closely with the child, diluting parental discipline.

Within the family model, we often work initially with the parents, providing basic educational information concerning ADHD, including school issues, then moving to behavioral training modules based on Barkley's 10-step program (Barkley, 1987). These modules cover attending and ignoring skills, reward systems, response cost, and timeouts. Once some control over the child's behavior is established, parents often feel an increase in competence and self-esteem and view their child's behavior as less extreme (Anastoupouls, Barkley, & Shelton, 1996). Homework assignments are a critical part of this process since the aim is to develop individualized programs, carefully crafted with feedback from parents after implementing them at home. This initial phase of treatment can often occur in a group setting. We have found that parents find it particularly helpful and supportive to interact with others experiencing the same kind of problems. Within the context of the behavioral management modules, children, the identified patient, and siblings are brought in to develop a sense of family commitment to improving functioning.

Several other types of intervention have proved successful in reducing conflict within families and can be incorporated into the family behavioral therapy approach. Robin and Foster (1989) promote a problem-solving communication training program which helps family members generate multiple solutions to conflict and evaluate them reasonably, learn more direct, unambiguous means of communication, and identify and reframe irrational beliefs about each other. Since boundary issues and unhealthy alliances are a common feature of ADHD families, structural therapy techniques have been used successfully to alter alignments.

Besides family conflict, peer rejection and disapproval have been shown to be strongly predictive of later maladaptation in ADHD children and children in general (Parker & Asher, 1987). In social skills training, cognitive-behavioral techniques, such as self-monitoring and self-evaluation, have been used to increase the awareness of ADHD children of their own negative and aggressive behavior with others and to promote more proso-cial acts. Hinshaw (1996) developed a group procedure in which children earn reinforce-ment by the closeness of a match between their rating of their attainment of a criterion level of social behavior with that of an adult observer. Although developed for use in a group context, the program can be transferred to school and home situations. Social behavior can also be advanced through cognitive-behavioral anger management training, because ADHD children are often the recipients of a great deal of teasing. Hinshaw points out that the feedback and reinforcement from adults are important therapeutic components of these programs.

Educational Intervention

The high incidence of academic underachievement and school behavior problems in ADHD youngsters demands significant outreach into the schools in the form of teacher consultation on behavioral management, efforts to improve peer relationships, and involve-ment in the development of individual educational plans. One of the first tasks is to promote a more positive teacher-student relationship, which often has degenerated into negative commands and a sense of frustration on both sides. This process often begins with provid-ing information on ADHD to improve the teacher's grasp of the nature, course, outcome, and etiology of the disorder. Erroneous information can often lead to teachers' views that disruptive behavior is completely intentional, caused by a lack of home discipline, and/or only modifiable by medication. There are many brief and accessible publications aimed at teachers as well as videotape presentations. Goldstein (1994) provided detailed suggestions for the development of school-based behavioral interventions.

Behavioral interventions have been used to modify disruptive and off-task activity; however, to be successful, these must be tailored to the specific target behaviors of the child and the demands of the particular classroom. Interventions that require close moni-toring and record keeping and the delivery of frequent rewards may not be possible in a classroom of 40 children. To begin with, frequent contact between the outpatient thera-pist and the teacher may be necessary to train the teacher, provide support, and monitor implementation. Parents should be involved in the development of the behavioral plan in order to integrate with the program they have developed at home. An initial face-to-face meeting with teacher, parent, and child producing a written "contract" is a good way to ensure everyone's understanding of the plan. For older children, cognitive behavioral tech-niques, such as the self-monitoring and self-evaluation procedures outlined previously, can be included in the overall plan.

Pfiffner & Barkley (1990) lay out general classroom management principles for ADHD children and carefully outline teacher-and peer-administered behavioral interven-tions as well as home-based programs to help at school. The latter interventions are par-ticularly important because they promote parent investment in the school program and open communication lines between parents and teachers. In a typical program, a daily or weekly report (formal or informal) indicating whether goals for the occurrence of positive behaviors and non-occurrence of negative behaviors has been met. Targets may be aca-demic (e.g., completion of work), behavioral (e.g., staying in seat) or social (e.g., playing appropriately) and parents reward achievement of goals. These home-based contingencies are less taxing on teachers' time; however, the combination of classroom and home-based contingencies has proven most effective.

ADHD children often are in need of special services (academic resource help, occupational therapy, speech and language services); however, these needs may not be recognized because of the salience of the behavioral problems they present. Therefore, it is critical that a child displaying academic underachievement be fully evaluated for possible learning disabilities. Parents need to be advised on how to pursue such evaluation. Without comorbid learning or emotional difficulties, an ADHD child is unlikely to qualify for special education services as the regulations are currently constituted. In some school districts, ADHD qualifies as a handicap under section 504 of the 1990 Individuals with Disabilities Education Act (IDEA) and a specific educational plan can be written to mandate reasonable accommodations in terms of class materials (e.g., assignments provided in advance), physical facilities (e.g., preferential seating), teaching modifications (e.g., more time to complete tasks), and necessary related services (e.g., guidance services, reading resource help).

CONCLUSION

Conceptualization of ADHD has progressed from a narrow view of problems of overactivity and inattention confined to latency-age children to one recognizing the lifelong nature of the disorder, the significance of the many associated problems to prognosis, and the complicating presence of various comorbid conditions. Assessment procedures in the outpatient setting must reflect this broader view, employing a comprehensive approach and well-developed behavioral assessment instruments in order to adequately describe and classify the often complicated symptom picture. Treatment of ADHD children and adolescents has also progressed, albeit in a slower fashion, from a focus on stimulant medications or single psychosocial interventions to one acknowledging the need for a broad-based and intensive approach. Therapists must extend traditional notions of intervention and use family and group modalities and make significant outreach efforts to modify school and home environments.

REFERENCES

Abidin, R. R. (1986). The Parenting Stress Index (2nd ed.). Charlottesville, VA: Pediatric Psychology Press.

Abikoff, H. (1991). Cognitive training in ADHD children: Less to it than meets the eye. *Journal of Learning Disabilities, 24*, 205–209.

Abikoff, H., Courtney, M., Pelham, W. E., & Koplewicz, H. S. (1993). Teachers' ratings of disruptive behaviors: The influence of halo effects. *Journal of Abnormal Child Psychology, 21*, 519–533.

Achenbach, T. M. (1991a). Manual for the Child Behavior Checklist/4-18 and 1991 profile. Burlington, VT: University of Vermont, Department of Psychiatry.

Anastopoulos, A. D., Barkley, R. A., & Shelton, T. L. (1996). Family-based treatment: Psychosocial intervention for children and adolescents with Attention Deficit Hyperactivity Disorder. In E. D. Hibbs & P. S. Jensen (Eds.), *Psychosocial treatments for child and adolescent disorders* (pp. 267–284). Washington, DC: American Psychological Association.

American Psychiatric Association [APA]. (1994). *Diagnostic and statistical manual of mental disorders (DSM-IV)* (4th ed.). Washington, DC: the Association.

Asher, S. R., & Coie, J. D. (1990). *Peer rejection in childhood.* New York: Cambridge University Press.

Barkley, R. A. (1987). *Defiant children: A clinician's manual for parent training.* New York: Guilford Press.

Barkley, R. A. (1990). *Attention deficit hyperactivity disorder: A handbook for diagnosis and treatment.* New York: Guilford Press.

Barkley, R. A. (1991). *Attention-deficit hyperactivity disorder. A clinical workbook.* New York: Guilford Press.

Barkley, R. A., Anastopoulos, A. D., Guevremont, D. C., & Fletcher, K. E. (1991). Adolescents with attention deficit hyperactivity disorder: Patterns of behavioral adjustment, academic functioning, and treatment utilization. *Journal of the American Academy of Child and Adolescent Psychiatry, 30*, 752–761.

Biederman, J., Newcorn, J., & Sprich, S. (1991). Comorbidity of attention deficit hyperactivity disorder with conduct, depressive, anxiety, and other disorders. *American Journal of Psychiatry, 148*, 564–577.

Biederman, J., Faraone, S., Milberger, S., Curis, S., Chen, L., Marrs, A., Ouellette, C., Moore, P., & Spencer, T. (1996). Predictors of persistence and remission of ADHD in adolescence: Results from a four-year prospective follow-up study. *Journal of the American Academy of Child and Adolescent Psychiatry, 35*, 343–351.

Carlson, G.A. (1984). Classification issues of bipolar disorders in childhood. *Psychiatric Developments, 2*, 273–285.

Conners, C. K. (1993). *Conners' Abbreviated Symptom Questionnaire Parent and Teacher.* North Tonawanda, NY: MHS.

Conners, C. K. (1994). *Conners' Continuous Performance Test.* North Tonawanda, NY: MHS.

Elia, J., Borcherding, B. J., Rapoport, J. L., & Keysor, C. S. (1991). Methylphenidate and dextroamphetamine treatments of hyperactivity: Are there true nonresponders? *Psychiatry Research, 36*, 141–155.

Goldstein, S. (1994). *Understanding and Managing Children's Classroom Behavior.* New York: John Wiley.

Gordon, M. (1983). *The Gordon Diagnostic System.* Boulder, CO: Clinical Diagnostic Systems.

Hechtman, L., Weiss, G., Perlman, R., & Amsel, R. (1984). Hyperactives as young adults: Initial predictors of outcome. *Journal of the American Academy of Child Psychiatry, 23*, 250–260.

Henker, B., & Whalen, C. K. (1989). Hyperactivity and attention deficits. *American Psychologist, 44*, 216–223.

Hinshaw, S. P. (1996). Enhancing social competence: Integrating self-management strategies with behavioral procedures for children with ADHD. In E. D. Hibbs & P. S. Jensen (Eds.), *Psychosocial treatments for child and adolescent disorders* (pp. 285–309). Washington, DC: American Psychological Association.

Hunt, R. D., Arnsten, A. F. T., & Asbell, M. D. (1995). An open trial of guanfacine in the treatment of attention-deficit hyperactivity disorder. *Journal of the American Academy of Child and Adolescent Psychiatry, 34*, 50–54.

Kwasman, A., Tinsley, B. J., & Lepper, H. S. (1995). Pediatricians' knowledge and attitudes concerning diagnosis and treatment of attention deficit and hyperactivity disorders: A national survey approach. *Archives of Pediatric and Adolescent Medicine, 149*, 1211–1216.

Lambert, N., Hartsough, C., & Sandoval, J. (1990). *Children's Attention and Adjustment Survey.* Minneapolis, MN: American Guidance Service.

Leonard, H. L., Meyer, M. C., Swedo, S. E., Richter, D., Hamburger, S. D., Allen, A. J., Rapoport, J. L., & Tucker, E. (1995). Electrocardiographic changes during desipramine and clomipromine treatment in children and adolescents. *Journal of the American Academy of Child and Adolescent Psychiatry, 34*, 1460–1468.

Loney, J., & Milich, R. (1982). Hyperactivity, inattention, and aggression in clinical practice. In M. Wolraich, & D. K. Routh (Eds.), *Advances in developmental and behavioral pediatrics* (Vol. 3). Greenwich, CT: JAI Press.

Mayes, S., Crites, D., Bixler, E., Humphrey, F., & Mattison, R. (1994). Methylphenidate and ADHD: Influence of age, IQ, and neurodevelopmental status. *Developmental Medicine and Child Neurology, 36*, 1099–1107.

McCarney, S. B., & Bauer, A. M. (1989). *Attention Deficit Disorders Evaluation Scale.* Columbia, MO: Hawthorne Educational Services.

Mirsky, A. F., Anthony, B. J., Duncan, C. C., Ahearn, M. B., & Kellam, S. G. (1991). Analysis of the elements of attention: A neuropsychological approach. *Neuropsychology Review, 2*, 109–145.

Moos, R. H., & Moos, B. S. (1974). Manual for the Family Environment Scale. Palo Alto, CA: Consulting Psychologists Press.

Morgan, A. E., Hynd, G. W., Riccio, C. A., & Hall, J. (1996). Validity of DSM-IV ADHD predominantly inattentive and combined types: Relationship to previous DSM diagnoses/subtype differences. *Journal of the American Academy of Child and Adolescent Psychiatry, 35*, 325–333.

Parker, J. G., & Asher, S. R. (1987). Peer relations and later personal adjustment: Are low-accepted children at risk? *Psychological Bulletin, 102*, 357–389.

Pelham, W. E., & Bender, M. E. (1982). Peer relationships in hyperactive children: Description and treatment. In K. Gadow & I. Bialer (Eds.), *Advances in learning and behavioral disabilities* (Vol. 1, pp. 365–436). Greenwich, CT: JAI Press.

Pelham, W. E., Swanson, J. M., Furman, M. B., & Schwindt, H. (1995). Pemoline effects on children with ADHD: A time-response by dose-response analysis on classroom measures. *Journal of the American Academy of Child and Adolescent Psychiatry, 34*, 1504–1513.

Pfiffner, L. J., & Barkley, R. A. (1990). Educational placement and classroom management. In R. A. Barkley, *Attention deficit hyperactivity disorder: A handbook for diagnosis and treatment* (pp. 498–539). New York: Guilford Press.

Popper, C. W. (1988). Disorders usually first evident in infancy, childhood, or adolescence. In J. A. Talbott, R. E. Hales, & S. C. Yudofsky (Eds.), *Textbook of psychiatry* (pp. 649–735). Washington, DC: American Psychiatric Press.

Richters, J. E., Arnold, L. E., Jensen, P. S., Abikoff, H., Conners, C. K., Greenhill, L. L., Hechtman, L., Hinshaw, S. P., Pelham, W. E., & Swanson, J. M. (1995). NIMH collaborative multisite multimodal treatment study of children with ADHD: I. Background and rationale. *Journal of the American Academy of Child and Adolescent Psychiatry, 34*, 987–1000.

Robin, A. L., & Foster, S. (1989). *Negotiating parent-adolescent conflict.* New York: Guilford Press.

Satterfield, J. H., Satterfield, B. T., & Cantwell, D. P. (1981). Three-year multi-modality treatment study of 100 hyperactive boys. *Journal of Pediatrics, 98*, 650–655.

Schachar, R., & Tannock, R. (1993). Childhood hyperactivity and psychostimulants: A review of extended treatment studies. *Journal of Child and Adolescent Psychopharmacology, 3*, 81–97.

Spencer, T., Biederman, J., Wilens, T., Harding, M., O'Donnell, D., & Griffin, S. (1996). Pharmacotherapy of attention-deficit hyperactivity disorder across the life cycle. *Journal of the American Academy of Child and Adolescent Psychiatry, 35*, 409–432.

Taylor, E., Sandberg, S., Thorley, G., & Giles, S. (1991). The epidemiology of childhood hyperactivity. New York: Oxford University Press.

Ullman, R. K., Sleator, E. K., & Sprague, R. L. (1991). *ADD-H Comprehensive Teacher's Rating Scale—2nd Edition.* Chicago: Riverside Publishing Co.

Wilcox, C. L., Anthony, B. J., Feldstein, S., Rebok, G. W., & Mirsky, A. F. (1997). The relationship between attention and social status. Manuscript submitted for publication.

Wolraich, M. L., Hannah, J. N., Pinnock, T. Y., Baumgaertel, A., & Brown, J. (1996). Comparison of diagnostic criteria for attention-deficit hyperactivity disorder in a county-wide sample. *Journal of the American Academy of Child and Adolescent Psychiatry, 35*, 319–324.

Wozniak, J., Biederman, J., Kiely, K., Ablon, J. S., Faraone, S. V., Mundy, E., & Mendin, D. (1995). Mania-like symptoms suggestive of childhood-onset bipolar disorder in clinically referred children. *Journal of the American Academy of Child and Adolescent Psychiatry, 34*, 867–876.

Chapter 14

Conduct and Oppositional Defiant Disorders

Harinder S. Ghuman, M.D.

HISTORICAL NOTE

Prichard (1837) used the term moral insanity to designate patients with recurrent anti-social behaviors who were not blatantly psychotic. Healy and Bronner (1926) described delinquents as having "psychic constitutional deficiency." Bowlby (1944) described various types of delinquent boys including affectionless character, the most common. Jenkins and Hewitt (1944) developed their theoretical frame of reference employing psychoanalytic concepts and identified three types of conduct disorders including unsocialized aggressive reaction, socialized delinquent reaction, and overanxious reaction.

In the *Diagnostic and Statistical Manual (DSM-I)* (1952) there was no separate diagnosis describing behavior disorders in children and adolescents. The diagnosis of "sociopathic personality: antisocial reaction" was codified. In *DSM-II* (1968), a new set of diagnoses under the category of behavior disorders of childhood and adolescence, was designed. This category was divided into three diagnoses: (a) runaway reaction, (b) unsocialized aggressive reaction, and (c) group delinquent reaction of childhood (adolescence). In *DSM-III* (1980), conduct disorder was identified as a diagnosis in describing children and adolescents who showed repetitive and persistent patterns of conduct in which either the basic rights of others or major age-appropriate societal norms or rules were violated. This disorder was divided into four subtypes: (a) undersocialized, aggressive; (b) undersocialized, non-aggressive; (c) socialized, aggressive; and (d) socialized, non-aggressive. The diagnosis of oppositional disorder was offered for the first time in describing children and adolescents with a pattern of disobedient, negativistic, and provocative opposition to authority figures but without violation of basic rights of others or major age-appropriate societal norms or rules.

In *DSM-III-R* (1987), the four subtypes of conduct disorder were replaced by three subtypes: (a) solitary aggressive type, (b) group type, and (c) undifferentiated type. The severity was rated as mild, moderate, or severe. The diagnosis of Oppositional Disorder was renamed as Oppositional Defiant Disorder with a revised criteria comprised of a single index of symptoms selected to describe the various manifestations of this disorder better.

CONDUCT DISORDER

In *DSM-IV* (1994), Conduct Disorder has been defined as a repetitive and persistent pattern of behavior of a person in which the basic rights of others or major age-appropriate societal norms or rules are violated. These behaviors are further grouped into four categories: (a) aggression to people and animals, (b) destruction of property, (c) deceitfulness or theft, and (d) serious violation of rules. The disturbance in behavior must cause clinically significant impairment in social, academic, or occupational functioning. Conduct disorder is divided into childhood-onset type and adolescent type. Conduct disorder can be further specified as mild, moderate, or severe depending upon the severity of conduct problems.

Prevalence

- Males under age 18 years range from 6 percent to 16 percent; for females, 2 percent to 9 percent (*DSM-IV*).
- Rutter, Tizard, and Whitmore in 1970 reported prevalence rate of 4.2 percent among 10-11 years olds in the Isle of Wight study, and the rate was four times higher in boys than in girls.
- Offord, Boyle, and Racine (1991) studied children from 4 to 16 years old in the Province of Ontario, Canada and found an overall rate of 5.5 percent of conduct disorder; male to female ratio was 4:1.

Clinical Presentation

Typically, conduct disorder patients are brought for evaluation by their parents as a result of concerns regarding the child's behavior problems at home and/or school, poor performance in school, and/or legal involvement. Other conduct disorder patients are referred by juvenile services for psychiatric evaluation and treatment. In some of these latter cases it is not unusual to notice the absence of parental involvement, frequent placements of the child outside the home, and/or denial or lack of understanding of the child's problems by the parents.

Common presenting behavior problems include aggression toward peers, teachers, and family members, truancy from school, not following parental directions and staying out late at night, running away, stealing, destruction of property, car theft, and substance abuse. Other behavior problems include fire setting, cruelty to animals, rape, aggression, and, occasionally, murder. The behavioral manifestation of conduct disorder varies with age as the individual acquires physical strength, mobility, and cognitive and sexual abilities. There is gender variation in the presentation of behavior problems in conduct disorder. Males with conduct disorder commonly present with aggression, stealing, and discipline problems in school whereas females are more likely to present with lying, truancy, running away, substance abuse, and prostitution.

During the interview, conduct-disordered children and adolescents often come across as obnoxious, unmotivated, challenging, threatening, boasting about their acting-out behavior, and sometime openly aggressive toward the clinician. This behavior often results in the clinician spending less time with the patient and thereby potentially missing various vulnerabilities and comorbid conditions. Lewis (1991) warned that the clinician must be especially careful not to allow a negative transference to get in the way of performing a thorough, unbiased evaluation.

There is a need for careful and thorough information collection regarding family, medical, and developmental history. Family history is frequently positive for substance abuse, psychiatric illness, and legal problems. Often these children are born to unwed teenage mothers. The majority are unplanned and some unwanted. During pregnancy, there may be history of substance abuse by the mother and often poor prenatal care. A history of neglect, abuse, abandonments, and losses with frequent changes in caregivers and multiple placements including early institutionalization is not uncommon. Developmental milestones are often delayed. And a history of hyperactivity, attentional, and learning problems is not uncommon with conduct-disordered patients. The clinician should look for a history of birth trauma, lead poisoning, head injury, and seizure disorder.

During the interview, the clinician needs to pay attention to signs and symptoms of organic, affective, and psychotic disorders even if these signs and symptoms fail to meet criteria for these disorders. Many conduct-disordered patients have been noted to suffer from borderline psychosis, paranoid ideation, mood disorders, substance abuse, borderline intelligence, and learning disorders. The clinician should carefully assess the suicidal and homicidal potential of conduct-disordered patients. Shaffer (1974) reported antisocial behavior in 75 percent of the adolescents who had committed suicide in his psychological postmortem study.

Etiology and Pathogenesis

Social and Family Factors   Sociological theories attempting to explain antisocial behavior include: (a) Socioeconomic disadvantages turn the person to crime, and (b) Antisocial behavior reflects the values of a delinquent subculture (however, studies on gangs seems to contradict this second theory.). Friedman, Mann, and Friedman (1975) reported that the most powerful predictor of gang membership was violent behavior of the youngster prior to joining a gang.

Parental factors include sociopathy and alcoholism in parents, especially the father (Robins, 1966; Rutter 1984), level of aggressiveness of the father (Huesmann, Eron, Lefkowitz, & Walder, 1984), psychoses in parents (Lewis, Shanok, & Balla, 1981), inconsistent discipline by parents, and a chaotic home situation. Often, the histories of conduct-disordered children reveal physical and sexual abuse by caregivers. These parental factors often interfere in a child's ability to trust and to develop close relationships, a value system, and the capacity to delay gratification or impulse and not to act out.

Biological Factors   Genetic studies report higher rates of 47 XYY (Jacobs, Price, Richmond, & Ratcliff, 1971) and XXY Klinefelter's syndrome (Nielsen & Fischer, 1965) in institutionalized offender population. Hutching and Mednick (1974) studied the records of adopted-away offspring of criminal and noncriminal fathers and found that offspring of criminal fathers reared apart from the biological fathers were more likely to become antisocial; the children at greatest risk, however were those with criminal biological and adoptive fathers.

Hormonal studies have looked at the relationship of testosterone levels and aggressive behavior in males. Mattsson, Schalling, Olwens, Low, & Svensson, (1980) reported slightly higher levels of testosterone in incarcerated recidivist juvenile delinquent males. Biochemical studies indicate an association between a decreased amount of serotonin in the CNS and aggressive behavior (Virkkunen, DeJong, Bartko, Goodwin, & Linnoila, 1989). Lewis (1991) wrote about the likelihood of adverse medical histories in delinquent youngsters including head trauma, seizures, and abnormal EEG findings.

Diagnostic Evaluation

A comprehensive psychiatric evaluation is necessary before making a diagnosis of conduct disorder because of clinical, social, and prognostic implications of this disorder as well as the complexity of comorbid diagnoses including ADHD, depressive disorders, and learning disorders, among others. It is important to know the nature and circumstances under which the behavior occurs, and how much control the child has over the behavior. There is need for careful assessment of family structure and role of the family in the child's behavior and what interventions have been tried and the outcome of these interventions.

A detailed medical history including history of seizure, injuries, and abuse is essential. A neurological workup, head CT and MRI, and EEG may be necessary if there is a history of head injury and a possibility of seizure activity. Psychological testing can be helpful to assess cognitive functioning and to rule out other disorders. Because exposure to lead contributes to behavior problems, it is important to obtain a lead level. Urine drug screen may be necessary if drug abuse is suspected.

Differential Diagnosis

Attention-Deficit/Hyperactivity disorder children may show disruptive behavior as a result of their hyperactivity and impulsivity but they do not generally violate age-appropriate societal norms and engage in aggressive behavior. Manic episodes in children and adolescents can be distinguished from conduct disorder based on the episodic course and symptoms of a manic episode including abnormality of mood, grandiosity, decreased need for sleep, flight of ideas, distractabilty, psychomotor agitation, and other factors.

Oppositional defiant disorder children show disobedience and opposition to adult authority, and difficulty getting along with peers but they do not usually engage in severe aggression and violation of societal norms or rules. Adjustment disorder with disturbance of conduct should be considered if behavioral problems are time-limited and developed in clear association with the onset of a psychosocial stressor.

CLINICAL COURSE AND PROGNOSIS

Several studies have looked at predictors, prognostic signs, and outcome of conduct disorder. Richman, Stevenson, and Graham (1982) reported that high levels of activity and management difficulties at age 4 years were associated with conduct disorder at age 8 years. Lefkowitz, Eron, Walder, & Huesmann (1977) reported that aggressive behavior at age 8 years was one of the best predictors of adolescent aggression. West & Farrington (1973) found 27 percent of children rated by peers and teachers as having troublesome behavior at age 8 years and 10 years became delinquent during adolescence compared to 0.7 percent not perceived as troublesome. White, Moffitt, and Silva (1989) indicated the presence of above-average intellectual functioning and achievement as a good prognostic sign.

Rutter's (1984) review of follow-up studies indicated that a minority of conduct disturbances in childhood become antisocial personality disorders as adults. Robins' (1966)

30-year follow-up study of all the behavior-disordered children referred to the child guidance clinic at St. Louis found that only 28 percent were later diagnosed as sociopathic as adults. Robins (1966) and Loeber & Dishion (1983) reported early age of onset to be related to more serious and persistent antisocial behavior. Robins found that children whose conduct disorder onset occurs before age 11 years were twice as likely to receive a diagnosis of antisocial personality disorder in adulthood as those with an onset after age 11.

According to Lewis (1991), youngsters under 18 years of age commit a disproportionate number of crimes. In 1987, of all arrests five percent were children under 15 years of age, 16 percent under age 18 years, and 29 percent of arrests for crime considered most serious by the FBI were committed by children under 18 years of age. Yeager and Lewis (1990) found that the death rate for 118 incarcerated delinquents in a seven-year follow-up study was 58 times the expected rate and all seven deaths were from violent causes.

TREATMENT

It is important to decide whether the treatment should take place in an outpatient, inpatient, residential, or day hospital setting. This depends upon the severity of the patient's behavior and the family's ability to provide structure and support to the child. If the child is involved with the juvenile justice system, the probation officer and in relevant cases the juvenile master/judge must be contacted. For those children who are court-referred, the clinician must set clear guidelines regarding treatment and behavioral expectation from the child and parents. The clinician should also coordinate care with the probation officer and court to support the implementation of these guidelines. A close alliance between the clinician and probation officer as well as a balance of optimal consequence for the child's antisocial behavior and treatment interventions is absolutely essential to maximize a successful outcome.

Because of the complexity of biopsychosocial factors, a multimodal treatment approach in treating children and adolescents with conduct disorder is necessary. This includes several factors examined in the following discussion.

Psychotherapy

The goal of individual psychotherapy goal is to help conduct-disordered children establish a close, warm, and trusting relationship with an adult, something they often are lacking. As a result of their past traumatic experiences with adults, these children have a great deal of difficulty developing close relationships despite their overwhelming need for them. Therapists often get overwhelmed and distracted by the conduct-disordered child's behavior and by their own countertransference feelings. If the therapist is able to establish a relationship with a conduct-disordered child, however rudimentary it may be, the therapy can gradually be expanded to include identification and expression of various feelings, worries, and needs, to develop coping skills and an understanding of reasons for the acting out behavior, the short- and long-term consequences of behaviors, alternatives to acting out, and developing a value system. A functional family therapy approach has been applied in treating conduct-disordered children, adolescents, and their families. This approach is to improve direct communication, to create supportive behavior among family members, and to utilize positive reinforcement of socially acceptable behavior.

Behavioral Interventions

Parent Management Training   Several parent training programs have been found effective in changing aggressive antisocial behavior, especially in younger children (Kazdin, 1985). In these programs parents of conduct-disordered children are asked to describe the child's positive and aversive behavior, to make a record of the frequency of this behavior, and to respond contingently and consistently. The clinician can teach parents by using various means including interviewing, role playing, modeling, problem solving, guided practice, and homework assignments. Parents are taught positive and negative reinforcement, ignoring and distraction, and contingency contracting techniques. These techniques can be taught individually, in groups, and in a variety of settings including the child's home.

Social Skill Training   In social skill training programs, children are asked to practice pro-social skills, for example, how to deal with common social situations like resisting peer pressure, and are provided training in communication skills necessary for positive relationships (Bierman, Miller, & Stabb, 1987).

Problem-Solving Skills   Based on considerable evidence that conduct-disordered children tend to distort social reality and do not make proper use of their cognitive abilities, problem-solving skills training is directed toward modifying children's thought processes and their self-statements (Meichenbaum & Goodman, 1971), identifying problems, understanding causation and consequences, and considering alternatives. Comprehensive and multifaceted interventions like multisystemic treatment (Henggeler & Borduin, 1990) have been found useful in treating conduct-disordered youngsters. Interventions are present-focused and action-oriented, and address intrapersonal and systemic factors.

Medication

The choice of a psychopharmacological agent in the treatment of conduct-disordered patients is entirely based on controlling aggressive behavior and/or symptoms of comorbid diagnoses. There is no specific medication, in contrast to affective disorder and ADHD, for example. Various neuroleptic agents including chlorpromazine, thioridazine, haloperidol, molindone, and, more recently, risperidone and clozapine have been found effective in controlling aggressive behavior in children and adolescents (Stoewe, Kruesi, & Lelio, 1995). Neuroleptic agents in low dosage maintenance may be more effective with conduct-disordered patients who show paranoid presentation, some impairment in reality testing, and, often, bordering psychosis. Neuroleptic agents in higher dosages are also useful during acute agitated states. The risk of tardive dyskinesia, cognitive blunting, neuroleptic malignant syndrome, and various other side effects must be weighed against the consequences of the aggression and the use of alternative medication.

Clonidine is becoming increasingly popular in the treatment of aggression in children and adolescents and has shown promising results (Kemph, Devane, Levin, Jarecke, & Miller, 1993). Lithium carbonate has been found effective in treating explosively aggressive conduct disordered children (Campbell, Small, Green, Jennings, Perry, Bennett, & Anderson, 1984). Buspirone has been found effective in dealing with aggression in adult mentally retarded and neurologically impaired cases as well as in one case report of an 8-year-old male with conduct disorder and ADHD (Quaison, Ward, & Kitchen, 1991). Anticonvulsants including phenytoin, carbamazepine, and valproic acid have been used in treating aggression in children and adolescents and these may be more effective in treating conduct-disordered patients with seizure disorder or borderline EEG and neurological findings. Stimulants are useful in treating aggression along with ADHD symptoms. Depression is often a comorbid disorder with conduct disorder and these patients may respond to the use of antidepressants.

OPPOSITIONAL DEFIANT DISORDER

In *DSM-IV*, Oppositional Defiant Disorder has been defined as a recurrent pattern of negativistic, hostile, and defiant behavior toward authority figures lasting at least six months. The disturbance causes significant impairment in social, academic, or occupational functioning. The behaviors do not occur exclusively during the course of a psychotic or mood disorder.

Prevalence

The rate of oppositional defiant disorder in children and adolescents has not been carefully studied. Rates of 2 percent to 16 percent have been reported in the past (*DSM-IV*). The disorder is more common in males before the onset of puberty.

Clinical Presentation

The oppositional defiant child is often brought by the child's parents because of their concerns regarding the child's behavior and or concerns of the child's teacher. The common presenting behavior problems include frequent loss of temper, excessive arguments with the parents and teachers, persistent testing of limits, and actively defying or refusing to comply with the requests or rules of the parents and teachers.

In addition, these patients are often provocative and deliberately annoying with their verbal and physical interaction to peers, siblings, and adults which sometime can lead to fights. They are not, however, generally involved in serious physical aggression as observed in conduct disorder. They show poor or erratic academic performance and as they grow old, there are often interpersonal problems, especially difficulty in following directions, leading to poor work skills and performance.

Defiance and oppositional behavior to a certain extent is common in the 18- to 36-month-old child and again during adolescence as a part of normal development when the child or adolescent is faced with conflicting desires regarding autonomy, control, and dependency. A diagnosis of oppositional disorder is made only if the behavior is extreme.

During the interview, the oppositional defiant child may not follow the clinician's directions, may get easily annoyed, and is sometime provocative by actively defying rules and limits of the office or clinic. There are times that symptoms of this disorder may not be obvious in the presence of or in interactions with the clinician who is a stranger to the child. As in conduct disorder, the clinician has to be careful not to allow negative feelings to get in the way of a thorough evaluation.

Etiology and Pathogenesis

Psychosocial Factors   Oppositional defiant disorder, especially in males, tends to be more common among those who, in the preschool years, have difficult temperament or high motor activity. Reid and Hendrick (1973) reported that parents of the oppositional child tend to be more irritable than parents of either normal or conduct-problem children. They talk with each other less than do normals and frequently behave as if the other person has not interacted with them when, in fact, they have. They are also more irritable when they talk to each other. One can hypothesize that this combination of a difficult, temperamental child and an irritable parent, especially during developmental periods when a child is more defiant and oppositional, sets up a vicious cycle in which the parent and child bring out the worst in each other. Often, parents of the oppositional child respond with punitive anger, thereby running the risk of reinforcing the child's defiance. Oppositional disorder is more common in families in which child care has been disrupted, child rearing practices are harsh, inconsistent, or neglectful, and there is serious marital discord.

Biological Factors   There is little information regarding genetic, hormonal, biochemical, or neurological factors affecting oppositional defiant disorder.

Diagnostic Evaluation

In addition to obtaining a comprehensive present, past, family, medical, and developmental history, it is important to get information from the parents and teachers regarding the frequency of each symptom and the setting in which these symptoms occur. It is also important to know what, if any, intervention has been tried, for how long, and its results. One can use the child behavior checklist (CBCL) and parent's and teacher's daily or weekly report to evaluate and monitor the child's behavior. During the interview, the clinician should carefully evaluate and determine that the oppositional behavior is not a result of, or part of, other serious psychopathology such as mood disorders, psychosis, or conduct disorder.

The child's family needs to be carefully assessed about child rearing practices, parental consistency or inconsistency in setting limits, and parental conflicts regarding separation, autonomy, and controls.

Psychological and educational testing, and medical workup may be necessary in cases where there is the possibility of a comorbid diagnosis complicating the clinical picture.

Differential Diagnosis   Conduct disorder can be distinguished from oppositional disorder by the more severe nature of behavior problems including violence toward people and animals and serious violation of societal rules and individual rights of others.

Attention-Deficit/Hyperactivity disorder often demonstrates disruptive behavior in children because of inattention and impulsivity, and often co-occurs with oppositional defiant disorder.

Oppositional defiant behavior is a common associated feature of mood and psychotic disorders and should not be diagnosed separately if symptoms occur exclusively during a mood disorder or psychotic episode. Oppositional defiant disorder should also be distinguished from oppositional behavior which occurs as a part of the normal developmental stages of early childhood and adolescence.

Course

Oppositional defiant disorder is usually evident before age 8 years with gradual onset of symptoms at home. Later on, symptoms occur in school and other settings. A significant number of cases turn out to be conduct disorder over time. In a four-year follow-up study of childhood disorders, Cantwell and Baker (1989) reported the poorest recovery rate for oppositional disorder.

Treatment

Behavioral Interventions   The clinician should work with the child and parents in developing a behavior program by defining the troublesome behaviors in a simple and concrete manner, selecting one or two target behaviors, generating a list of small tangible rewards the child can pick for points earned on a daily or weekly basis, and setting up a behavior charting system. The parents should be advised to combine praise and encouragement with points and rewards. Brief time-outs, if used appropriately, can be useful in reducing the frequency and intensity of problem behaviors.

Psychotherapy   Individual psychotherapy can be useful in gaining the child's trust, helping the child express feelings appropriately, improving self-esteem, and helping the child learn new ways to assert himself or herself in a nonoppositional fashion. Family therapy can be useful when parents are conflated about issues of autonomy and control, and inconsistent in setting limits.

CONCLUSION

Conduct disorder continues to be a controversial diagnosis and presents a challenge to child and adolescent psychiatrists because of poorly understood etiology, the role of racial and socioeconomic factors, the poor response to traditional treatment interventions, a resistance by some health providers to treating the disorder, poorly coordinated interventions by departments of juvenile justice and mental health providers, and insurance companies' reluctance or refusal to reimburse for treatment. The clinician needs to carefully assess conduct-disordered youngsters for comorbid disorders and be acutely aware of bias and countertransference issues in working with conduct-disordered children and adolescents. Treatment must be comprehensive, addressing biopsychosocial needs of the patient; the crux of the treatment is to provide structure, set limits, and support and coordinate services among the various agencies involved.

Oppositional defiant disorder has been considered a milder form of conduct disorder. It seems that a number of children and adolescents with oppositional defiant disorder become conduct-disordered. There is a need for improved clarification regarding the relationship of these two disorders as well as their relationship to personality disorders. A major focus in the treatment of oppositional defiant disorder is behavioral and family interventions.

REFERENCES

American Psychiatric Association. (1952), (1968), (1980), (1987), and (1994). *Diagnostic and statistical manual of mental disorders* (1st, 2nd, 3rd, 3rd-rev., 4th eds.). Washington, DC: the Association.

Bierman, K. L., Miller, C. L., & Stabb, S. D. (1987). Improving the social behavior and peer acceptance of rejected boys: Effects of social skills training with instructions and prohibitions. *Journal of Consulting and Clinical Psychology, 55*, 194–200.

Bowlby, J. (1944). Forty four juvenile thieves: Their characters and home life. *International Journal of Psychoanalysis, 25*, 19–53.

Eyberg, S., & Boggs, S. R. (1989). Parent training for oppositional-defiant preschoolers. In C. E. Schaefer & J. M. Briesmeister (Eds.), *Handbook of parent training: Parents as cotherapists for children's behavior problems* (pp. 105–132). New York: John Wiley & Sons.

Campbell, M., Small, A., Green, W., Jennings, S. J., Perry, R., Bennett, W. G., & Anderson, L. (1984). Behavioral efficacy of haloperidol and lithium carbonate – a comparison in hospitalized aggressive children with conduct disorder. *Archives of General Psychiatry, 41*, 650–656.

Cantwell, D. P., & Baker, L. (1989). Stability and natural history of DSM-III childhood diagnosis. *Journal of the American Academy of Child and Adolescent Psychiatry, 28*, 691–700.

Friedman, C. J., Mann, F. & Friedman, A. S. (1975). A profile of juvenile street gang members. *Adolescence, 40*, 563–607.

Healy, W. & Bronner, A. F. (1926). *Delinquents and criminals, their making and unmaking. Studies in two American cities.* New York: Macmillan.

Henggeler, S. W., & Borduin, C. M. (1990). *Family therapy and beyond: A multisystemic approach to treating the behavior problems of children and adolescents.* Pacific Grove: Brooks/Cole.

Huesmann, L. R., Eron, L. D., Lefkowitz, M. M., & Walder, L. O. (1984). Stability of aggression over time and generation. *Developmental Psychology, 20*, 1120–1134.

Hutching, B., & Mednick, S. A. (1974). Registered criminality in the adoptive and biological parents of registered male criminal adoptees. In S. A. Mednick, F. Schulsinger, J. Higgins, & Bell, B. (Eds.), *Genetics, environment and psychopathology.* Amsterdam: Elsevier.

Jacobs, P. A., Price, W., Richmond, S., & Ratcliff, R. A. W. (1971). Chromosome surveys in penal institutions and approved schools. *Journal of Medical Genetics, 8*, 49–53.

Jenkins, R. L., & Hewitt, L. (1944). Types of personality structure encountered in child guidance clinics. *American Journal of Orthopsychiatry, 14*, 84–94.

Kazdin, A. E. (1985). *Treatment of antisocial behavior in children and adolescents.* Homewood, IL: Dorsey.

Kemph, J., Devane, C., Levin, G., Jarecke, R., & Miller, R. L. (1993). Treatment of aggressive children with clonidine: Results of an open pilot study. *Journal of the American Academy of Child and Adolescent Psychiatry, 32*, 577–581.

Lefkowitz, M. M., Eron, L. D., Walder, L. O., & Huesmann, L. R. (1977). *Growing up to be violent: A longitudinal study of aggression.* Oxford: Pergamon Press.

Lewis, D. O. (1991). Conduct disorder. In M. Lewis (Ed.), *Child and adolescent psychiatry* (pp. 561–572). Baltimore: Williams & Wilkins.

Lewis, D.O., Shanok, S., & Balla, D.A. (1981). Parents of delinquents. In D. O. Lewis (Ed.), *Vulnerabilities to delinquency* (pp. 265–295). New York: Spectrum.

Loeber, R., & Dishion,T. J. (1983). Early predictors of male delinquency: A review. *Psychological Bulletin, 94*, 68–99.

Mattsson, A., Schalling, D., Olweus, D., Low, H., & Svensson, J. (1980). Plasma testosterone, aggressive behavior and personality dimensions in young male delinquents. *Journal of the American Academy of Child Psychiatry, 19*, 476–491.

Meichenbaum, D. H., & Goodman, J. (1971). Training impulsive children to talk to themselves: A means of developing self-control. *Journal of Abnormal Psychology, 77*, 115–126.

Nielsen, J., & Fischer, M. (1965). Sex-chromatin and sex abnormalities in male hypogonadal mental patients. *British Journal of Psychiatry, 111*, 641–647.

Offord, D. R., Boyle, M. C., & Racine, Y. A. (1991). The epidemiology of antisocial behavior in childhood and adolescence. In D. J. Pepler & K. H. Rubin (Eds.), *The development and treatment of childhood aggression* (pp. 31–54). Hillside, NJ: Lawrence Erlbaum.

Prichard, J. C. (1837). *A treatise on insanity and other disorders affecting the mind.* Philadelphia: Haswell, Barrington and Haswell.

Quaison, N., Ward, D., & Kitchen, T. (1991). Buspirone for aggression. *Journal of the American Academy of Child and Adolescent Psychiatry, 30*, 1026.

Reid, J. B., & Hendricks, A. F. C. J. (1973). A preliminary analysis of the effectiveness of direct home intervention for treatment of predelinquent boys who steal. In L. Hamerlynck, L. Handy, & E. Mash (Eds.), *Behavior therapy: Methodology, concepts, and practice.* Champaign, IL: Research Press.

Richman, N., Stevenson, J., & Graham, P. J. (1982). *Pre-school to school: A behavioral study.* London: Academic Press.

Robins, L. N. (1966). *Deviant children grown up.* Baltimore: Williams & Wilkins.

Rutter, M., Tizard, J., & Whitmore K. (1970). *Education, health and behavior.* London: Longmans.

Rutter, M. (1984). Family and school influences: Meaning, mechanisms and implications. In R. A. Nicol (Ed.), *Longitudinal studies in child psychology and psychiatry: Practical lessons from research experiences* (pp. 357–403). Chichester, England: Wiley.

Shaffer D. (1974). Suicide in childhood and early adolescence. *Journal of Child Psychology and Psychiatry, 15,* 275–291.

Stoewe, J. K., Kruesi, J. P., & Lelio, D. F. (1995). Psychopharmacology of aggressive states and feature of conduct disorder. *Child and Adolescent Psychiatric Clinics of North America, 4,* 2, 359–379.

Virkkunen, M., DeJong, J., Bartko, J., Goodwin, F. K., & Linnoila, M. (1989). Relationship of psychobiological variables to recidivism in violent offenders and impulse fire setters. *Archives of General Psychiatry, 46,* 600–603.

Yeager, C. A., & Lewis, D. O. (1990). Mortality in a group of formerly incarcerated juvenile delinquents. *American Journal of Psychiatry, 147,* 612–614.

West, D. J., & Farrington, D. P. (1973). *Who becomes delinquent?* London: Heinemann Educational.

White, J. L., Moffitt, T. E., & Silva, P. A. (1989). A prospective replication of the protective effects of IQ in subjects at high risk for juvenile delinquency. *Journal of Clinical and Consulting Psychology, 57,* 719–724.

Chapter 15

Alcohol and Substance Abuse in Children and Adolescents

Steven L. Jaffe, M.D. and Robin J. Mogul, M.D.

INTRODUCTION AND EPIDEMIOLOGY

Following a downward trend from the 1980s through 1992, adolescent alcohol and substance abuse is on the rise. According to a 1994 survey by the National Institute on Drug Abuse (NIDA)(Johnston, O'Malley, & Bachman, 1993, 1995), the peak annual prevalence rate (i.e., the use of any illicit drug one or more times in the prior 12 months) among high-school seniors in 1979 was 54 percent, and in 1992 was 27 percent.

Specifically for marijuana, the peak annual prevalence rates were 51 percent and 22 percent respectively. In 1994 the peak annual prevalence rate increased to 32 percent, while marijuana increased even further to 40 percent, with 3.6 percent of the students admitting to daily use. In the two years from 1992 to 1994 alone, a 66 percent increase in the marijuana-use prevalence among 10th graders was reported, as was a 45 percent increase among 8th graders, with 0.7 percent admitting to daily use. By 1995 almost one in twenty (4.6%) of high school seniors reported daily use.

There has indeed been a sharp increase in marijuana use, but most alarming is the increase in all illicit drug use by the early adolescent population. The peak annual prevalence rate for 8th graders is now almost double that of 1991. The substances most abused by adolescents include alcohol, tobacco, marijuana, cocaine, stimulants, LSD, and inhalants, with alcohol being the most abused. Over 90 percent of high school students have admitted to at least trying alcohol; moreover, approximately 28 percent of high school seniors, 24 percent of 10th graders, and 14.5 percent of 8th graders admitted to heavy drinking (i.e., having imbibed five or more consecutive drinks on at least one occasion in the two weeks prior to the survey). In 1994 the rates of recent use (use within the past 30 days) for 12th, 10th, and 8th graders was 50 percent, 39 percent, and 26 percent, respectively. From surveys of problem drinking, approximately 30 percent of adolescent males report patterns of problem drinking, and 26 percent of 8th graders report having been drunk at least once. Alcohol use still seems to be the highest, however, among college students and young adults.

Cocaine use peaked in 1986, perhaps related to the advent of crack cocaine in 1985, but has subsequently decreased. There has been a slight increase in adolescent abuse between 1994 and 1995; however its use is highest among young adults (Chatlos, 1996). LSD, while epidemic in the 1960s, decreased in use secondary to severe, detrimental reactions. A newer, less potent form called blotter acid, however, has led to its resurgence. A single sheet of blotter paper may contain one hundred "hits" of acid selling between $2.00 and $5.00/hit, named for its color (for example blue, yellow, or red blotter) or for its image (such as tulip, happy face, or even Christian crosses). Increases in annual prevalence rates for 8th, 10th, and 12th graders in the years 1991 to 1993 are as follows: 1.7 percent to 2.4 percent, 3.7 percent to 5.2 percent, and 5.2 percent to 6.9 percent, respectively. This translates to a 41 percent increase in use among 8th and 10th graders, and a 33 percent increase among 12th graders. Overall, 1 percent of 8th graders, 2 percent of 10th graders, and 3 percent of 12th graders have used LSD.

Use of inhalants, such as glue, solvents, gasoline, fluorocarbons (freon), Scotch-guard®, and even household bleach has also risen in recent years with use highest among 8th graders. According to the NIDA survey, 11.7 percent of 8th graders in 1994 admitted to inhalant use in the past year, an increase from 9 percent in 1991. The 1994 rates of recent use among 8th, 10th, and 12th graders were 6 percent, 4 percent, and 3 percent, respectively. Inhalants are associated with many serious medical complications ranging from "sudden sniffing death" to encephalopathy, diffuse brain atrophy, and dementia (Dell, 1996).

The most frequently used substance is tobacco. In 1993, use among 8th graders was at 8 percent, 10th graders at 14 percent, and 12th graders at 19 percent. As with tobacco use, adolescents tend to use alcohol and drugs in an inverse relationship to their recognition and understanding of the risk of harm. There also is an age-related progression with substances of abuse. Adolescents typically move from beer and wine/wine coolers to hard liquor, to marijuana followed by other illicit substances (Kandel, 1975). Since early use directly correlates with later degree of use and with the use of more than one drug, the increase in use of all substances by 8th graders is an alarming trend.

Geographic and socioeconomic status (SES) appears to have little to do with drug use, with two exceptions: higher SESs tend to use more marijuana than lower SESs and the highest SESs have LSD prevalence rates twice that of the lowest SESs.

DIAGNOSIS

Adolescent substance abuse differs from that of adults because adolescents almost invariably abuse multiple drugs. They are also 40 percent to 90 percent more likely to have co-morbid psychiatric disorders when compared to the general adolescent population. Disruptive behavior disorders such as oppositional defiant disorder, conduct disorder, and ADHD accompany substance abuse more often than not. Mood disorders, anxiety disorders (especially phobias and panic), PTSD, bulimia nervosa, and schizophrenia often coexist as well (Bukstein, Brent, & Kaminer, 1989). This is not surprising since substance abuse is one of the many disorders manifesting in adolescence and/or early adulthood.

In a study of hospitalized substance abusing youths, 82 percent had comorbid diagnoses not necessarily recognized at admission; specifically, 61 percent suffered mood disorders, 54 percent conduct disorder, 43 percent oppositional defiant disorder, 8 percent ADHD, and 3 percent schizophrenia (Stowell & Estroff, 1992). Thus, one cannot expect to treat substance abuse/dependency without treating the comorbid psychiatric disorders and vice-versa.

The definition of substance abuse and dependence is provided by the *Diagnostic and Statistical Manual, 4th Edition (DSM-IV)* (American Psychiatric Association [APA], 1994). While this is a useful guide in identifying adolescents with patterns of substance abuse/dependence, it is important to recognize that the criteria were actually based on and developed for the adult population. The diagnosis of substance abuse requires a maladaptive pattern of recurrent use resulting in significant levels of distress or impairment in functioning resulting in failure to meet major role obligations. Substance dependence involves larger amounts of required substances as tolerance increases, despite physical or psychosocial problems caused or exacerbated by the substance (APA, 1994). Adolescents, unlike adults, rarely exhibit withdrawal symptoms (Martin, Kaczynski, Maisto, Bukstein, & Moss, 1995). Increasing preoccupation with obtaining, using, and recovering from the substance often is evidenced by giving up previously important activities and spending more time in use-related activities.

Abuse must be differentiated from use. The use and/or possession of illicit substances although illegal does not equate with abuse/dependence. Substance use by adolescents is not a disorder, despite the substance-induced intoxication that often leads to changes in mood (from depressive to euphoric), cognition (from impaired attention and concentration to delusions), and behavior (such as disinhibition, agitation, hypervigilance, and somnolence) (Jaffe, 1990). Substance use can lead to family and interpersonal conflicts as well as academic failures. It can also lead to risk-taking behaviors such as driving while inebriated, stoned on marijuana, or tripping on LSD, not to mention early and promiscuous sexual behaviors which put adolescents at risk for both pregnancy and sexually transmitted diseases including HIV. Legal problems often ensue as well. Although not necessarily pathological, substance use can interfere with the developmental tasks of adolescence (Baumrind & Moselle, 1985).

FACTORS INFLUENCING ABUSE

Adolescents appear to be particularly at risk for substance abuse. The National Institute of Mental Health (NIMH)-sponsored Epidemiologic Catchment Area (ECA) community survey determined a 13.5 percent lifetime prevalence rate for alcohol abuse or dependence and a 6.1 percent rate for other drug abuse or dependence. The probability of onset for drug/alcohol abuse or dependence peaked in the 15-to 19-year-old range with a median age of drug use onset at 18 and alcohol use onset at 21 years.

There are risk factors that predispose adolescents to substance abuse, with perhaps the foremost being the developmental task of adolescence itself. In the process of forming their own identity, preparing for individual and societal relationships encompassing marriage, parenthood, and jobs, adolescents experiment with, or "try on" a variety of attitudes and behaviors including experimenting with psychoactive substances (commonly alcohol and cigarettes, known as "gateway" substances) in a social context. Most adolescents will experiment with gateway substances, with some advancing to more serious levels of substance use, a process known as "progression" (Kandel, 1975). In contrast to adults, teenagers often do not give up the drug of the previous stage but continue to use it along with the new drug. One exception to this pattern of staged progression is the use of inhalants by 8th graders, which peaks in the 8th grade. Donovan and Jessor (1983) have elaborated on the stages of progressive use to range from non-use of drugs or alcohol to non-problem use of alcohol, to use of marijuana, to involvement in problem drinking, to use of one or more pills (amphetamines, barbiturates, or hallucinogens) and to use of hard drugs (cocaine or heroin). Depressive mood has been found to be related to the onset of marijuana use and has predicted the use of other drugs by marijuana users.

The Federal Anti-Drug Abuse Act of 1986 (amended in 1988), outlined the following as predisposing risk factors to substance abuse: parental substance abuse, teenage pregnancy, mental health problems, victims of physical, sexual, or psychological abuse, attempted suicide, involvement in violent or delinquent acts, dropping out of school, being homeless or a runaway, and being economically disadvantaged (Chatlos, 1996). Other important risk factors include parental tolerance of use, poor attachment between parent and child/adolescent, lack of parental involvement in the child's/adolescent's life, peer substance abuse or peer tolerance of use, greater orientation of the child/adolescent to peers instead of parents, difficult temperament with early childhood disruptive behavior problems (especially aggressive, impulsive, and risk-taking behaviors), poor academic achievement, school failure, poor self-esteem, low SES, high population density with high crime rate, and physical deterioration of the community.

Genetic and biochemical, physiological, and neurodevelopmental factors are equally important. There is a 54 percent concordance rate for alcoholism in identical twins compared to a 28 percent rate in fraternal twins. Adopted sons of biological alcoholic fathers are four times more likely to develop alcoholism than controls. Only 20 percent of biological sons of alcoholics become alcoholics themselves however; thus the genetics are multifactorial (Donovan, 1986). Alcohol elimination rates, activity levels of alcohol dehydrogenase, and EEG differences have also been found suggesting that substance abusing individuals obtain different levels of reinforcement from their drugs of choice as compared to controls (Pihl, Peterson, & Finn, 1990).

MANIFESTATIONS OF ABUSE

As originally outlined by MacDonald (1984), the progression of drug use in adolescents follows four stages:

- Stage 1: Experimental use
- Stage 2: Regular use
- Stage 3: Preoccupation with use/Substance abuse
- Stage 4: Substance dependence/Compulsive use

Experimental use often begins in junior high school with associated peer pressure to just "try" alcohol (usually beer), marijuana, or inhalants. The setting can be virtually anyplace (home, school, party) or simply "hanging out." After getting high on a small amount of the drug, the adolescent returns to a normal mood without difficulty. The adolescent has learned, however, that drugs can affect mood, and now associates drug use with activation of the pleasure centers of the brain.

Regular use often progresses to hard liquor or drinking to get drunk as a means of coping or activating the pleasure centers of their brains again. Drinking now occurs midweek, and more alcohol is required as tolerance develops; missing school or work as a result of hangovers is not uncommon. Different drugs including hallucinogens and pills are tried and non-using friends are dropped. Money may be stolen from family to buy drugs, and lying ensues to cover up drug use. Mood changes are rapid and interest in normal activities change.

By the substance abusing stage, problems have arisen in many areas of the adolescent's life. Preoccupation with drug use results in failures at home, school, work, and play, oftentimes leading to legal problems. Despite the negative inter-/intrapersonal consequences caused by or worsened by drugs, repeated use continues. Mood and behavior changes fluctuate because of drug cravings.

Substance dependence involves increased tolerance and larger amounts of drug use and/or harder drugs. Preoccupation with drug use intensifies as do problems in the adolescent's life. Attempts to cut down or quit fail, and use occurs simply to feel normal. Use is now compulsive and out of control. Most adolescents fortunately do not progress to stage four; however, stages one through three can be equally as debilitating and potentially fatal when one considers that 80 percent of teenage deaths are a result of accidents, homicides, and suicides with 50 percent of these being drug- or alcohol-related.

TREATMENT AND MANAGEMENT

The primary goal in treating adolescents with substance use/abuse disorders is abstinence, although there is some debate regarding controlled use similar to adult alcoholics and controlled drinking. Treatment must involve much more than just abstinence or even controlled use however; for even if the drug is removed, the learned drug behaviors such as mistrust, cravings, and impulsiveness still persist, as do the intra-/interpersonal problems or comorbid psychiatric disorders which affect virtually every domain of the adolescent's life. Treatment programs that deal with all the coexisting problems associated with substance use/abuse have, not surprisingly, improved abstinence and lower relapse rates (Friedman & Beschner, 1985).

Unlike adult programs, treatment for adolescents must be geared toward their cognitive and social developmental tasks; peer orientation is crucial, as is the dependent status of the adolescent within his or her family system. Treatment should encourage family involvement as well as improved communication and parenting skills in a culturally and socioeconomically sensitive fashion. The adolescents and their families need to work together in developing an alcohol- and drug-free lifestyle which necessitates uncovering and treating parental addiction as well.

There are four basic treatment settings: acute/intensive inpatient (either hospital or freestanding rehabilitation-based), residential (either group homes or long-term therapeutic communities), intensive outpatient/partial hospitalization programs (PHP), or outpatient and community-based programs. The "decision tree" or criteria considered in determining the appropriate treatment setting is dependent not only on the stage of addiction or progression, but the ability and motivation of the adolescent to work and remain safe within the least restrictive environment. This is directly related to his or her individual need for structure and limit-setting, family and social supports, and comorbid psychiatric disorders.

Outpatient Treatment: The Least Restrictive

The adolescent who is only involved in experimental or social use of substances does not fulfill diagnostic criteria for abuse but is at high risk, and therefore, requires education and counseling. Education is for both the adolescent and his or her parents and should include accurate drug and alcohol information including the detrimental effects, as well as the addiction process itself, encompassing predisposing risk factors, identifying enabling systems, and determining at what stage of progression the adolescent resides. Counseling, generally once or twice weekly, should target the adolescent's drug use and, in conjunction with education, should clarify misinformation and demystify myths; facilitating alternative choices and behaviors so that the adolescent will be able to remain alcohol-, tobacco-, and drug-free. Any coexisting psychiatric disorders identified in the evaluation process should be addressed by a mental health professional as well. Family counseling is needed so that parents set appropriate limits and modify/reinforce appropriate behaviors leading to abstinence.

Outpatient Treatment: More Restrictive

The adolescent who has progressed to more regular use requires an abstinence contract, usually for one month, in which he or she agrees to abstinence from drugs and drug behaviors (i.e,. drug paraphernalia, violation of curfew, and so on) and regular urine drug screening. Also known as an "honest look contract," this contract affords the adolescent who claims he or she "will have no problem stopping" an opportunity to confirm or refute the need for additional treatment (Bailey, 1996). Because the adolescent's lack of motivation is often tied to a systemic enabling system, a failed abstinence contract helps break the circle of denial and encourages the entire family to seek help. Family therapy in addition to individual and group therapy is integral to treatment at this stage (even in the absence of a familial enabling system) because the adolescent is a part of a family system. (Kaufman, 1979).

Partial/Day Hospitalization

By the time an adolescent is preoccupied with substance use, he or she meets diagnostic criteria for substance abuse and, in addition to earlier described interventions, requires a more intensive outpatient treatment setting. Partial/day hospitalization provides the same level of care as inpatient hospitalization without having the adolescent stay overnight. This proves ideal for adolescents having stable family or social supports in place.

Adolescents in partial hospitalization will usually attend self-support groups as part of their treatment including 12-step programs such as CA (Cocaine Anonymous), AA (Alcoholics Anonymous) and/or NA (Narcotics Anonymous) which introduce the adolescent to the self-support group process available in their communities. This serves to remind the adolescent of the negative consequences of use/relapse and the benefits of abstinence, but even more importantly provides him or her with a new peer group that includes those in recovery, as well as older members who can serve as role models and sponsors. The 12-step philosophy is grounded in the belief that an addict must first recognize his or her problem with substances and acknowledge that he or she cannot overcome the addiction without the help of spiritual awareness and growth. Components of the program include lectures and assignments based on the 12-step work and group therapy. Once again, as with all adolescent treatment, the work must be relevant to their developmental tasks and concerns. *The Step Workbook for Adolescent Chemical Dependency Recovery-A Guide to the First Five Steps* does this not only for substance abuse but for dual diagnosis as well (Jaffe, 1990). This workbook provides concrete questions that the adolescent answers in written form as they work their steps. These answers are then verbalized and discussed in individual and group therapies.

When Outpatient Treatment Fails: Inpatient Treatment

Adolescents meeting criteria for chemical dependency often require intensive inpatient treatment. Failure of previous intensive outpatient settings, such as a partial hospitalization program, necessitates a higher degree of support and structure in assessing and treating the adolescent because a deeper level of resistance, denial, or even an acute crisis might be in play, perhaps compounded by an unsupportive family or sabotaging social system, and/or even a more serious underlying psychiatric or psychosocial problem. Furthermore, although rare in adolescents, physical addiction to alcohol, sedatives, and minor tranquilizers can lead to a potentially life-threatening withdrawal syndrome necessitating detoxification. Adolescents generally do not require detoxification however, despite a 50 percent increase in tolerance, because they tend to be in better physical health than most adults, abuse multiple drugs, and the drugs they most commonly abuse (i.e., marijuana, LSD, and cocaine) do not require psychopharmacological interventions. In addition, abuse of alcohol is generally episodic which does not lead to the development of physical addiction. Nonetheless, the need for detoxification must be ruled out. Finally, it is important to assess the psychiatric status of the patient, especially those with comorbid disorders for if acutely psychotic, suicidal, homicidal, or dangerous, they would require a dual disorder program.

Residential Treatment: Longer-Term

Longer-term residential treatment settings (including group homes and halfway houses) are appropriate for adolescents with complex psychiatric and psychosocial problems. Such treatment can follow acute inpatient hospitalizations as a means of facilitating the adolescent's successful transition back into the community. Adolescents with significant histories of previous treatment failures, particularly inpatient hospitalizations, are ideal candidates for this type of treatment. Residential treatment is less restrictive than an inpatient setting yet provides a high degree of structure and support affording the adolescent an opportunity to establish stable social supports and an improved living situation (home, school, and/or employment). The duration of treatment is individually tailored to the adolescent and is dependent on his or her demonstrated motivation and ability to utilize other less-intensive treatment settings (i.e., outpatient and/or community treatment), as well as remaining abstinent and psychiatrically stable. This proves to be a very effective treatment setting in that the length of stay in residential treatment is favorably related to decreased drug and alcohol use, a similar finding to that in adult therapeutic communities.

Psychotherapeutic Interventions

Outpatient treatment encompasses individual, group, family, and multifamily therapy and generally is limited to a few sessions per week with a focus on a specific problem related to substance use/abuse and education. As previously discussed, it is an equally appropriate treatment modality for the highly motivated adolescent, with or without psychiatric comorbidity, who comes from a stable, supportive family, as well as the less fortunate adolescent with a history of previous treatment failures following intensive inpatient and/or residential treatment.

There are several different theoretical approaches to individual psychotherapy, however, Cognitive Behavioral and Psychodynamic or Interpersonal therapies are generally

used in treating addiction. Cognitive psychotherapeutic interventions have been successful in treating adolescents with depression, and although not yet systematically studied
in the adolescent substance abusing population, should prove useful in identifying cognitive distortions and negative thoughts, particularly internalized self-statements which may
lead to negative feelings and subsequent substance use/abuse behaviors (Lewinson, Clarke,
Hops, & Andrews, 1990). Cognitive-behavioral interventions have been effective in building skills for relapse prevention, substance refusal, anger control, problem solving, communication skills, and time management. For example, in relapse prevention, the adolescent
must first identify the internal and external stressors that trigger his or her substance use,
then develop coping skills to prevent relapse. Through self-awareness adolescents learn
control (Bukstein, 1993).

There are no controlled studies of psychodynamic/interpersonal psychotherapeutic
methods in substance abusing adolescents; however, interpersonal therapy appears to be
efficacious in adult cocaine and opioid users and gestalt techniques are especially effective
in substance abusing adults with personality-disordered features (Zarcone, 1980, 1984).
Regardless of the therapeutic technique used, the ingredient for success probably includes
the warmth, empathetic understanding, and unconditional regard for the patient by the therapist.

Behavioral therapy or, more specifically, operant conditioning, is used in inpatient,
residential and partial hospitalization programs. In this type of program a contract is designed in which positive reinforcers are rewarded for the attainment of prosocial behavioral
goals and abstinence, and negative consequences are established for violation of rules.
This programming provides the structure and support for the adolescent to focus on his
or her specific treatment goals and prepares him or her for contracting with parents when
discharged to home, thereby ensuring continued monitoring of the adolescent's behavior.
Parent education is obviously needed for the home contract.

There are several different theoretical orientations for group therapy as well, but
whether geared toward a deeper understanding of behavior (i.e., psychodynamic/interper-
sonal) or toward altering behavior (cognitive-behavioral), they are all grounded in the
group dynamic which affords a safe and reliable opportunity to explore relationships, dysfunctional behaviors, and unconscious processes in the "here and now." Group therapy is
ideal for adolescent treatment because groups are inherent to their developmental stage;
namely, adolescents must belong to groups and use peer relationships to validate their
thoughts and feelings, develop values and socialization skills, and grapple with autonomy
and independence in separating from parental authority into the outside world. There is
probably no other time in development where groups are as powerful in influencing the
developing self, for groups are the social reality in which adolescence takes place (Cramer
Azima & Richmond, 1989).

There are different approaches to family therapy as well, including narrative, strategic, structural, and systemic frameworks, which have been described by others. All family
therapies directed at treating substance abusing adolescents, however, despite their theoretical perspectives share common goals, namely to break down resistances to treatment and
denial about the problem (i.e., substance abuse), to facilitate abstinence by getting the adolescent into treatment, to improve communication and functioning among family members,
and to help the parents establish parental influence (i.e., structure, limit setting, monitoring of the adolescent's activities and behaviors). Family therapy also serves to uncover
and/or confront parental addiction, other family psychopathology including physical, sexual, emotional, and spousal abuse, and sabotaging coalitions. Multi-family group therapy
is another approach which serves an educational and therapeutic function.

Community Treatment

Community treatment is another branch of outpatient treatment which encompasses school-based programs, self-and/or peer-support groups (e.g., AA, NA), and day programs, which offer prosocial, supervised, drug-free recreational activities like sporting and wilderness experiences which also serve to foster a drug-free lifestyle. Self-help groups such as Al-Anon, and Parents of Teenage Alcohol & Drug Abusers (POTADA) are also available to friends and families of adolescents with substance abuse problems which, in addition, to providing support and education, also serve to lessen systemic maladaptive enabling behaviors. Regardless of the type or combination of psychotherapy used, national studies of treatment efficacy have shown outpatient treatment to be helpful (Sells & Simpson, 1979).

CONCLUSION

According to Bailey (1996), "adolescents are complex... frustrating... gratifying... obstinate... pliable, resistant and workable, fragile and resilient, exhausting and energizing, defeating and uplifting, and at all times a true challenge.... To be successful, the clinician must truly like adolescents... enjoy working with them... and must never lose sight of the fact that most adolescents who engage in treatment do so because they trust the clinician. Anything short of this may result in less than optimal treatment success." It is not clear which type of treatment ultimately works best for the adolescent substance abuser because there are few well-controlled studies comparing specific types of treatment in the adolescent literature; however, some treatment is better than none, and as Bailey alluded to so eloquently, the therapeutic relationship is the essential ingredient, proven through clinical experience and objective research.

Treatment success factors have been identified and include not only the aforementioned staff attitude(s) and training, but the availability of services, family participation, and the length of time in treatment. Conversely, failure to complete treatment has been associated with younger age of onset, abuse of multiple substances (including serious alcohol use), and deviant behavior(s); although risk factors for relapse involve thoughts, feelings, and cravings about alcohol, less involvement with school and/or work and less satisfaction with recreational activities (Catalono, Hawkins, Wells, Miller, & Brewer, 1990–1991). Keeping these risk factors in mind, treatment should be comprehensive and patient-specific, designed not only for the stage of abuse, but with consideration for the adolescent's level of motivation, familial/social supports, psychiatric comorbidity, and other psychosocial factors. Further, different outpatient treatment modalities and levels of care can be combined to provide the least restrictive setting while still affording an opportunity for success. With so many adolescents using and abusing alcohol and drugs, it is essential that clinicians working with teenagers be knowledgeable and proficient in these treatment modalities.

REFERENCES

American Psychiatric Association (APA) (1994). *Diagnostic and statistic manual of mental disorders* (4th ed.) *(DSM-IV)*. Washington, DC: the Association.

Bailey, G. (1996).Helping the resistant adolescent enter substance abuse treatment: The office intervention. In S. Jaffe (Guest Ed.), *Child and adolescent psychiatric clinics of North America, adolescent substance abuse and dual disorders* (pp.149–164.). Philadelphia: W. B. Saunders.

Baumrind, D., & Moselle, K. (1985). A developmental perspective on adolescent drug abuse. *Advances in Alcohol and Substance Abuse, 4,* 41–67.

Bukstein, O., Brent, D., & Kaminer, Y. (1989). Comorbidity of substance abuse and other psychiatric disorders in adolescents. *American Journal of Psychiatry, 146* (9), 1131–1141.

Bukstein, O. G., Van Hasselt, V. B. (1993). Alcohol and drug abuse. In Bellack A. S., Hersen (Eds.), Handbook of Behavior Therapy in the Psychiatric Setting (pp. 453–475). New York: Plenum Press.

Catalono, R., Hawkins, J., Wells, E., Miller, J., & Brewer, D. (1990–1991). Evaluation of the effectiveness of adolescent drug abuse treatment, assessment of risks for relapse, and promising approaches for relapse prevention. *The International Journal of the Addictions, 25* (9A & 10A), 1085–1140.

Chatlos, J. (1996). Recent trends and a developmental approach to substance abuse in adolescents. In S. Jaffe (Guest Ed.), *Child and adolescent psychiatric clinics of North America, adolescent substance abuse and dual disorders* (pp.1–27). Philadelphia: W. B. Saunders.

Cramer Azima, F., & Richmond, L. (1989). Preface. In F. Cramer Azima & L. Richmond (Eds.), *Adolescent group therapy*, American Group Psychotherapy Association monograph series monograph 4 (p. ix). Madison, Connecticut: International University Press, Inc.

Dell, M. (1996). Medical considerations in child and adolescent substance abuse: Medical complications, pain management, and emergency treatment. In S. Jaffe (Guest Ed.), *Child and adolescent psychiatric clinics of North America, adolescent substance abuse and dual disorders* (pp.123–147). Philadelphia: W. B. Saunders.

Donovan, J. (1986). An etiologic model of alcoholism. *American Journal of Psychiatry, 143* (1), 1–11.

Donovan, J., & Jessor, R. (1983). Problem drinking and the dimension of involvement with drugs: A Guttman Scalogram analysis of adolescent drug use. *American Journal of Public Health, 73* (5), 543–551.

Freidman, A., & Beschner, G. (Eds.) (1985). *Treatment services for adolescent substance abusers.* U.S. Department Health and Human Services Pub. No. (ADM) 85-1342, Washington, DC: U.S. Government Printing Office.

Jaffe, J. (1990). Drug addiction and drug abuse. In L. Goodman & A. Gilman (Eds.), *The pharmacological basis of therapeutics* (pp.522–573). New York: Pergamon Press.

Jaffe, S. (1990). *Step workbook for adolescent chemical dependency recovery: A guide to the first five steps.* Washington, DC: American Psychiatric Press.

Johnston, L., O'Malley, P., & Bachman, J. (1993). *National survey results on drug use from the Monitoring the Future Study, 1975–1992.* U.S. Department of Health and Human Services, National Institute on Drug Abuse. Washington, DC: U.S. Government Printing Office.

Johnston, L., O'Malley, P., & Bachman, J. (1995). *National survey results on drug use from the Monitoring the Future Study, 1975–1994.* U.S. Department of Health and Human Services, National Institute on Drug Abuse. Washington, DC: U.S. Government Printing Office.

Kandel, D. (1975). Stages in adolescent involvement in drug use. *Science, 190,* 912–914.

Kaufmann, P. (1979). Family therapy with adolescent substance abusers. In E. Kaufman & P. Kaufmann (Eds.), *Family therapy of drug and alcohol abuse* (pp. 71–70). New York: Gardner Press.

Lewinson, P., Clarke, G., Hops, H., & Andrews, J. (1990). Cognitive-Behavioral treatment for depressed adolescents. *Behavior Therapy, 21,* 385–401.

Martin, C., Kaczynski, N., Maisto, S., Bukstein, O., & Moss, H. (1995). Patterns of DSM-IV alcohol abuse and dependence symptoms in adolescent drinkers. *Journal of Studies on Alcohol, 56,* 672–680.

Pihl, R., Peterson, J., & Finn, P. (1990). Inherited predisposition to alcoholism: Characteristics of sons of male alcoholics. *Journal of Abnormal Psychology, 99* (3), 291–301.

Sells, S., & Simpson, D. (1979). Evaluation of treatment outcome for youths in the drug abuse reporting program (DARP): A follow-up study. In G. Beschner & A. Friedman (Eds.), *Youth drug abuse* (pp. 571–628). Lexington, MA: Lexington Books.

Stowell, J., & Estroff, T. (1992). Psychiatric disorders in substance abusing adolescent inpatients: A pilot study. *Journal of the American Academy of Child and Adolescent Psychiatry, 31,* 1036–1040.

Zarcone, V. (1980). An eclectic therapeutic community for the treatment of addiction. *The International Journal of the Addictions, 15* (4), 515–527.

Zarcone, V. (1984). Gestalt techniques in a therapeutic community for the treatment of addicts. *Journal of Psychoactive Drugs, 16* (1), 43–46.

Chapter 16

Pervasive Developmental Disorders and Learning Disorders

Harinder S. Ghuman, M.D., Jaswinder K. Ghuman, M.D., and
Laurence W. Ford, M.Ed.

HISTORICAL NOTE

The concept of autism originated with Kanner's 1943 publication of his classic paper, *Autistic Disturbance of Affective Contact*, in which he described detailed histories of 11 children and noted that these children showed extreme autistic aloneness, abnormalities of language, anxiously obsessive desire for the maintenance of sameness, and limitation in a variety of spontaneous activity.

In 1908, Heller reported six cases with "dementia infantilis" and in 1930 described this condition in children who—without preceding illness—had become conspicuous in their third and fourth years by becoming moody, whinny, negativistic, disobedient, and often raging without reason. In addition, he noted that these children experienced cognitive and neurological regression leading to complete loss of speech, to complete idiocy, and with many becoming incontinent.

In 1944, Asperger described a number of patients who showed severe and characteristic difficulties of social integration, unusual aspects of nonverbal communication and voice quality, unusual interests, and clumsiness of gait and gross motor functions and introduced the term "autistic psychopathy" for these children.

In 1966, Rett described a disorder confined to females who were apparently normal until age 6 to 12 months and subsequently developed a progressive loss of motor and cognitive skills, inappropriate social interactions, absence of an ability to communicate, and deceleration of head growth.

DIAGNOSTIC CLASSIFICATION

In the *Diagnostic and Statistical Manual of Mental Disorders* (1st and 2nd editions) (*DSM-I*, *DSM-II*), these disorders were diagnosed under "schizophrenic reaction, childhood type" (*DSM-I*) and "schizophrenia, childhood type" (*DSM-II*). In 1980 the concept of pervasive development disorder was introduced in *DSM-III* and categorized into infantile autism, childhood-onset pervasive development disorder, and atypical pervasive developmental disorder. In 1987, *DSM-III-R* combined the first two categories into a single category of autistic disorder and the last category was renamed as pervasive developmental disorder not otherwise specified (NOS).

In 1994, *DSM-IV* (American Psychiatric Association [APA], 1994) categorized pervasive development disorders into autistic disorder, Rett's disorder, childhood disintegrative disorder, Asperger's disorder, and pervasive development disorder, NOS.

CLINICAL PRESENTATION

Autism

According to *DSM-IV* (APA, 1994), the three major diagnostic criteria for autistic disorder include qualitative impairment in social interaction and communication, and restricted repetitive and stereotyped patterns of behavior, interest, and activities. In addition, there is a delay or abnormal functioning in at least one of the following areas prior to age 3 years: (a) social interaction, (b) language as used in social communication, or (c) symbolic or imaginative play.

Social Interaction   One of the most important clinical feature of autism is impairment in reciprocal social interaction which is manifested early and differently depending on the age of the child. For example, during infancy, autistic children may not show interest in attachment behaviors like other children who enjoy physical closeness and being picked up by their parents. Kanner mentioned that these children's fail to assume anticipatory posture preparatory to being picked up and an inability to adjust their body to the posture of the person holding them. As toddlers, these children may not follow their parents in the house, not go to their parents to seek comfort when upset or hurt, and often do not develop the bedtime kiss and cuddle routine (Rutter, 1985). These children may not manifest stranger or separation anxiety. Some of these children have been described to be happiest when left alone and easy to take care of as a babies.

As they grow up and come in contact with their peers, autistic children fail to develop age- appropriate peer relationships. They may show lack of interest in sharing activities and enjoyment or achievements with others. They may treat others as tools or mechanical aids and fail to perceive other's feelings or needs. There is lack of social or emotional reciprocity. In addition, autistic children show impairment in the use of nonverbal behavior for social interaction, particularly lack of eye-to-eye gaze.

Communication   There is marked impairment in verbal and nonverbal communication in children with autism. Autistic children may show a total lack of or a delay in the development of speech and an abnormal pattern of language development as well as language use. Alternate modes of communication such as gestures, pointing with the index finger, and mime are absent or minimal. And autistic children often fail to show social imitation and engage in imitative games like pat-a-cake.

Autistic children who speak may show marked impairment in the ability to initiate, and to engage in and sustain meaningful conversation. Their speech is often stereotyped in form and marked by I/you pronominal reversal, immediate and delayed echolalia, and idiosyncratic word usage. The speech is marked by abnormality in pitch, intonation, rate, rhythm, or stress. Autistic children show impairment in understanding spoken language and may not comprehend simple directions and questions. There is a failure to use speech for social communication and a lack of head nods, facial expressions, and gestures ordinarily used in conversational exchange.

Play   Children with autism may show play patterns with little variety or imagination and rarely involve themselves in spontaneous make-believe games or social imitative play appropriate to their developmental level.

Behavior, Interest, and Activities   Autistic children show restricted repetitive and stereotyped patterns of behavior, interests, and activities. These children may endlessly line up items or collect curious objects such as stones, rubber bands, or cans. They may spend inordinate amounts of time on one activity—e.g., collecting bus routes and train timetables or on stereotyped, repetitive movements such as finger flicking, clapping, rocking, twisting, and spinning. These children are fascinated with movements like spinning wheels of a toy car or watching electric fan movements. They insist on sameness in the environment and become extremely upset if household items are moved or if there is a change in routine. There is often an unusual interest in the smell or feel of objects. Extreme food fads are common.

Associated Features   About 75 percent of children with autism function at an intellectually retarded level and in most cases the retardation is in the moderate range (IQ 35–50). There is uneven development in cognitive skills and deficits are marked in verbal skills, especially in language comprehension. Many of these children show hyperactivity, impulsivity, short attention span, temper tantrums, aggressiveness, and self-injurious behavior. They may show high pain thresholds, an oversensitivity to sound and touch, and an exaggerated reaction to light or odors. There are abnormalities of mood and affect and inappropriate reaction to real danger and other life situations.

Autism is sometimes associated with a neurological or other general medical condition—e.g., congenital rubella, infantile spasms, tuberous sclerosis, fragile x syndrome, encephalitis, or phenylketouria. The incidence of major motor seizures in autistic children is 25 percent to 35 percent and onset of seizures is most common in early childhood, with a second peak of onset during adolescence.

CHILDHOOD DISINTEGRATIVE DISORDER

The *DSM-IV* (APA, 1994) diagnostic criteria for childhood disintegrative disorder include a normal developmental period of the child for at least the first two years followed then by a marked regression in multiple areas of functioning and a clinically significant loss of previously acquired skills. According to Rutter (1985) often there is a premonitory period of vague illness and the child then becomes restive, irritable, anxious, and overactive. This loss is marked in at least two of the following areas: expressive or receptive language, social skills or adaptive behavior, bowel or bladder control, play, or motor skills. There is qualitative impairment in social interaction, in communication, and restricted, repetitive, and stereotyped patterns of behavior, interests, and activities, including motor stereotypies and mannerisms.

Children suffering from childhood disintegrative disorder show a marked decline in intellectual functioning, often to a severe mental retardation level. Other associated features include seizure disorder and an increased frequency of EEG abnormalities. This disorder is occasionally seen in association with medical conditions such as metachromatic leukodys-trophy and Schilder's disease.

ASPERGER'S DISORDER

The diagnostic criteria for Asperger's disorder include qualitative impairment in social in-teractions and the development of restricted repetitive and stereotyped patterns of behavior, interests, and activities as described previously under autistic disorder. The children with Asperger's disorder, however, differ from autistic children in that there is no clinically sig-nificant delay in language (e.g., single words used by age 2 years, communicative phrases used by age 3 years) and in cognitive development or in the development of age-appropriate self-help skills, adaptive behavior (other than in social interaction), and curiosity about the environment in childhood. Associated features include delayed motor milestones, motor clumsiness, and various nonspecific neurological symptoms or signs.

Asperger's initial description of what he termed autistic psychopathy included abnor-malities in social interaction, "shutting off of relations between self and the outside world from start," nonverbal communication—e.g., lack of integrated gaze, posture and poverty of gesture, and a lack of feelings for others.

RETT'S DISORDER

The essential diagnostic features of Rett's disorder include developmental regression in multiple areas following a period of normal functioning after birth. Head growth deceler-ates between ages 5 and 48 months, and there is loss of previously acquired purposeful hand skills between ages 5 and 30 months with subsequent development of stereotyped midline hand movements such as hand-wringing or hand washing. There is loss of interest in the social environment early on, although social interaction may develop later. There is appearance of poorly coordinated gait or trunk movements and severe impairment in expressive and receptive language development with severe psychomotor retardation.

This disorder is often associated with severe or profound mental retardation and there may be increased frequency of EEG abnormalities and seizure disorder in about 70 percent to 80 percent of cases. Hyperreflexia, choreoathetosis, dystonia, growth retardation, and subsequent development of scoliosis has been reported (Trevathan & Naidu, 1988).

DIFFERENTIAL DIAGNOSIS

Schizophrenia arises in childhood after years of normal, or near normal development and these children show relatively normal social reciprocity. Active-phase symptoms include thought disorder and prominent delusions or hallucinations that last for at least one month.

In selective mutism, the child may be socially withdrawn but speaks normally in some situations and does not have severe impairment in social interactions and play as well as restricted patterns of behavior associated with pervasive development disorders.

In development language disorders, language impairment is not associated with im-pairment in social interactions and restricted, repetitive, and stereotyped patterns of behav-ior.

Childhood disintegrative disorder should be differentiated from dementia which often occurs as a consequence of a direct physiological effect of a general medical condition such as with head trauma.

Asperger's disorder needs to be distinguished from obsessive-compulsive disorder and schizoid personality disorder. The child with obsessive-compulsive disorder does show repetitive and stereotyped patterns of behavior but not qualitative impairment in social interactions and restricted pattern of interest and activities as seen in Asperger's disorder. Asperger's disorder is characterized by stereotyped behaviors, interests, and activities and much more severely impaired social interaction than schizoid personality disorder.

It may be difficult to determine whether additional diagnosis of autistic disorder is required in severe or profound mental retardation. If there are qualitative deficits in social and communication skills and the specific behavioral characteristics of pervasive developmental disorders are present, an additional diagnosis of pervasive developmental disorders can be considered.

EPIDEMIOLOGY

Most epidemiological studies of autistic children suggest worldwide prevalence rates of 4 to 5 cases per 10,000. Autism is more frequent in boys, with a sex ratio of 3 to 1. Girls with autism may be more severely affected and are more likely to have a family history of learning and language problems. Information on the prevalence of Rett's disorder, childhood disintegrative disorder, and Asperger's disorder is limited. Rett's disorder has been reported only in females whereas childhood disintegrative disorder and Asperger's disorder are more common in males.

DIAGNOSTIC ASSESSMENT

History and Examination

A detailed history should be obtained regarding pregnancy, birth, and development milestones. The parents should be specifically asked about maternal infections during pregnancy, perinatal or postnatal insult to the brain, meningitis, encephalitis, or seizures in the patients. In addition to obtaining routine family history of psychiatric illness, inquiries should be made into family history of autism, schizophrenia, and other genetic and development disorders. The child should be observed in a one-to-one setting as well as with the family, and if possible in a group setting like nursery or classroom.

There are several rating instruments available for the assessment of autistic children, including parent or teacher checklists (Krug, Arick, & Almond, 1978; Rimland 1984), instruments based on the interview of the parents (LeCouteur, Rutter, Lord, Rios, Robertson, Haldgrafer, & McLenan, 1989b; Wing & Gould 1978) and instruments based on a structured observation of the child (Lord et al., 1989).

Psychological Testing

Assessment of cognitive functioning is essential to aid in diagnostic formulation and to plan appropriate interventions and determine prognosis. Children with autism usually perform much lower on verbal scales than performance scales. Standard test batteries such as Wechsler Intelligence Scale for Pre-school Children, the Wechsler Intelligence Scale for Children-Revised and the Stanford-Binet: 4th edition should be used whenever possible. Alternative test batteries like Kaufman-Assessment Battery for Children (K-ABC) and the Leiter International Performance Scale should be considered in children with limited linguistic and cognitive skills.

Language Assessment   A speech and language evaluation by a speech and language specialist should be done to assess the formal aspects of language (e.g., articulation, vocabulary, and syntax), intonation, inflection of voice, pragmatics, narrative-discourse performance (in higher functioning verbal children), and nonverbal communication.

Educational Assessment   The educational assessment should be helpful in developing an individualized educational plan and in planning specific interventions to be used in the classroom setting by the teacher and aides.

Behavioral Assessment   A formal assessment by a behavioral specialist may be necessary to develop specific behavioral interventions/strategies to be used at home and/or in the classroom.

Assessment of Adaptive Functioning   It is necessary to determine the child's ability to adapt to environmental demands. The most frequently used instrument to assess adaptive functioning is the Vineland Adaptive Behavior Scales.

Physical Examination

A thorough physical examination is necessary with special attention to any dysmorphic features and signs of specific disorders such as tuberous sclerosis, fragile X syndrome, Rett's disorder, congenital rubella, or other genetic disorders that may be responsible for the child's symptomatology. Neurological examination may reveal sensorimotor deficits and soft neurological signs.

Medical Investigation

Chromosome analysis and Fragile X screening (DNA testing if possible) are indicated as a result of genetic implications especially when there is a history of mental retardation in the child or in the family. Wake and sleep EEG should be considered if the history is suggestive of seizures, behavioral regression, or loss of language. Metabolic screening, amino acid chromatography, tests for serum copper and ceruloplasmin, and serological evidence of intrauterine infections such as toxoplasmosis or cytomegalic disease are indicated if symptoms appeared after age 3 years or are progressive. Routine MRI, CT, or PET scanning is not warranted. Hearing should be tested, especially if there is speech delay.

ETIOLOGY

Psychological Basis

Kanner's initial description of parents of autistic children as cold, methodical, distant, and obsessive led to speculation of a parental role in the pathogenesis despite Kanner's emphasis on a constitutionally based inborn disturbance in autism. Initially, a great deal of consideration was given to psychotherapeutically treating the supposed deleterious effects of the cold "refrigerator mother." Many psychoanalysts have attempted to provide understanding of autism. Klein (1946) commented upon the primitive projective identification underlying the child's feeling of omnipotently controlling the world; Bettelheim (1967) suggested the absence of the internal organization for experiencing and interacting with the external world; Mahler (1965) pinpointed inborn constitutional defects resulting in the inability to perceive and utilize the mothering agent; and Mendelsohn (1987) emphasized the autistic child's remarkable sensitivity to unempathic stimuli.

Biological Basis

Cerebellar Abnormalities   There have been reports of selective hypoplasia of the neocerebellar vermis on midsagittal MR images (Courchesne, Yeung-Courchesne, Press, Hesselink, & Jernigan, 1988); Autopsy studies have reported 25 percent to 30 percent evenly distributed Purkinje neuron loss in the vermis (Arin, Bauman, & Kemper, 1991).

Cortical and Intracerebral Abnormalities   In autism, various abnormal cortical findings have been reported including cortical gyral malformations suggesting developmental errors in neuronal migration (Piven, Berthier, Starkstein, Nehme, Pearlson, & Folstein, 1990a); an increase in cerebral cortex volume (Filipek et al., 1992); a decrease in parietal lobe volume (Courchesne, Press, & Yeung-Courchesne, 1992); cytoarchitectonic abnormalities consisting of increased cell-packing density in the hippocampus, amygdala, entorhinal cortex, mammillary body and septum bilaterally (Bauman & Kemper, 1994); and decreased complexity and extent of the dendritic arbors in some pyramidal neurons of the hippocampus (Raymond, Bauman, & Kemper, 1989).

Brainstem Abnormalities   The persistence of a fetal pattern of circuitry in olivo-cerebellar pathways has been reported in neuropathological studies of individuals with autism (Bauman & Kemper, 1989). There have also been reports of a smaller pons and total brainstem area in an autistic group (Gaffney, Kuperman, Tsai, & Minchin, 1988). On the other hand, absence of pontine abnormalities was reported by Hsu and colleagues (1991).

In summary, variable findings have been reported in various brain regions. This neuroanatomical heterogeneity most likely reflects etiological heterogeneity.

Neurochemistry   Elevated levels of whole blood serotonin have been found in 25 percent to 40 percent of autistic patients (Anderson et al., 1987); however, this finding is not specific to autism. Increased dopamine functioning has been suggested in autism based on the finding of elevated mean basal cerebrospinal fluid (CSF) levels of the primary metabolite of brain dopamine, homovanillic acid (HVA), in medication-free autistic children in comparison to matched controls (Gillberg & Svenerholm, 1987). However, Narayan, Srinath, Anderson, & Meundi in 1993 reported normal CSF HVA levels in autistic individuals.

Elevated levels of plasma norepinephrine (NE) have been reported in autistic individuals (Lake, Ziegler, & Murphy, 1977), but other studies have found no group differences in plasma 3-methoxy-4-hydroxyphenyl-glycol (MHPG) and urinary NE, MHPG, and vanillyl-mandilic acid (VMA) between autistic and control subjects, and have reported normal CSF levels of MHPG in the autistic individuals (Gillberg & Svenerholm,1987).

Neuropeptide Function   Reports of elevated CSF endorphin levels in autistic children have led to the speculation that a defect in a maturation of the brain endorphin system may underlie some of the symptoms of autism (Gillberg, Terenius, & Lonnerholm, 1985).

Prenatal and Perinatal Factors

An association has been reported between congenital rubella and autism, and between congenital cytomegalovirus infection and autism (Chess, 1971). Studies examining prenatal and perinatal factors in autism have found evidence of more problems in children with autism than controls (Folstein & Rutter, 1977; Gillberg & Gillberg, 1983a). However, a recent study failed to identify increased frequency of any pre- or perinatal pathogenic factors among an autistic group compared to a nonautistic sibling control group (Mason-Brothers, Ritvo, Pingree, Peterson, Jenson, McMahon, Freeman, Jorde, Spencer, Mo, & Ritvo, 1990).

Genetic Influence

The prevalence of autism in the siblings of autistic probands has been estimated to be 50 to 100 times greater than expected (2–3/100 vs. 4–5/10,000) (Stefenberg & Gillberg, 1986). An early population-based twin study in Great Britain found 36 percent concordance for autism in monozygotic (MZ) pairs compared to no concordance in dizygotic (DZ) pairs, and 82 percent concordance for a variety of cognitive and social deficits in the nonautistic MZ co-twins as compared to 10 percent in the nonautistic DZ co-twins (Folstein & Rutter, 1977).

Certain cognitive deficits (reading, spelling, executive function, and mental retardation), specific language abnormalities (especially social use of pragmatic language and narrative discourse), personality characteristics (e.g., social deficits), and psychiatric disorders (e.g., anxiety and affective disorder) are found more commonly in family members of affected probands compared to individuals with other developmental disabilities.

Some genetic conditions have been reported to be associated with autism. Features of autistic disorder have been described as part of the neuropsychiatric presentation in males with fragile X syndrome, certain single-gene disorders including tuberous sclerosis, untreated phenylketonuria, and possibly neurofibromatosis.

PROGNOSIS

Autism is a lifelong disorder and about two-thirds of adults with autism remain severely handicapped, often requiring institutional support. About 40 percent to 50 percent acquire useful speech early on in their life but continue to show abnormalities in language usages and speech delivery. Behavior problems often become more prominent during elementary school years. There may be either a severe regression or a marked gain in skills and behavior in some individuals during adolescence. Deterioration reported during adolescence in 12 percent of autistic subjects may be explained by the onset of major motor or complex partial seizures (Lockyer & Rutter, 1970).

Only one-third of autistic individuals are able to achieve partial self-sufficiency and independence, and 1 percent to 2 percent are able to live fully independent. Of these higher functioning autistic adults, 5 percent to 17 percent may live independently with minimum supervision and may be able to participate in "supported employment."

The best prognosis is in the cases with the presence of communicative speech by age 5 years, and normal nonverbal intellectual skills and communicative language.

MANAGEMENT

Autism and other pervasive developmental disorders require a comprehensive treatment program. There is a need to start the treatment program as early as possible instead of waiting for a lengthy assessment to take place. Rutter (1985) advocated five goals of treatment including fostering normal development, promoting cognitive language and social learning, reducing rigidity and stereotypy, eliminating nonspecific maladaptive behaviors, and alleviating family distress.

To address the lack of communicative ability and social interactions, parents may be asked to set aside regularly scheduled short periods of "floor time" (Greenspan & Greenspan, 1989) to play with their autistic child, with emphasis on promoting purposeful reciprocal social exchange through "any and all forms of communication and not just speech per se" (Rutter, 1985). Because of the autistic child's tendency to be engrossed in solitary play or activity, avoiding eye contact and human interaction, parents may have to introject themselves to force a response from the child (Ghuman & Kates, 1992).

Direct speech training is most effective when there is evidence of some limited language or prelinguistic skills, and alternative modes of communication (sign language, augmented communication) can be introduced if there is little or no progress in speech. Autistic children often need direct social skills training to help them address their social incapacity.

Appropriate individualized educational programs are the main focus of management in autistic children. The autistic child is in need of structured teaching as a result of lack of self-direction, and limiting the prompts to only essential cues has been advocated (Lovaas, Koegel, & Schreibman, 1979; Schopler, 1994). It is important to break the learning task into a series of small steps and to organize these steps in such a way that the child is successful in achieving them.

Areas of particular attention include more specialized academic/cognitive intervention, vocational counseling and supported employment for the higher functioning autistic individuals (with direct attention paid to the autistic individuals' inability to generalize learned skills to new situations), self-help skills for the more severely affected individual, and structured exposure to other children who do not have similar communication and socialization deficits.

Behavioral therapy approaches are the mainstay of treatment to reduce rigidity, stereotypy, and perseveration and to eliminate maladaptive behaviors such as tantrums, aggression, and self-injurious behavior. Various behavior techniques can be applied after careful analysis of behavior. Supportive psychotherapy and, occasionally, insight-oriented therapy, especially in the higher functioning individual can be helpful. The goal of therapy should be to help the patient deal with their limitations and emotions, and to improve expression of their needs and feelings to others.

Because the impact on families can be devastating, it is important to alleviate family distress by helping the family gain an understanding of their child's behavior. The parents should be engaged as co-therapists in the child's treatment and fully participate in the child's education, language and socialization development, and behavior management. Families will also need support to help them deal with their excessive denial, guilt, frustration with slow or seeming no progress, to advocate for their child's educational needs, financial needs for various therapeutic interventions, financial/disability eligibility, and respite care to enable them to attend to other members of the family. Information regarding self-help and support groups is available through the local branches of the National Society of Autism.

PHARMACOTHERAPY

Pharmacological intervention in autism is usually target, symptom-oriented with emphasis placed on aggression, ritualistic/stereotypic/self-injurious behavior, attentional problems, and seizures.

Dopamine antagonists have been the most commonly employed psychopharmacological agents in the treatment of autism. The D2 antagonists, haloperidol, at .25–4 mg/day (Anderson, Campbell, Adams, Small, Perry, & Shell, 1989; Campbell, Anderson, Meier, Cohen, Small, Samit, & Sachar, 1978; Joshi, Capozzoli, & Coyle, 1988) and pimozide, at 1–9 mg/day (Naruse, Naghata, Nakane, Shirahashi, Takesada, & Yamazaki, 1982) have been shown to decrease symptoms of withdrawal, stereotypes, hyperactivity, fidgetiness, negativism, and angry affect. They have also been shown to increase relatedness and facilitate discrimination learning as a result of their effects on attentional mechanisms.

Based on the findings of dysregulation in 5-HT function in some patients with autism, several drugs affecting this system have been studied. Fenfluramine is an indirect 5-HT agonist that releases 5-HT presynaptically and blocks its reuptake from 5-HT neurons. Ritvo, Freeman, Geller, and Yuwiler in 1983 reported improvement in social and sensory function and a decrease in abnormal motor movements with fenfluramine. Subsequent studies with fenfluramine have not shown consistent clinical improvement in stereotypies or in the core symptoms of autism as compared to placebo, while many side effects such as weight loss, excessive sedation, loose stools, and irritability have been reported (Campbell, Adams, Small, Curren, Overall, Anderson, Lynch, & Perry, 1988).

Potent 5-HT reuptake inhibitors, clomipramine, fluoxetine, fluvoxamine, and sertraline, have been studied in autism. Fluvoxamine at 150–300 mg/day in adults (McDougle, Naylor, Goodman, Volkmar, Cohen, & Price, 1993); clomipramine at 90-170 mg/day in children (Gordon, Rapoport, Hamburger, State, & Mannheim, 1992); flouxetine at 20 mg every other day to 80 mg/day in children and adults (Cook, Rowlett, Jaselskis, & Leventhal, 1992); and sertraline at 50–200 mg/day in adults (McDougle, 1993) have been shown to improve repetitive behaviors, obsessive-compulsive symptomatology, and aggression in individuals with autism.

Stimulants can be helpful for short attention span, hyperactivity, and impulsivity; however, close followup is needed as stimulants can worsen the behavior and stereotypies in some autistic individuals. Anticonvulsants are used to treat seizures, mood lability, and aggression in children with autism in the same way they are in children without autism.

LEARNING DISORDERS

This section will provide an overview of Developmental Disabilities, with particular emphasis on Learning Disorders, formerly, Academic Skills Disorders, as identified in *DSM-IV* (APA, 1994). The chapter will include basic definitions, diagnostic criteria, and protocols used in the identification of the disorders.

The term Developmental Disability/Disorders (DD) has undergone significant changes over the past 20 years. In 1970, P.L. 91-517 defined DD as:

> ... a disability attributable to mental retardation, cerebral palsy, epilepsy or another neurological condition of an individual... closely related to mental retardation... which originated before such individual reaches age 18... (which) can be expected to continue indefinitely, and which constitutes a substantial handicap for the individual.

In 1975, **P.L. 94-103** revised the definition to include dyslexia and autism. In 1978, P.L. 95-602 further revised the definition to include:

> ... any severe disability, whether mental or physical, or a combination thereof, which is manifest before age 22 and which results in substantial functional limitations in certain specified areas of life activity, requiring lifelong services....

The term Learning Disorders, which in this chapter will be synonymous with Learning Disabilities (LD), continues to undergo change as consensus among professionals concerning an acceptable definition has not been satisfactorily achieved. Presently, a definition widely regarded and adopted by many Local Educational Agencies (LEA) was formulated by the National Joint Committee for Learning Disabilities (1989) as follows:

> LD is a generic term that refers to a heterogeneous group of disorders manifested by significant difficulties in the acquisition and use of listening, speaking, reading, writing, reasoning and mathematical abilities. These disorders are intrinsic to the individual and presumed to be due to central nervous system dysfunction. Even though a learning disability may occur concomitantly with other handicapping conditions (e.g. sensory impairment, mental retardation, social and emotional disturbance), or environmental influence... it is not the direct result of those conditions.

The learning (academic) disorders identified by *DSM-IV* (APA, 1994) include Reading Disorder, Mathematics Disorder, Disorder of Written Expression, and Learning Disorder, Not Otherwise Specified (NOS).

For the clinician, the disorders share relatively similar diagnostic criteria:

- "... achievement, as measured by individually administered standardized tests... is substantially below that expected given the person's chronological age, measured intelligence, and age-appropriate education..."
- "... the disturbance significantly interferes with academic achievement or activities of daily living..."
- "... if a sensory deficit is present, the difficulties... are in excess of those usually associated with it."

Definitions of LD employed by educators and psychologists share much in common with the language of *DSM-IV* (APA, 1994). However, traditional educational/psychological definitions of LD are considered more explicit. Tables 1 and 2 describe in universal terms the major types of LD typically understood by psychologists and special education teachers.

DSM-IV (APA, 1994) is clearly less-than-specific in the choice of its terms "substantially" and "significantly." Considerable debate exists among physicians, psychologists, parents, teachers, and students regarding diagnosis, treatment, and the rights guaranteed to those with disabilities. Although the physician can render a medical, *DSM-IV* (APA, 1994) diagnosis, clarification of such is traditionally sought from trained psychologists and special educational teachers. When the diagnosis is needed for special education funding or programming, the importance of each discipline becomes much more apparent.

Table 1   Disorders of Written Language (Writing and Reading)

WRITING

DYSGRAPHIA: inability to learn appropriate motor patterns for the act of writing
RECALL DEFICITS: inability to revisualize or copy letters from memory (even when they can be named)
FORMULATIVE/SYNTACTIC DEFICIT: inability to produce coherent sentences, or paragraphs observing the established rules for conventional (style, punctuation, capitalization) and linguistic (syntactic and semantic elements) expression

SPELLING

AUDITORY CHANNEL DEFICITS:
  substitutions- t for d, f for v,
  omissions- plsh for polish,
  vowel confusion- bit for bet
VISUAL CHANNEL DEFICITS:
  omissions- hapy for happy,
  reversals- s for a, b for d, on for no *phonetic spellings-* tuff for tough

READING

DYSLEXIA: a language disorder characterized by deficits in phonological processing... segmentation, phoneme awareness and phonological coding of written language.
Problems commonly associated with Dyslexia include:
  ...a history of delayed language development
  ...spatial and directional confusion
  ...reversing of letters and numbers
  ...slow, word by word reading
  ...mispronouncements of "mastered" words

When the diagnostician is asked to evaluate a student to determine the existence of a learning disability, a relatively standard protocol is invoked. Typically, a "battery" of tests such as those listed in Table 3, is administered. From the list, the examiner chooses one test from each group, depending on the depth and breadth of information needed.

Scores from the individually administered tests are recorded and then compared. Essential to the identification and assignment of handicapping condition such as LD is the

Table 2   Disorders of Arithmetic

Mathematical dysfunction, which is not attributable to MR or other factors is defined as DYSCALCULIA.
Problems commonly associated with DYSCALCULIA include:
  ...inability to establish 1 to 1 correspondence
  ...difficulty being able to count meaningfully, the relationship between symbol and quantity is not established or maintained
  ...problems visualizing clusters of objects in a group (all must be counted)
  ...difficulties grasping conservation of quantity (ten cents can be two nickels, ten pennies, one dime, or 1 gallon is the same as 4 quarts)
  ...inability performing arithmetic functions
  ...inconsistently recalling/understanding process signs
  ...difficulty understanding the arrangement of the numbers on a page
  ...difficulty choosing process(es) for problem solving, isolating essential information, and sequencing steps in operations

Table 3

TESTS OF INTELLIGENCE/COGNITIVE ABILITY
The Wechsler Intelligence Scale
The Kaufman Assessment Battery for Children
The Stanford-Binet Intelligence Scale

INDIVIDUALIZED TESTS OF ACADEMIC ACHIEVEMENT
The Woodcock-Johnson Psychoeducational Battery
The Kaufman Test of Educational Achievement
The Wecshler Individual Achievement Test

OTHER INDIVIDUALIZED TESTS FOR SPECIFIC AREAS
The Beery Test of Visual Motor Integration
The Woodcock Language Proficiency Battery
The Gray Oral Reading Test
The Test of Language Development
The Test of Written Spelling

---

establishment of a *severe discrepancy* between academic achievement and cognitive ability. Guidelines are available to assist the diagnostician in rendering the diagnosis. Table 4 is such a guide, commonly used for comparative purposes. It is based on *age-based, standard scores* (mean 100, standard deviation 15).

Example

John, with a posted IQ score of 108, is expected to achieve reading, math and written language scores in the 100 to 105 range. Should John's score fall in the 77 to 82 range, he may be considered severely discrepant and experiencing a learning disability in the specific area or areas. Furthermore, in assigning the handicapping condition of LD, the clinician must be convinced that the severe discrepancy is not attributed to emotional disturbances, hearing, visual, motor handicaps, environmental disadvantages, cultural differences,or economic detriments. These conditions can, however, exist simultaneously with the LD.

It is not uncommon for evaluators to face diagnostic dilemmas. Scores could be thought of as an "underestimate" of ability or possibly invalid as a result of any one or more of the following possibilities:

- The student's educational history may have been inappropriate or inconsistent.
- English may be a second language.

Table 4   Severe Discrepancy Guidelines

IQ range	Expectancy range	Severe disc.
130–139	118–123	95–100
120–129	112–117	89–94
110–119	106–111	83–88
100–109	100–105	77–82
90–99	94–99	71–76
80–89	88–93	65–70
70–79	82–87	59–64

- Test rapport was thought to be poorly established.
- The student's motivation may have been adversely affected by depression, concentrational deficits, and performance anxiety.

At these junctures, the diagnostician must employ his or her best clinical judgment, attempting to obtain as much historically relevant information as possible and integrating it with the test data.

CONCLUSION

The complexity of learning disabilities presents formidable challenges to the clinician. Although much has been advanced in the field, the central nervous system and how it processes information retain their mysterious character, a dialectic defying logical interpretation, confused by medical and educational jargon and retaining its illusive nature; a phenomenon not always as it appears. In brief, those who pursue a greater understanding of LD agree that:

- Its etiology is probably multifactorial.
- Successful informational processing involves focused attention, concentration. associative ability, decoding, verbal comprehension and general intelligence.
- Clinical and psychoeducational considerations must come together in a diagnosis of learning disability.

REFERENCES

American Psychiatric Association. (1980). *Diagnostic and Statistical Manual of Mental Disorders* (3rd ed.) Washington, DC: the Association.

American Psychiatric Association (APA). (1994). *Diagnostic and statistical manual of mental disorders* (4th. ed.) *(DSM-IV)*. Washington, DC: the Association.

Anderson, G. M., Freedman, C. X., Cohen, D. J., Volkmar, F. R., Hoder, E. L., McPhedran, P., Minderaa, R. B., Hansen, C. R., & Young, J. G. (1987). Whole blood serotonin in autistic and normal subjects. *Journal of Child Psychology and Psychiatry, 28,* 885–900.

Anderson, L. T., Campbell, M., Adams, P., Small, A. M., Perry, R., and Shell, J. (1989). The effects of haloperidol discrimination learning and behavioral symptoms in autistic children. *Journal of Autism and Developmental Disorders, 19,* 227–239.

Arin, D. M., Bauman, M. L., & Kemper, T. L. (1991). The distribution of Purkinje cell loss in the cerebellum in autism. *Neurology, 41,* 307 (abstract).

Asperger, H. Die "autistichen Psychopathen" Kindesalter. (1944). *Archchive Psychiatrika Nervenkranz, 117,* 76–136.

Bauman, M. L., & Kemper, T. L. (1989). Abnormal cerebellar circuitry in autism? *Neurology, 39* (suppl 1), 186.

Bauman, M., & Kemper, T. (1994). Neuroanatomic observations of the brain in autism. In M. Bauman & T. Kemper (Eds.), *The Neurobiology of Autism* (pp. 119–145). Baltimore, and London: Johns Hopkins University Press.

Bettelheim, B. (1967). *The empty fortress.* Toronto: Collier-Macmillian Canada Ltd.

Campbell, M., Adams, P., Small, A., Curren, E. L., Overall, J. E., Anderson, L. T., Lynch, N., & Perry, R. (1988). Efficacy and safety of fenfluramine in autistic children. *Journal of the American Academy of Child and Adolescent Psychiatry, 27,* 434–439.

Campbell, M., Anderson, L.I., Meier, M., Cohen, I., Small, A., Samit, C., and Sachar, E. (1978). A comparison of haloperidol, behavior therapy and their interaction in autistic children. *Journal of the American Academy of Child Psychiatry, 17,* 640–655.

Chess, S. (1971). Autism in children with congenital rubella. *Journal of Autism and Childhood Schizophrenia, 1,* 33–47.

Cook, E. H., Rowlett, R., Jaselskis, C., & Leventhal, B. L. (1992). Fluoxetine treatment of children and adults with autistic disorder and mental retardation. *Journal of the American Academy of Child and Adolescent Psychiatry, 31*, 739–745.

Courchesne, E., Press, G. A., & Yeung-Courchesne, R. (1992). Parietal lobe abnormalities detected by magnetic resonance in patients with infantile autism. *Society for Neuroscience Abstracts, 18*, 332.

Courchesne, E., Yeung-Courchesne, R., Press, G. A., Hesselink, J. R., & Jernigan, T.L. (1988). Hypoplasia of cerebellar lobules VI and VII in infantile autism. *New England Journal of Medicine, 318*, 1349-1354.

Developmental Disabilities Service and Construction Act (P. L. 91-517). 1970. Washington, DC: Federal Register Developmental Disabilities Assistance and Bill of Rights (P. L. 94-103). 1975. Washington, DC: Federal Register.

Filipek, P. A., Richelime, C., Kennedy, D. N., Rademacher, J., Pitcher, D. A., Zidel, S., & Caviness, V. S. (1992). Morphometric analysis of the brain in developmental language disorders and autism. *Annals of Neurology, 32*, 475 (abstract).

Folstein, S. E., & Rutter, M. L. (1977). Infantile autism: A genetic study of 21 twin pairs. *Journal of Child Psychology and Psychiatry, 18*, 297–321.

Gaffney, G. R., Kuperman, S., Tsai, L. Y., & Minchin, S. (1988). Morphological evidence of brainstem involvement in infantile autism. *Biological Psychiatry, 24*, 578–586.

Ghuman, J. K., & Kates, W. (1992). Approaches to the development of social communication in foster children with pervasive developmental disorder. *Zero to Three, 13* (2), 27–31.

Gillberg, C., & Gillberg, I. C. (1983a). Infantile autism: a total population study of reduced optimality in the pre-, peri-and neonatal period. *Journal of Autism and Developmental Disorders, 13*, 153–166.

Gillberg, C., & Svennerholm, L. (1987). CSF monoamines in autistic syndromes and other pervasive developmental disorders of early childhood. *British Journal of Psychiatry, 151*, 89–94.

Gillberg, C., Terenius, L., & Lonnerholm, G. (1985). Endorphin activity in childhood psychosis. *Archives of General Psychiatry, 42*, 780–783.

Gordon, C. T., Rapoport, J. L., Hamburger, S. D., State, R., & Mannheim, G. B. (1992). Differential response of seven subjects with autistic disorder to clomipramine and desipramine. *American Journal of Psychiatry, 149*, 363–366.

Greenspan, S., & Greenspan, N. (1989). Floortime: From the ground up. In S. Greenspan & N. Greenspan (Eds.), *The Essential Partnership: How parents and children can meet the emotional challenges of infancy and childhood* (19–62). New York, Viking Penguin.

Heller, T., (1908). Dementia infantilis. Zeitschrift fur die Erforschung und Behandlung des Jugenlichen Schwachsinns 2:141–165, 1908.

Kanner, L. (1943). Autistic disturbances of affective contact. *Nervous Child, 2*, 217–250.

Heller, T. (1930). Uber Dementia infantalis. *Zeitschrift Fur Kinderforschung.* 37: 661–667

Hsu, M., Yeung-Courchesne, R., Courchesne, E., & Press, G. A. (1991). Absence of magnetic resonance imaging evidence of pontine abnormality in infantile autism. *Archives of Neurology, 48*, 1160–1163.

Joshi, P. T., Capozzoli, J. A., & Coyle, J. T. (1988). Low dose neuroleptic therapy for children with childhood onset pervasive developmental disorder. *American Journal of Psychiatry, 145*, 335–338.

Kanner, L. (1943). Autistic disturbance of affective contact. *Nervous Child, 2*, 217–250.

Kaufman, A. S. (1994). *Intelligence testing with the Wisc-III.* New York: John Wiley & Sons.

Klein, M. (1946). *Notes on some schizoid mechanisms. Envy and gratitude.* New York: Delacorte Press.

Krug, D. A., Arick, J. R., & Almond, P. J. (1978). *Autism behavior Checklist.* Pro-ed, Inc., Austin: Texas.

Lake, C. R., Ziegler, M. G., & Murphy, D. L. (1977). Increased norepinephrine levels and decreased dopamine-beta-hydroxylase activity in primary autism. *Archives of General Psychiatry, 34*, 553–556.

LeCouteur, A., Rutter, M., Lord, C., Rios, P., Robertson, S., Haldgrafer, M., & McLennan, J. (1989b). Autism diagnostic interview: A standardized investigator-based instrument. *Journal of Autism and Developmental Disorders, 19* (3), 363–387.

Lockyer, L., & Rutter, M. (1970). A five to fifteen year follow-up study of infantile psychosis: patterns of cognitive ability. *British Journal of Social and Clinical Psychology, 9*, 152–163.

Lord, C., Rutter, M., Goode, S., Heemsbergan, J., Jordan, H., Mawhood, L., & Schopler, E. (1989). Autism diagnostic observation schedule: A standardized observation of communicative and social behavior. *Journal of Autism and Developmental Disorders, 19* (2), 185–212.

Lovaas, O., Koegel, R., & Schreibman, L. (1979). Stimulus overselectivity in autism: A review of research. *Psychology Bulletin, 86*, 1236–1254.

Mahler, M. S. (1965). On early infantile psychosis, the symbiotic and autistic syndrome: Infant psychiatry. *Journal of the Academy of Child Psychiatry, 94*, 554.

Mason-Brothers, A., Ritvo, E. R., Pingree, C., Peterson, P. B., Jenson, W. R., McMahon, W. M., Freeman, B. J., Jorde, L. B., Spencer, M. J., Mo, A., & Ritvo, A. (1990). The UCLA University of Utah epidemiologic survey of autism: Prenatal, perinatal, and postnatal factors. *Pediatrics*, *86*, 514–519.

McDougle, C. J., Naylor, S. T., Goodman, W. K., Volkmar, F. R., Cohen, D. J., & Price, L. H. (1993). Acute tryptophan depletion in autistic disorder: A controlled case study. *Biological Psychiatry*, *33*, 547–550.

Mendelsohn, R. M. (1987). *The synthesis of self* (vol. 3). New York: Plenum.

Narayan, M., Srinath, S., Anderson, G. M., & Meundi, D. B. (1993). Cerebrospinal fluid levels of homovanillic acid and 5-hydroxyindoleacetic acid in autism. *Biological Psychiatry*, *33*, 630–635.

Naruse, H., Nagahata, M., Nakane, Y., Shirahashi, K., Takesada, M., and Yamazaki, K. (1982). A multi-center double-blind trial of pimozide (Orap), haloperidol and placebo in children with behavior disorders, using cross-over design. *Acta Paedopsychiatrica*, *48*, 173–184.

National Joint Committee on Learning Disabilities. (1989). Letter from NJCLD to member organizations, Modifications to the NJCLD definition of learning disabilities. Washington, DC.

Piven, J., Berthier, M. L., Starkstein, S. E., Nehme, E., Pearlson, G., & Folstein, S. (1990a). Magnetic resonance imaging evidence for a defect of cerebral cortical development in autism. *American Journal of Psychiatry*, *147* (6), 734–739.

Raymond, G, Bauman, M. I., & Kemper, T. L. (1989). The hippocampus in autism: Golgi analysis. *Annals of Neurology*, *26*, 483–484.

Rehabilitation, comprehensive services, and developmental disabilities act (P.L. 95-602). (1978). Washington DC: Federal Register.

Rett, A. (1966). *Uber ein cerebral-atropnisches syndrom bei hyperammonaemie*. Wien: Bruder Hollinek.

Rimland, B. (1984). Diagnostic checklist form E2: A reply to Parks. *Journal of Autism and Developmental Disorders*, *13*, 255–267.

Ritvo, E. R., Freeman, B. J., Gellar, E., Yuwiler, A. (1983). Effects of Fenfluramine on 14 outpatients with the syndrome of autism. *Journal of the American Academy of Child and Adolescent Psychiatry*, *22*, 549–558.

Rutter, M. (1985). Infantile autism. In D. Shaffer, A. A. Ehrhardt, & L. L. Greenhill (Eds.), *The clinical guide to child psychiatry* (pp. 48–78). New York: the Free Press.

Schopler, E. A. (1994). Statewide program for the treatment and education of autistic and related communication handicapped children (TEACCH). In F. Volkmar (Ed.), *Child and adolescent psychiatric clinics of North America: Psychoses and pervasive developmental disorders* (91–103). Philadelphia: W. B. Sanders.

Steffenberg, S., & Gillberg, C. (1986). Autism and autistic-like conditions in Swedish rural and urban areas: A population study. *British Journal of Psychiatry*, *149*, 81–87.

Trevathan, E., & Naidu, S. (1988). The clinical recognition and differential diagnosis of Rett syndrome. *Journal of Child Neurology*, *3*, S6–S16.

Wing, L., & Gould, J. (1978). Systematic recording of behaviors and skills of retarded and psychotic children. *Journal of Autism and Childhood Schizophrenia*, *8*, 79–97.

Part 4

Therapeutic Interventions

Chapter 17

Pharmacotherapy in Children and Adolescents

Paramjit T. Joshi, M.D.

HISTORY

Pharmacotherapy in the treatment of psychiatrically disturbed children dates back to 1937 when amphetamines were first introduced in the treatment of a heterogeneous group of institutionalized children with behavior disorders. Soon after there were reports of improvement in children who had symptoms of short attention span, increased motor activity, and poor organizational skills when treated with Benzedrine. Over the next two decades, there was considerable controversy about the use of pharmacological agents in the treatment of psychiatric illnesses in children and adolescents. In the 1950s, phenothiazine became available and was used primarily in the management of institutionalized, severely behaviorally disordered and brain-damaged children. With the remarkable increase in the number and type of drugs available, paradoxically, the field of pediatric psychopharmacology has been plagued with many difficulties. In addition to the stigma attached to treat childhood psychiatric disorders, many of the early studies designed to assess efficacy have been limited. The childhood psychiatric disturbances have often been poorly defined; diagnostic classifications have varied over time, and a relatively small number of subjects has been included in most clinical trials. Most of the studies have been poorly designed, with methodological difficulties including lack of standardized rating scales, outcome measures, and the lack of control groups in most studies.

However, over the last 10 years, there has been an enormous increase in both the quality and number of studies examining the use of psychopharmacological agents in the treatment of psychiatric disorders in children and adolescents. The development of a descriptively based diagnostic classification system has led to clinicians becoming more reliable in classifying childhood psychopathology. This has had a positive effect on the field of childhood psychopharmacology, which has expanded in diversity and methodological sophistication.

The Food and Drug Administration (FDA) has provided explicit approval for only a limited number of medications for the treatment of psychiatric disorders in children and adolescents. Historically most studies examining the efficacy of psychopharmacological agents have been conducted in adults. Therefore, the field of pediatric pharmacology was left behind, but it has made important strides recently toward establishing the role of pharmacotherapy in the treatment of childhood psychiatric disorders. In fact, despite the lack of officially recognized labeling, psychotropics are prescribed to children and adolescents for a variety of psychiatric disorders (Weiner & Jaffe, 1996). This off-label use is widespread and there are indications that it has been on the increase. To address this problem there has been an explosion in both the quantity and quality of studies examining the use and efficacy of various pharmacological agents for the treatment of psychiatric disorders in children. These efforts are important and timely to better understand the pharmacokinetics and efficacy of psychotropics and to delineate appropriate indications and contraindications of these drugs for children and adolescents

Pharmacotherapy in children and adolescents is only one aspect of a biopsychosocial treatment model. Youngsters often have comorbid conditions, making treatment complex and difficult. Pharmacotherapy is usually considered in the primary treatment of children and adolescents with major depressive disorders, childhood schizophrenia, attention deficit disorder, anxiety disorders, obsessive compulsive disorders, and Tourette's syndrome (Joshi, Coyle, & Walkup, 1994). In other instances, medications are used to reduce symptoms such as aggression, anxiety, perseveration, and self-mutilation, as seen in children with pervasive development disorder. The reduction of aggressive and markedly disruptive behaviors with psychotropic medications is sometimes controversial, since some view it as a "chemical restraint." Nevertheless, controlled studies are now providing evidence of the efficacy of certain medications in trials, where patients are selected based on the presence of symptoms, rather than diagnosis, in severely disturbed children and adolescents. This may reflect, in part, the current limitations of diagnostic nosology, but is also analogous to the effectiveness of antipsychotics on delusions and hallucinations, regardless of whether they occur in the context of schizophrenia or psychotic depression.

The remainder of this chapter is devoted to a discussion of groups of medications commonly utilized to treat psychiatric symptoms and disorders in children and adolescents. Emphasis is on indication for initiating treatment, dosage titration, measuring outcome, followup, and the identification and management of adverse side effects. It is of utmost importance when undertaking pharmacological treatment of minors to discuss in detail, with the parents or the legal guardian, the purpose of treatment, expectations, potential risks, and side effects, and to address any fears that the patient and parents may harbor. It is perhaps advisable to obtain written consent from the parents, not only to increase their awareness of medication usage but also to decrease the potential for misunderstandings and future litigious actions. A discussion of the advantages and disadvantages of particular medications with parents will not only enhance the communication between the psychiatrist and the caregiving adults, but also serve to improve compliance with the medication after discharge from the hospital. The poorer the understanding parents have of medications, the greater the likelihood of noncompliance. Handouts describing the medications, dosage, and side effects may be an additional source of information.

STIMULANTS

The psychostimulants are the drugs of choice in the treatment of attention deficit disorder with hyperactivity. These include the following:

- Amphetamines (Dexedrine and Benzedrine)
- Methylphenidate (Ritalin)
- Magnesium pemoline (Cylert)

The treatment of ADHD with stimulants should be part of an individually designed multimodal treatment plan to address target symptoms. It often includes behavior modification both at home and school, and educational assistance or special education, along with appropriate school placement. Some children with ADHD also require social skills training, family therapy, and individual therapy to address specific issues. These recommendations are based on the severity of symptoms, the ability of the school and classroom teacher to manage the child's distractibility and short attention span, the degree of disruption that the symptoms cause, interference in learning, and the views of the parents and the child about taking medication. The decision is also based on the results of previous treatment modalities employed.

Before the institution of stimulant treatment, a careful psychiatric and physical examination is essential. In addition, baseline ratings of the patient's behavior on the Connors' Teacher Rating Scale should be compared to ratings obtained while the child's dosage is being titrated to the desired balance between optimal clinical response and adverse drug effects. Preferably, teachers should be unaware as to whether the child is on medication, to avoid bias as they make their observations on the rating scales. Parent rating scales are available as well. However, because of the relatively short duration of action, and end-of-dose exacerbation in some children, the desired clinical effect is rarely seen in the late afternoon after a noontime dose.

Parents can become discouraged and demoralized about the lack of change in behavior at home. Therefore, they need to be educated and advised about the nature and timing of the effects of stimulants in their children to avoid noncompliance based on unrealistic expectations. Because of the appetite suppressant effects of stimulants, consideration of restricting treatment to school days should be considered, depending upon the ability of the parent or caretaker to tolerate the behaviors at home.

All these drugs are prescribed orally with good absorption, easily cross the blood brain barrier, and cause significant central nervous systemic excitation. With the amphetamines, peak plasma levels are achieved within 2 to 3 hours, with a half-life of 4 to 6 hours in children. Clinical response is usually seen at 1 to 3 hours. A steady state half-life of 10 hours is usually achieved after the patient has been on the drug regularly for approximately 6 months. Methylphenidate remains the most commonly prescribed medication for ADHD because of the relatively low incidence of side effects. Peak plasma levels are reached in one to two hours with a half-life of 2 to 3 hours. A long-acting preparation of (SR) is also available and fairly widely used, but treatment with Ritalin SR has been shown to have inconsistent effects over time. Magnesium pemoline reaches peak serum levels in 2 to 4 hours but has a much longer half-life of 12 hours. Significant clinical improvement may not be noted for up to 3 to 4 weeks (Greenhill, 1992).

Dosage

For methylphenidate the recommended dosage is 0.3 to 0.6 mg/kg, usually given in two dosages, morning and noon. However, it may be necessary to rearrange dosage schedules depending on the particular needs of the child as it pertains to time of onset, duration of effect, and schedule of classes and work assignments. There is evidence suggesting that the lower dosages selectively improve attention (0.2–0.4 mg/kg) while higher dosages (0.5–1.0 mg/kg) affect behavior and may not improve attention.

Adverse Effects

The most frequent and annoying early and usually temporary, side effects are gastrointestinal: including anorexia, nausea, abdominal cramps or pain, thirst, and vomiting. Cardiovascular side effects, such as tachycardia and elevated blood pressure, can sometimes persist after the first few weeks of treatment. Central nervous system (CNS) side effects reported are insomnia, lability of mood, irritability, sadness, and dysphoria. Long-term consequences of stimulant treatment are potentially inhibition in growth, both height and weight, with reduction in growth velocity during active treatment with stimulants. However, this is sometimes compensated for by an accelerated rate of growth or "rebound growth" after the stimulants are discontinued. This phenomenon supports the utility of "drug holidays" on weekends and vacations. Some children are more vulnerable to these side effects of growth suppression than others.

Measurements of height, weight, blood pressure, and pulse rate should be taken approximately every 4 to 6 weeks. Stimulants can precipitate tics, especially in those who are predisposed to a tic disorder, and controversy exists over whether stimulants are totally contraindicated in such cases. Hepatotoxicity is of special concern with the use of pemoline, with elevated liver enzymes reported in 1 percent to 3 percent of children treated with this drug, normalizing after discontinuing the medication. It is therefore essential to monitor liver function tests in children being treated with magnesium pemoline throughout the duration of therapy (Medical Economics, 1996). To minimize untoward side effects, one should titrate the dosage schedule slowly, with the goal of achieving the most effective dose with the fewest untoward effects.

Stimulant dosages seem to have a "creeping effect" where at times children receive methylphenidate dosages of up to 80 mgs/day. This has usually taken place after poor response to standard doses, in an attempt to get a therapeutic effect. It is uncommon to achieve a good effect at such high doses and unwanted drug effects of dysphoria, even delirium, are often seen, and appetite suppression is usually profound. In such cases, there are often comorbid conditions such as mental retardation or anxiety, which may indicate treatment with other drugs besides stimulants. A common myth that parents usually have about the use of stimulants is subsequent predilection for substance abuse as adults. Without minimizing the severe problems and prevalence of substance abuse in youngsters with a history of attention deficit hyperactivity disorder, studies do not suggest an increase in the rate of substance abuse in those children who have been treated with stimulants.

ANTIDEPRESSANTS

The use of antidepressants specifically for the treatment of affective disorders has already been discussed in some detail in the chapter on affective disorders in children and adolescents. However, antidepressant medications are also used for disorders other than mood disorders. Three main groups of antidepressants that are used in the treatment of children and adolescents for a variety of conditions include the tricyclics (TCAs), the most widely used group, the monoamine oxidase inhibitors (MAOIs), and the serotonin selective reuptake inhibitors (SSRIs). However, in the last few years there have been several other antidepressants introduced that do not belong to any particular class of antidepressants. These are discussed individually in this chapter.

Efficacy Studies

There have been only eight randomized placebo-controlled TCA studies published involving 218 subjects in children and adolescents compared to over a 100 in adults, one-third of which were negative. Efficacy of the TCAs for the treatment of major depression in children and adolescents has not been definitively established, even though antidepressants continue to be used in large numbers of depressed young patients with reported good clinical response in most of the open studies.

Decision Making in Selecting an Antidepressant

The following should be examined when selecting an antidepressant for any given patient:

- previous history of response
- previous history of untoward side effects
- family history of affective disorder and response to specific antidepressants
- medical history limiting use of a specific antidepressant—i.e. cardiac disease, hypertension undesirable side effects which the patient wants to avoid—i.e. weight gain with TCA, especially in adolescent females.
- avoiding plasma levels in patients phobic of needle sticks and therefore decreasing compliance
- comorbid psychiatric disorders—i.e. affective disorder and anxiety disorders may be more responsive to the TCAs as would affective disorders and ADHD. On the other hand, comorbid OCD with affective disorder may be more responsive to an SSRI. Patients with neurally mediated hypotension seen in chronic fatigue syndrome along with an affective disorder would be better treated with an SSRI.

It is highly recommended to obtain informed consent once a decision has been made to use a particular antidepressant.

Tricyclic Antidepressants

The most commonly prescribed tricyclic antidepressants are:

- Imipramine (Tofranil)
- Desipramine (Norpramine)
- Nortriptyline (Pamelor or Aventyl)
- Chlomipramine (Anafranil)

The newer generation of heterocyclic antidepressants such as amoxapine (Asendin) and trazadone (Desyrel), are seldom used in children, and this section focuses only on the most commonly used ones. The use of chlomipramine will be discussed separately.

Pretreatment Workup   Patients should have a physical examination, including an EKG and blood pressure and pulse rate recordings both in the prone and supine positions, before initiating treatment with any of the tricyclic antidepressants. The cardiovascular effects of tricyclic antidepressants include a slight but significant lengthening of the PR and QRS intervals occurring at doses of 5 mg/kg and greater. It has been suggested that the greatest lengthening of the PR interval during imipramine therapy occurs among children with the shortest PR intervals to begin with and that this effect may be protective. It has also been indicated that a relatively longer PR interval within itself is not a contraindication to receiving tricyclic medication. Other tests recommended prior to treatment with the tricyclic antidepressants include thyroid and liver function tests.

The following EKG parameters are recommended:

- Do not start treatment with a TCA if the baseline parameters are:
  - PR interval > 0.21 sec
  - QRS complex > 0.12 sec
  - QTc > 0.425 sec

- Decrease dose or stop treatment if the parameters during treatment are:
  - PR interval > 0.21 sec
  - QRS > 30% from baseline
  - QTc > 0.425 sec
  - Resting heart rate > 100/min
  - Standing heart rate > 120/min
  - BP > 130 mm/Hg systolic
  - BP > 90 mm/Hg diastolic

Dosing Regimen   Starting dose of 10–25 mg/d depending on the age of the child (approximately 1 mg/kg and gradually titrated over a period of 4 to 5 days by approximately 25 percent. It is advisable not to exceed more than 5 mg/kg of nortriptyline).

Ongoing Medical Monitoring   Plasma levels should be obtained regularly with increase in the dose plasma levels of 50–150 ng/ml desirable for Nortriptyline and between 150–250 ng/ml of either imipramine or a combination of imipramine and desipramine. The advantage of obtaining plasma levels is threefold: guide dosing regimen, determine compliance, and recognize those patients who are slow metabolizers (approximately. 10%).

Repeat ECG when steady plasma levels are obtained if the baseline ECG is normal. Repeat ECGs are recommended every 3 to 6 months if the patient is doing well and tolerating the TCA without any side effects.

Periodic weight measurements are also recommended.

Adverse Effects   Adverse effects include the early and annoying ones that include dryness of the mouth, constipation, blurred vision, postural dizziness, and sedation. Middle and moderate adverse side effects are weight gain and an increase in the PR, QRS, and QTc intervals, tachycardia, and hypertension. Late and serious side effects requiring immediate attention are cardiac toxicity and atropinic delirium (with higher plasma levels), especially with desipramine.

(Some patients complain of "flu-like" withdrawal symptoms when being tapered off TCAs.)

Indications for Tricyclics   These include enuresis, attention deficit hyperactivity disorder, panic disorder and agoraphobia, depression, and obsessive-compulsive disorder.

Pharmacotherapy is used in the treatment of enuresis only when behavioral approaches have failed. Imipramine was first described as useful in the treatment of enuresis in 1960. Despite the fact that imipramine stops or reduces bed-wetting in many children, enuresis can recur when the medication is discontinued. The mechanism of action of imipramine in the treatment of enuresis remains unclear, although its potent muscarinic receptor antagonistic action which interferes with parasympathetic function is thought to contribute to its efficacy. Its anti-enuretic action is usually unrelated to its antidepressant effects, and usually commences within 48 hours after starting a low dose in the order of 0.5–1.5 mg/kg. The initial dosage in children between the ages of 6 to 12 years is 25 mg, administered about an hour before bedtime. If the desired response is not obtained, the dose can be increased to 50 mg at bedtime. In children over the age of 12 years, the dose can be increased up to 75 mg.

Although most studies find stimulants superior to tricyclic antidepressants, the latter have been shown to be effective treatments for ADHD. They may be used as an alternative to stimulants in those patients who have either a poor response to stimulants or develop intolerable side effects. Tricyclics should also be considered in patients who are at high risk for developing tics. Since the tricyclics have a much longer half-life than stimulants, they can also be useful in patients who develop such severe rebound hyperactivity on stimulants that they are unmanageable at home in the late afternoon or evenings. Since the FDA has so far not approved the use of tricyclics in the treatment of ADHD, there are no recommended dosage guidelines. However, based on published scientific reports, it is recommended that patients start on a low dose of 0.5 mg/kg or 10–25 mg per day with gradual titration upward to a dose not to exceed 3 mg/kg.

Imipramine has been found to be effective in the treatment of adult patients with agoraphobia and panic attacks. Similar results have been reported in some children with separation anxiety disorder and school refusal. However, the reports are not conclusive and therefore it is recommended that TCAs not be precluded from consideration in the management of separation anxiety disorder.

The treatment of depression with the tricyclic antidepressants began in the early 1960s, long before there was any nosological consensus about what constitutes depression in children. With the advent of diagnostic criteria, followed by the publication of the *Diagnostic and Statistical Manual of Mental Disorders (3rd edition) (DSM-III)* in 1980, several studies appeared in the literature in which tricyclic antidepressants were used for the treatment of childhood depression. Most of these early studies, which demonstrated promising results, were open trials. More rigorous and better controlled research designs have not confirmed significant therapeutic effects of antidepressants in child or adolescent depression. However, as stated above, the number of patients studied in this manner are few compared to the adult studies. In addition, the study patients often have a chronic, unremitting course of depressive illness, with a high percentage of positive family histories of depressive disorder, alcoholism, suicidality, and a high rate of comorbidity. Adult study samples with a high degree of comorbidity and severity have also been reported to be resistant to treatment with tricyclics

The apparent lack of significant efficacy of antidepressants in the treatment of major depressive disorder of children and adolescents observed in recent well-controlled studies raises some interesting issues. It is presumed that they are suffering from the same type of disorder as occurs in adults that has reportedly been demonstrated to be responsive to antidepressants. This assumption has genetic underpinnings, and is based in part on phenomenological similarities between adult- and childhood-onset depression, and in part on the fact that the children and adolescents often have parents with medication-responsive depression. However, these assumptions may be inadequate: early age of onset may signal a more severe form of affective illness, and treatment refractiveness may be related to severity. Alternatively, the immature brain may not be synaptically capable of responding to antidepressant action in a way that reverses an episode of depression in the child or adolescent. This may necessitate the exploration of novel or combined treatment strategies.

Clomipramine (Anafranil) is a tricyclic antidepressant which has been well studied for the treatment of obsessive-compulsive disorder (OCD). Several well-designed studies have established the efficacy of clomipramine in the treatment of OCD in children and adolescents. The usual recommended starting dose is 25 mg/day, gradually increasing in increments of 25 mg/day up to 3mg/kg/day or 200 mg/day in divided doses. The side effect profile of clomipramine is similar to the other tricyclic antidepressants described previously, thus mandating the same pretreatment evaluation, especially cardiovascular status.

Monoamine Oxidase Inhibitors

With the advent of several newer and relatively safer antidepressants, especially the SSRIs there has been a marked decrease in the prescribing of the monoamine oxidase inhibitors (MAOIs). The use of MAOIs for the treatment of depressive disorders in children and adolescents is therefore limited, as are scientific studies examining their efficacy. Resistance to the use of this group of antidepressants stems primarily from the required dietary restrictions which are difficult to enforce in children and adolescents, especially in outpatient treatment. The two most commonly used drugs are phenelzine (Nardil) and tranylcypromine (Parnate).

Studies have shown efficacy for the treatment of major depression in adolescents, especially those with atypical features (Ryan et al., 1988). However, the side effects and dietary restrictions make the MAOIs less user-friendly and more cumbersome. The drug interactions can cause serious difficulties, especially hypertensive crises which can be lethal. MAOIs should be prescribed with particular caution. If one is compelled to use this group of medications, it is advisable to select the patients very carefully, restricting use to patients who are reliable, compliant, and do not indulge in substance abuse or impulsive behaviors.

Selective Serotonergic Reuptake Inhibitors

Since fluoxetine (Prozac) was introduced in the United States as the first SSRI antidepressant, it has received wide publicity, ranging from its description as a "cure-all" and "miracle drug" to one that allegedly causes patients to indulge in severe aggression and suicidal behavior. Since then, several other SSRIs have been introduced with reportedly effective antidepressant properties.

In the United States the following SSRIs are now available:

- Fluoxetine (Prozac)
- Sertraline (Zoloft)
- Paroxetine (Paxil)
- Fluvoxamine (Luvox)

Efficacy Studies   The experience with the selective serotonergic reuptake inhibitors (SSRIs) is limited. However, a recent large study by Emslie and colleagues (1997) demonstrated the efficacy of Fluoxetine in a double-blind controlled trial, using an "intent-to-treat" model. They report approximately 80 percent success in 96 children and adolescents, of whom 56 percent were randomized to active drug.

Characteristics of the SSRIs   Fluoxetine is a potent and highly selective sero-tonin reuptake inhibitor. It was introduced for the treatment of depression and obsessive-compulsive disorder in adults. To date, fluoxetine has not been approved for use in children and adolescents. Its side effect profile makes it a very attractive choice for the treatment of depression in adults, children, and adolescents. Unlike the tricyclic antidepressants and the MAOIs, it has minimal cardiac, anticholinergic, and antihistaminic side effects. Two newer serotonergic antidepressants are now available for the treatment of depression in adults. Both of these, fluvoxamine and sertraline, have a shorter half-life than fluoxetine. Fluvoxamine has fewer noradrenergic effects and can be administered at bedtime since it does not disrupt sleep. The half-life of fluvoxamine is 14 to 15 hours in healthy adults, and 17 to 22 hours in adult patients after multiple dosing. There are now a few reports in the literature of the use of these two drugs in youngsters, though controlled studies are still underway.

Pretreatment Workup   A recent physical examination is recommended before start-ing the patient on a SSRI. No specific laboratory tests are essential because none of the fac-tors tested are known to be altered during treatment. The author however suggests routine laboratory tests as indicated in the individual patient.

Dosing Regimen: Fluoxetine   The starting dose for Fluoxetine varies from 5 to 20 mg depending on the age of the child. It is infrequent for a patient with major de-pression to receive more than 40 mg of fluoxetine. There are reports of patients becoming disinhibited and irritable, hyperactive and self-destructive at higher dosages. It is perhaps possible that some patients are receiving too much fluoxetine, resulting in a serotoner-gic overload, causing disinhibiton, hyperactivity, and impulsiveness, with consequent poor judgment and self-destructive behaviors. These complications result from a rapidly rising blood level caused by the long half-life of fluoxetine. This outcome is particularly likely when doctors and patients become impatient in waiting 6 to 8 weeks for a clinical response, and increase the dose too rapidly. In our experience, children and adolescents do better on lower dosages (i.e., 5 mg/day or 10 mg every other day). Increasing dosage slowly avoids some of the above unwanted effects, while maintaining clinical improvement. Fluoxetine is now available in liquid form, making it easier to administer smaller dosages.

Dosing Regimen: Sertraline   The recommended starting dose of sertraline is usu-ally 25 mg daily, titrating up to a 100 mg/day dose depending on the desired clinical re-sponse, not exceeding 200 mg/d. Because sertraline has a shorter half-life than fluoxetine, the dose can be increased sooner than with fluoxetine.

Dosing Regimen: Paroxetine   The dosing regimen for paroxetine is usually a start-ing dose of 10 mg/day titrating up to a maximum of 50 mg/day.

Dosing Regimen: Fuvoxamine   Open studies in adolescents suggests efficacy for major depression. It has a shorter half-life than Prozac (15 hours after multiple doses). Recommended dose is 100–300 mg/day starting at 50 mg/day.

Plasma Levels   There are no plasma levels that are of value in helping titrate dos-ing with the SSRIs. Therefore the dose is adjusted based entirely on the desired clinical response or the appearance of side effects.

Ongoing Medical Monitoring   There are no specific recommendations for ongoing medical monitoring of the patient while on any of the SSRIs.

Adverse Effects   Early side effects are usually gastrointestinal with symptoms of nausea, heartburn, and diarrhea. Later side effects include behavioral activation, disinhibition, and impulsiveness, often seen as hyperactivity in children and adolescents. Insomnia and occasionally hypersomnia, apathy, and loss of appetite can result as well. In the case of hypersomnia the dose is administered at bedtime rather than in the morning. Neurological side effects such as headaches can sometimes result in either decreasing the dose or discontinuation of the SSRI in some patients. Rarely, patients report the appearance of a tremor and akathesia. Delayed ejaculation can present a problem in male adolescents resulting in sexual dysfunction.

Despite reports of increased suicidality, the majority of data does not suggest a cause and effect relationship between the use of fluoxetine and suicidality. Evidence suggests that the rate of suicidality in fluoxetine-treated patients is no higher than in patients treated with other antidepressants. It appears, rather, to be an effect of the underlying vulnerability of patients with severe depression to suicidal ideation and behavior.

The SSRIs remain a promising group of antidepressants for the treatment of major depressive disorders in children and adolescents. They are especially favored by teenage girls who generally like to avoid the weight gain they may experience with the tricyclic antidepressants. Caution needs to be exercised when switching a patient from fluoxetine to a tricyclic antidepressant. Fluoxetine acts synergistically with tricyclics and can cause alarmingly high blood levels of the tricyclics, resulting in serious cardiotoxicity. Therefore, it is advisable to have at least a two weeks wash out period before starting the patient on a tricyclic antidepressant. The switching of a patient from a tricyclic to a SSRI is less of a problem.

Other Antidepressants

In addition to the tricyclics, selective serotonergic reuptake inhibitors, and monoamine oxidase inhibitors, the following are relatively new antidepressants are now being used in children and adolescents:

- Venlafaxine (Effexor)
- Bupropion (Wellbutrin)
- Buspirone (Buspar)
- Nefazodone (Serzone)

Venlafaxine (Effexor)   Venlafaxine strongly inhibits the uptake of both NE and 5-HT and, to a lesser extent, dopamine. It has a rapid onset of action that makes it unique among the antidepressants. There are no studies in children and adolescents to date except for anecdotal reports and clinical experience.

Dosing Schedule   The dosage ranges from 25 mg to not more than 200 mg/day in either BID or TID dosing prescribed in increments. Adult studies have not shown increased efficacy in dosages greater than 200 mg, even though dosages of up to 375 mg have been used. Plasma levels are not available. No pretreatment laboratory workup is recommended.

Adverse Effects   The side effects of Venlafaxine include the following:

- CNS: somnolence, dizziness, insomnia, nervousness, dry mouth, anxiety, and seizures
  - Gastrointestinal: nausea, loss of appetite, and weight loss
  - Urogenital: abnormal ejaculation reported in less than 1 percent of adults
  - Other: headaches, excessive sweating, and hypertension.

Bupropion (Wellbutrin)   Bupropion is a newer antidepressant which has been shown to be superior to placebo in randomized, double-blind placebo-controlled trials in adults. It is a weaker inhibitor of the neuronal uptake of serotonin and NE, and also inhibits the neuronal reuptake of dopamine to some extent. Bupropion is an attractive alternative to the tricyclic antidepressants in those patients who are unable to tolerate the side effects of the latter. There are anecdotal reports and a few open studies describing its efficacy in the treatment of major depression in children and adolescents. Bupropion is supplied in strengths of 75 and 100 mg tablets.

Dosing Schedule   The usual starting dose is 75 mg/d not to exceed a total of 450 mg/d in TID dosing. (No single dose of bupropion should exceed 150 mg.) Plasma levels are not available and pretreatment workup may include evaluation of the liver function tests, since hepatocellular damage has been reported in animal studies.

Adverse Effects   The most frequent and annoying side effects are as follows:

- CNS: including akathesia, agitation, sedation, insomnia, headaches, and tremors. The risk of seizures is 4/1000 patients. This is a fourfold increased risk compared to other antidepressants. Predisposing factors are a history of seizure disorder, head injury, CNS tumor, and sudden and large increments in the dose of bupropion.
  - Gastrointestinal: usually nausea and vomiting.
  - Dermatological: skin rashes
  - Cardiovascular: dizziness and tachycardia.
  - Others: fatigue, blurred vision, impotence, and menstrual cramps.

Buspirone (Buspar)   Buspirone is an anxiolytic agent with antidepressant properties. It is considered an effective and relatively safe alternative to the benzodiazepines in the treatment of anxiety disorders. There are case reports of its use in the treatment of anxiety disorder in adolescents. The recommended dose is 15 to 30 mg/d in divided dosage. No pretreatment workup is recommended. The side effect profile is reported to be relatively benign with a wide margin for safety and low abuse potential. The more commonly reported side effects are insomnia, dizziness, headaches, and gastrointestinal complaints. There is no established use of plasma levels.

Nefazodone (Serzone)   Nefazodone is one of the newest antidepressants, structurally different from the TCAs, SSRIs, and the MAOIs. There are no specific laboratory tests recommended. There are no case reports of its use in children and adolescents. No plasma levels are available. The dosing schedule follows (available in 100 mg and 150 mg tablets).

Dosing Schedule   Starting dose in adults is 100 mg BID

- Increments of 100 mg/day weekly
- Maximum recommended dose 600 mg/day
- Average dosing 300–600 mg/day

Adverse Effects   These infrequent in doses of less than 300 mg/day. They include the following and are usually dose-related.

- Gastrointestinal: dryness of the mouth, nausea, and constipation.
- CNS: headaches, somnolence and dizziness, and blurred vision.

MOOD STABILIZERS

Mood stabilizers have been used in children for a variety of conditions. These range from the treatment of bipolar disorders to the management of aggression, self-mutilating behaviors in autistic children, organic mood disorders, especially those secondary to closed head trauma, and hyperactivity. In addition, they have been shown to have a favorable antidepressant effect when used as an adjunct to antidepressants for the treatment of refractory major affective disorder.

The frequently used mood stabilizers include the following medications:

- Lithium (available in several preparations)
- Carbamazepine (Tegretol)
- Valproic acid (Depakene)

Lithium

Lithium is a monovalent cation from the alkali metal group. It is rapidly absorbed in the stomach and small intestine and is eliminated primarily by renal excretion. Pharmacokinetic studies have shown that the half-life is shorter and the renal clearance is usually greater in children than adults on the basis of body mass. Lithium has a tendency to concentrate in a few tissues, notably the thyroid gland and the renal medulla. Excretion of lithium depends on the glomerular filtration rate (GFR) and proximal reabsorption (Campbell, Perry, & Green, 1984; Delong & Aldershof, 1987).

Pretreatment Workup   Prior to initiating treatment with lithium, a thorough medical evaluation is mandatory, including an assessment of renal function, thyroid status, a baseline EKG, and serum electrolytes. There is currently disagreement over the necessity to carry out a quantitative assessment of the GFR by collecting 24-hour urine for creatinine clearance. This poses a practical problem, especially in younger children or seriously ill adolescents who are unable to cooperate fully with this procedure and in those children who have nighttime enuresis. The use of calculated creatinine clearance based on a single urine sample has been suggested by Cockcroft and Gault (1976).

Dosing Regimen   Lithium is available as lithium carbonate and lithium citrate. Lithobid, a coated form of lithium carbonate, is somewhat better tolerated and causes fewer initial gastrointestinal side effects. Lithium citrate is available in liquid form and is therefore useful in younger patients who require smaller or fractional dosages and in others for whom noncompliance by "cheeking" medications may be an issue.

The dosage regimen and scheduling in children over 5 years of age is similar to that of adults. A starting dose of 150–300 mg/day, depending on the age of the child, is recommended. Subsequently, the dose of lithium should be titrated every 4–5 days upwards obtaining lithium levels with each increase of the dose. Dosage requirements are determined by serum lithium levels and vary from one patient to another.

Plasma Levels   These should be obtained regularly to achieve and maintain a therapeutic lithium level of 0.7 meq/L to 1.2 meq/L. Serum levels should be drawn approximately 12 hours after the last lithium dose. In hospitalized patients, this is done effectively in the mornings. However, in outpatients, it may be more practical to obtain an afternoon or evening serum level, avoiding loss of school time that may be occasioned by a morning blood drawing.

Initially, serum levels are drawn about twice a week; as the patient stabilizes the frequency of serum levels can decrease. Our practice is to obtain serum levels every 2 to 3 months in those patients who are stable and not experiencing side effects.

Ongoing Medical Monitoring   Ongoing medical monitoring should include renal functions and thyroid function tests annually. Serum electrolytes should be done as needed, keeping in mind the unique needs of a particular patient. EKGs should be monitored regularly especially if the pretreatment EKG showed abnormalities.

Adverse Effects   The following side effects have been reported with the use of lithium:

Early and Mild   When treatment is initiated, patients may experience gastrointestinal symptoms such as nausea, diarrhea, and abdominal cramps. These tend to subside after stable serum levels are attained and can sometimes be alleviated by prescribing lithobid.

Middle and Moderate   The side effects associated with maintenance treatment with lithium are hand tremors which can be embarrassing or disabling to schoolage children, polyuria (possibly from nephrogenic diabetes insipidus), and hypothyroidism. These side effects must be addressed with the patient, because their presence can result in discouragement and noncompliance. The polyuria is accompanied by polydipsia and can sometimes precipitate the reemergence of enuresis. Weight gain and muscle weakness are other side effects which can be discouraging, especially the former.

Late and Serious   Symptoms of toxicity usually appear at serum levels above 1.5 meq/L. With rapidly rising lithium levels, hand tremors can reappear along with gastrointestinal symptoms. More severe toxicity is signaled by cardiac arrhythmias along with impairments in consciousness with lethargy, delirium, and stupor. Lithium toxicity is a serious but largely preventable complication if the patients are monitored closely and effectively.

Nonsteroidal anti-inflammatory agents, which are commonly used in youngsters, can interfere with renal excretion and can cause elevation in serum lithium, resulting in toxicity. Dehydration, caused by excessive sweating or febrile illness without fluid replacement, will elevate serum lithium levels. There has been concern about the effect of lithium on bone growth, since lithium is known to be deposited in the bone. At the present time, there is no evidence to support any growth impairment secondary to long-term lithium use. Facial acne may be exacerbated by lithium, which can undermine compliance, especially in adolescents. The acne can usually be effectively treated with antibiotics such as tetracyclines, with no known untoward effects.

Lithium is becoming an important psychopharmacological agent not only in the treatment and prophylaxis of depression and bipolar disorder, but also for aggression in children and adolescents. In many instances it is replacing neuroleptics for the management of aggressive and disruptive behaviors, avoiding cognitive dulling and the more serious long-term side effect, tardive dyskinesia, associated with neuroleptic treatment, especially in the mentally retarded.

Carbamazepine (Tegretol)

The most common anticonvulsant used in the treatment of psychiatric disorders in youngsters is carbamazepine. In the pediatric population, carbamazepine has been used mainly for controlling aggressive behaviors and for the treatment of patients with bipolar disorder. Carbamazepine is an iminodibenzyl derivative with a tricyclic structure similar to imipramine and chlorpromazine. Double-blind placebo-controlled studies in adults have shown anti-manic effects in neurologically normal bipolar patients. It has also been shown to be prophylactic in mania and depression in lithium-resistant patients, especially those with rapidly cycling bipolar disorder. In youngsters, carbamazepine has been reported to be effective in the treatment of explosive behaviors associated with temporal lobe epilepsy as well as in episodic dyscontrol. Other studies and case reports have shown carbamazepine to decrease impulsivity, agitation, aggression, and affective lability to varying degrees in youngsters.

Pretreatment Workup   This workup should include a complete blood count, including differential and platelet count, electrolytes, liver function tests, and an EKG.

Dosing Regimen   In children, the recommended starting dose is 100–300 mg/day in divided dosage depending on the age of the child. The dose should be titrated every 4 to 5 days upwards by 100 mg/day obtaining plasma levels with each increase to obtain therapeutic carbamazepine levels of 8–12 ug/ml. In adolescents, the dose ranges from approximately 400 to 800 mgs/day.

Ongoing Medical Monitoring   Ongoing medical monitoring should include blood counts every 3 months, electrolytes as needed, follow-up EKG if the pretreatment EKG shows abnormalities, and liver function tests annually.

Carbamazepine levels should be obtained with each increase in the dose and approximately every 8 to 12 weeks when therapeutic.

Adverse Effects

Early and Reversible   These include allergic skin rash, initial lethargy, drowsiness, ataxia, and dysarthria. Most of these can be eliminated by lowering the dosage.

Later and Serious   Other ill effects that have been reported and need to be closely monitored are elevated liver function tests, leucopenia, thrombocytopenia, and agranulocytosis.

Carbamazepine can be used synergistically with lithium, neuroleptics, and tricyclic antidepressants. Combination with MAOIs requires great caution, because of a substantial rise in the plasma concentration of carbamazepine causing potentially serious toxicity. Psychopharmacologically, carbamazepine is the second medication of choice after lithium as an anti-manic agent and for the prophylaxis of future episodes. It is considered especially useful for rapid cyclers—i.e., patients with four or more episodes of mania and/or depression each year. Carbamazepine is also useful for augmentation of an antidepressant.

Valproic Acid (Depakene)

Valproic acid is another anticonvulsant which has been widely used for the treatment of bipolar disorders in adults and which is gaining favor with child and adolescent psychiatrists as well.

Pretreatment Workup   This workup should include complete blood counts, serum electrolytes, and liver function tests.

Dosing Regimen   The recommended starting dose for valproic acid is 125 mg/day in divided dosage depending on the age of the child (15 mg/kg/day). The dose should be titrated at one-week intervals by 125 mg/day, obtaining plasma levels with each increase to obtain a therapeutic level of 50 to 100 mcg/ml. The maximum recommended dose should not exceed 60 mg/kg/day.

Ongoing Medical Monitoring   Medical monitoring should include blood counts every 3 months, serum electrolytes as needed, and depakene blood levels with each increase in the dose and approximately every 8 to 12 weeks when therapeutic.

Adverse Effects

Early and Reversible   These are usually gastrointestinal, skin rash, initial lethargy and drowsiness, dysarthria, and ataxia.

Later and Serious   These include elevated liver enzymes which may lead to hepatic failure in some patients. The occurrence of anemia, leucopenia, and thrombocytopenia need to be closely monitored.

From a psychopharmacological standpoint, valproic acid is now being considered as an important anti-manic agent along with lithium and carbamazepine. It is also being used clinically as an adjunct to lithium and/or carbamazepine for those patients who require double mood stabilization.

Neuroleptics

Neuroleptics, also known as "antipsychotic drugs" and "major tranquilizers," have been clinically available for over 40 years. In children and adolescents, they have been used to treat a number of psychiatric disorders, behavior problems, and symptoms. As in adults, they are most widely used specifically for the treatment of psychosis and severe agitation. In lower dosages, they have been used in the treatment of Tourette's disorder, attention deficit disorder with hyperactivity, and for the control of behavioral problems, especially in patients with mental retardation and pervasive developmental disorders. Neuroleptics are dopamine receptor antagonists. Post-synaptic receptor blockade in the mesolimbic system of the brain is thought to result in the desired therapeutic effect in psychosis, whereas similar blockade in the nigrostriatal dopamine pathway produces the unwanted extrapyramidal effects.

The most commonly used neuroleptics fall into three broad groups:

- Phenothiazines: Chlorpromazine (Thorazine), Thioridazine (Mellaril), Loxitane, Trifluperazine, and Fluphenazine (Prolixin)
- Thioxanthenes: Thiothixene and Taractan
- Butyrophenones: Haloperidol (Haldol) and Droperidol (Inapsine).

Among the variety of neuroleptics available, haloperidol has been relatively well studied by several investigators in the management of childhood disorders. In most of these studies, haloperidol proved to be significantly superior to placebo and was usually better than psychotropic medications from other classes, such as psychostimulants and lithium. Low doses of high-potency neuroleptics such as haloperidol and fluphenazine (0.5–4.0 mg/day) have been shown to be effective in reducing social withdrawal and stereotypic behaviors in autistic children and shown significant reductions in hyperactivity and aggressive symptoms, and significant improvement in peer relations in children with pervasive developmental disorders. The average dose used was 0.04 mg/kg per day of haloperidol or fluphenazine.

Current evidence does not suggest any clear superiority of a particular neuroleptic, once corrected for potency, in the management of psychotic symptoms. The incisive, high-potency neuroleptics such as haloperidol and fluphenazine are generally less sedating and thus interfere less with school performance. Review of the literature suggests that in most instances neuroleptics are generally well tolerated by youngsters without serious ill effects. Informed consent is recommended before starting any patient on a neuroleptic, especially in light of the potential for long-term deleterious side effects, such as tardive dyskinesia.

Adverse effects secondary to neuroleptic treatment can be described as early and late. The earlier side effects, which are reversible include sedation, dystonic reactions, restlessness, akathisia, parkinsonian symptoms, and postural hypotension. Most of these side effects are subjectively uncomfortable and in the case of a dystonic reaction, frightening to the patient. The extrapyramidal side effects can often be reversed by the administration of anticholinergic drugs, such as diphenhydramine (Benadryl) 25 m. orally or intramuscularly or benztropine (Cogentin) 0.5 to 2 mg given daily.

Withdrawal dyskinesia, choreoform movements which occur upon discontinuation of neuroleptics, are more frequent in children than in adults. Withdrawal dyskinesia subsides over a period of days to weeks and can be difficult to distinguish from tardive dyskinesia. Although tardive dyskinesia occurs more frequently in the elderly, it can develop in adolescents and young adults as a consequence of long-term and/or high-dose neuroleptic treatment. Though there is a belief that neuroleptics lower the seizure threshold, there are no systematic studies that demonstrate this. In our experience, neuroleptics can be safely used in patients with a seizure disorder, when monitored appropriately. Of particular importance to adolescents are the embarrassing side effects such as worsening of acne, weight gain, and easy sunburning.

Another potentially life-threatening disorder that affects up to 1 percent of patients receiving neuroleptics is the Neuroleptic Malignant Syndrome (NMS) (Joshi, Capozzoli, & Coyle, 1991). The proximate cause of the syndrome appears to be insufficient stimulation of CNS dopamine receptors, since a syndrome identical to NMS occurs in patients with Parkinson's disease who have their dopamine receptor agonists abruptly discontinued. The principal clinical features of NMS include striking rigidity, hyperthermia, diaphoresis, rhabdomyolysis, and delirium. Recent studies suggest that an underlying affective disorder may render individuals more vulnerable to developing NMS.

The risk for NMS may be increasing in the pediatric population, since psychotropic medications are assuming a greater role in the management of severe psychiatric disturbances in this age group. Neuroleptics are now being introduced early in the treatment of affective disorder with psychosis and childhood schizophrenia. There are case reports of youngsters who have developed NMS after having received neuroleptics. Usually the patients become seriously ill, needing treatment in the intensive care unit. The clinical symptoms of NMS can be reversed when treated with bromocriptine and/or dantrolene. Bromocriptine is a dopamine D-2 receptor agonist and is effective in reversing the acute extrapyramidal symptoms of profound rigidity and its secondary consequences, including hyperthermia and rhabdomyolysis. Dantrolene acts by enhancing intramuscular calcium sequestration. NMS should be considered in any patient presenting with fever of unknown origin, striking extrapyramidal symptoms, and current or recent treatment with neuroleptics.

OTHER MEDICATIONS

Clozapine (Clozaril)

Clozapine is an atypical neuroleptic that has been shown to be effective in a significant portion of chronic, treatment-resistant schizophrenics. The drug does not cause acute extrapyramidal side effects or tardive dyskinesia. A striking feature of the drug is its ability not only to reduce positive symptoms of schizophrenia but also to abate negative symptoms. Unfortunately, clozaril bears the serious, potential fatal risk of inducing aplastic anemia in up to 4 percent of treated patients. As a consequence, patients must be closely monitored with weekly white blood cell counts. The use of clozaril in the treatment of adolescents with schizophrenia, who had failed treatment with more conventional neuroleptics, has been described in the literature (Birmaher, Baker, Kapur, Quintana, & Ganguli, 1992). However, a number of new atypical neuroleptics without such toxicity are in clinical trials in the United States, and could prove useful in psychotic disorders in children and adolescents.

Risperidone (Risperdal)

Risperidone is now being used as an alternative to the traditional neuroleptic medication from the treatment of psychosis in adults, children, and adolescents. It is a serotonin/dopamine antagonist and is thought to decrease the incidence of tardive dyskinesia.

In adults it has been shown to be effective in the improvement of negative symptoms with lessened risk of extrapyramidal symptoms. This is thought to result from blockade of serotonin 5-HT, receptors, possibly through a modulatory effect on dopamine D2 activity in the frontal cortex and the basal ganglia. It is also shown to be effective in the improvement of positive symptoms as a result of blockade of dopamine D2 receptors in the limbic system. It is available in 1, 2, 3, and 4 mg. tablets.

The recommended starting dose is 0.5 mg BID with young children and increasing it in increments every 4 to 5 days. The maximum total dose recommended should not exceed 6 mg/day. The common adverse effects are initial sedation, orthostatic hypotension, and, in some patients, rigidity and cogwheeling. Not enough information is available at present on the concomitant use of risperdal and other antipsychotic medications. However, it is advisable to taper the previous neuroleptic before starting the risperdal, even though an overlap is sometimes necessary depending upon the severity of the patient's symptoms.

Clonidine (Catapress)

Clonidine is well known as an anti-hypertensive drug which was first used for the treatment of Tourette's syndrome. It is an alpha-2 adrenergic receptor agonist and acts by decreasing noradrenergic functioning. The results of several open and double-blind trials suggest that clonidine is effective in the reduction of tics in patients with Tourette's syndrome. However, clonidine has also been shown to be efficacious in the treatment of ADHD, especially with hyperarousal problems and PTSD. Several clinicians are now safely using a combination of stimulants and clonidine in those patients who do not respond adequately to either medication alone.

Pretreatment Workup   This should include a complete physical examination, paying special attention to the cardiovascular status and baseline pulse and blood pressure. A baseline EKG is recommended.

Dosing Schedule   The usual recommended starting dose of clonidine is 0.05 mg/day slowly titrated over several days and weeks to achieve the desired behavioral effect or reduction in tics. Dosages over 0.3 mg/day usually result in sedation and, thus, inattention in the class room. Clonidine has a slower onset of action than stimulants; therefore improvement in restlessness, attention span, or impulsiveness or diminution in tics may not be immediately evident.

Adverse Effects   These sometimes include hypotension with subjective dizziness, especially if the dose is increased rapidly. Because of the potential increase in the PR interval subsequent EKGs should be obtained regularly.

Guanfacine (Tenex)

Guanfacine is a relatively new medication that has been reported to be useful in the management of treatment-resistant ADHD. Guanfacine hydrochloride is a long-acting alpha-2 agonist. In open studies it has been shown to be highly effective with minimal side effects in patients ranging from 7 to 17 years of age. No specific pretreatment workup is recommended. The dose ranges from 0.5–3.0 mg/day. The only side effect reported in the open trials was mild sedation at the start of treatment. However, this was thought to be less of a problem than with clonidine.

Beta Blockers

The most commonly used beta adrenergic blocking agent in the treatment and management of psychiatric symptoms is propanalol. There have been reports in the literature of its effectiveness in the management of rage outbursts, aggressive and violent behaviors in youngsters. The dose range in adolescents is 80 to 280 mg/day in divided dosage. However, there are no well-controlled studies demonstrating its efficacy and safety. Propanalol acts on both the central nervous system and peripheral sympathetic system and is contraindicated in patients with asthma, diabetes mellitus, bradycardia, and hypotension. It is important to do an EKG and monitor the cardiac status by frequent measurement of the pulse rate and blood pressure.

CONCLUSION

The use of psychotropic medications in the treatment of psychiatric disturbances in children and adolescents has come to be common practice. It is therefore extremely important to have a rational approach to this mode of treatment and apply it rigorously.

It is not an easy task to extrapolate conclusions about efficacy and safety from adults to children when it comes to the use of psychopharmacological agents. The difficulties in demonstrating the efficacy of antidepressants in the treatment of child and adolescent major depressive disorders, for example, justifiably raises important questions about the facile assumption that knowledge gained in adult controlled studies can simply be extended to youth. The FDA generally does not provide endorsement to the pharmaceutical industry about the pediatric use of most of the medications that are currently being used. In fact, a general disclaimer is routinely inserted in the labeling, warning that "safety and efficacy have not been proven" in this age. It is imperative that pharmaceutical companies carry out well-controlled studies of the efficacy of new psychotropic medications on children, if it appears that the drug could be used in this age group. This development would certainly go far in advancing our knowledge of the rational use of psychotropic drugs in child and adolescent psychiatry.

As our understanding of psychotropic drug treatment in child and adolescent psychiatry advances, the real challenge will be to address ethical concerns that we face such as informed consent, use of placebo, and the definition of minimum risk. In addition, we remain challenged by some of the methodological obstacles in conducting well-controlled double-blind studies. It is abundantly clear that the judicious and responsible use of psychotropic medications in children and adolescents is a complex task. The next decade holds promise and excitement with the greater availability of a wide range of psychotropic medications. We in the mental health field need to keep pace and continue to become more sophisticated and skilled in the area of psychopharmacology.

REFERENCES

Birmaher, B., Baker, R., Kapur, S., Quintana, H., & Ganguli, R. (1992). Clozapine for the treatment of adolescents with schizophrenia. *Journal of the American Academy of Child and Adolescent Psychiatry, 31*, 1, 160–164.

Campbell, M., Perry, R., & Green, W. H. (1984). Use of lithium in children and adolescents. *Psychosomatics, 25*, 95–106.

Cockcroft, D. W., & Gault, M. H. (1976). Predictions of Creatinine clearance from Serum Creatinine: Nephron. 16: 31–41.

Delong, G. R., & Aldershof, A.L. (1987). Long term experience with lithium treatment in childhood: Correlation with clinical diagnosis. *Journal of the American Academy of Child and Adolescent Psychiatry, 26*, 389–394.

Emslie, G. H., Rush, A. J., Weinberg, W. A., Kowatch, R. A., Hughes, C. W., Carmody, T., & Rintelmann, J. (1997). A double blind, randomized placebo-controlled trial of Fluoxetine in depressed children and adolescents. *Journal of the American Academy of Child & Adolescent Psychiatry. 54*(11): 1025–1030.

Greenhill, L. L. (1992). Pharmacologic treatment of attention deficit disorder. *Pediatric Psychopharmacology: Psychiatric Clinics of North America, 15,* 1.

Joshi, P. T., Capozzoli, J. A., & Coyle, J. T. (1991). Neuroleptic malignant syndrome: A life-threatening complication of neuroleptic treatment in adolescents with affective disorder. *Pediatrics, 87* (2).

Joshi, P. T., Coyle, J. T., & Walkup, J. T. (1994). Pharmacotherapy in children and adolescents. In H. S. Ghuman & R. M. Sarles (Eds.), *Handbook of adolescent inpatient psychiatric treatment.* New York: Brunner/Mazel.

Medical Economics. (1996). *Physician's desk reference* (45th. ed.) Oradell, NJ: the Author.

Ryan, N. D., Puig-Antich J., Rabinovich H., Fied, J., Ambrosini, P. J., Meyer, V., Torres, D., Dachille, S., & Mazzie, D. (1988). MAOIs in adolescent major depression unresponsive to tricyclic antidepressants. *Journal of the American Academy of Child and Adolescent Psychiatry, 27,* 755–758.

Weiner, J. M., & Jaffe S. (1996). History of drug therapy in childhood and adolescent psychiatric disorders. In J. M. Weiner (Ed.), *Psychopharmacology in childhood and adolescence.* New York, Basic Books.

Chapter 18

Cognitive-Behavioral Therapy with Children and Adolescents

Mark D. Weist, Ph.D. and Jeffrey S. Danforth, Ph.D.

Cognitive-behavioral approaches are among the most widely used in assessment and treatment efforts with children, and their popularity has increased because of mounting pressures to provide services to youth more rapidly and efficiently. Diverse approaches may be characterized as cognitive-behavioral, with some focused primarily on modification of overt behavior such as parent-training in child behavior management, others focused mainly on modifying "inner characteristics" of the child such as changing "irrational" thoughts, and many others involving a combination of strategies focused on overt and covert behaviors. This chapter provides a brief review of the behavioral, and cognitive science underpinnings of cognitive-behavioral therapies, followed by a description of techniques, with illustrative case studies.

HISTORICAL AND THEORETICAL BACKGROUND

Behavior Therapy

Child behavior therapy has its roots in the historical case of Peter, a boy treated for his fear of furry objects by Mary Cover Jones (1924). Along with Jones, there were many other scientists (J. Stanley Gray, B. F. Skinner, Hans Eysenk, Joseph Wolpe) who were advancing the field of behavior therapy in the 1930s, 1940s, and 1950s. However, it was not until behavioral interventions were introduced in work with severely disturbed institutionalized children in the 1960s that child behavior therapy became widely used (Ross, 1981).

Learning theories relating to respondent conditioning (reflexive behavior elicited by stimuli) and operant learning (more purposive behavior shaped by its consequences; Skinner, 1938) were foundational to the development of child behavior therapy, with widely used techniques such as systematic desensitization, and positive reinforcement of behavior emanating from these respective theories. Progressively, approaches based on operant learning became more prominent as the effects of various schedules of reinforcement and punishment on behavior were elucidated. Beginning in the 1960s, the concepts of observational learning or modeling, as explicated by Bandura (1969), became an important part of the growing specialty of child behavior therapy.

Eschewing abstract conceptualizations, behavior therapists focus on overt and observable behavior, precisely measured before, during, and following treatment interventions. Target behaviors are assessed and modified along key dimensions of frequency, intensity, duration, and latency. Functional analysis is used to examine factors in the current environment that influence, or are functionally related to, the target behavior. Historical and individual features that may influence performance are considered when designing treatment plans, but the primary focus of the functional analysis is on the target behavior, its topography, its antecedents, and its consequences. The subsequent behavior therapy based on this analysis is aimed at increasing behaviors that are deficient, decreasing excessive behaviors, and facilitating the learning of important skills.

Cognitive Therapy

Cognitive therapy has a phenomenological conceptual basis which contends that the way individuals view themselves to a great extent determines how they feel and how they behave (Dattilio & Freeman, 1992). Aaron Beck played a pioneering role in the development of cognitive therapies through his studies on depression. Beck (1967) characterized the cognitive style of depressed patients as involving a triad; that is, thinking negatively about themselves, the world, and the future. Using an active and structured approach, the cognitive therapist assists the depressed patient in using a number of strategies to combat negative thoughts and emotional states. These include stopping automatic depressing thoughts, substituting more positive and objective cognitions for negative ones, and modifying dysfunctional belief systems that predispose individuals to depression.

Ellis (1962), in his rational-emotive therapy (RET), suggested an ABC model of negative emotion. In this model, activating events (A) are interpreted based on our beliefs (B), which influence the behavioral and emotional consequences (C) of the event. As such, it is our beliefs about events, versus the events themselves, that determine our emotional and behavioral reactions. Humans have a tendency to form irrational beliefs such as "one must be loved by everyone," or that mistakes are "catastrophic." These irrational beliefs then lead to negative behaviors and emotions. The essence of RET is on modifying these irrational beliefs.

Cognitive therapies of Beck (1967) and Ellis (1962) have in common their emphasis on the "automaticity" of thoughts, feelings, and behavior—that is, many patients believe they have no control over their feelings. An example is the patient who believes that problems at work directly cause him or her to become angry and depressed, and to lose control over his or her behavior. The essence of these cognitive therapies is to teach patients that they do in fact have control over their emotional and behavioral reactions; that events happen, are then interpreted, and these interpretations often dictate the way they subsequently act and feel. Thus, treatments emphasize training in forming more adaptive interpretations of themselves and events in their lives. Both approaches also include more behavioral elements, such as defining treatment goals in observable and measurable terms, assigning patients homework, and using an empirical approach to gauge the impact of psychotherapy.

Cognitive-Behavioral Therapy

Cognitive-behavioral therapy (CBT) involves elements of behavior therapy and cognitive therapy. Dysfunctional behavior is viewed as related to a complex interaction of cognitive factors including information processing style, problem solving and thought content, overt behaviors, and environmental experiences (Braswell & Kendall, 1988). An empirical approach is viewed as necessary to successful CBT. This involves collection of objective and reliable assessments from multiple sources including the child and his or her parents and teachers, and careful planning of interventions which are focused on empirically valid treatment targets (Weist, Ollendick, & Finney, 1991). Once interventions have begun, they are assessed carefully to determine whether they are having their intended effects. In assessment and treatment efforts, cognition and behavior are not viewed as dichotomous; rather, they are viewed as reciprocally determined, with cognition affecting behavior and vice-versa. The implication of this view is that all cognitive-behavioral strategies involve a focus on both observable behavior and cognitive factors, which is presumed to increase the potency of interventions beyond what could be accomplished by an exclusive behavioral or cognitive focus (Hart & Morgan, 1993). Essentially, there is a continuum of cognitive-behavioral approaches, with varying degrees of attention paid to cognitive factors relative to overt behaviors.

An Overview of Commonly Used CBT Strategies   In an early and extremely influential application of CBT, Meichenbaum and Goodman (1971) developed Self-Instructional Training (SIT) for use with impulsive children. The goal of this program was to teach these children in verbal self-coaching to guide their behavior through challenging situations. Using SIT, the therapist first works with the child and his or her family to identify situations in which behavioral problems or skill deficits are shown, such as working on math problems while other students are acting disruptive. The therapist then models for the child verbal self-coaching through the problem situation, like "Okay, this is a division problem, I can tell by the way the problem is presented. Let's see, I need to.... How am I doing?" In SIT, the therapist serves as a model who demonstrates "thinking aloud" for the child in therapy. In demonstrating these "thinking aloud" skills, the therapist models coping statements like "This isn't too hard, I can handle this." Following the therapist modeling, the child is guided through practice of SIT, first using self-coaching statements out loud, then whispering, then making such statements internally.

In our practices, we have been impressed by the power of this straightforward and fairly simple intervention. SIT provides training in a necessary skill of guiding behavior by thoughts that many children do not have. Often, adults make the implicit assumption that children think about their behavior; in reality, in many cases they do not, with their behavior functionally representing impulsive reactions to situations, with little, if any thinking actually going on. Training skills in thinking about behavior before, during, and after it occurs is a powerful intervention for most youth, even for those without emotional/behavioral disturbances.

There are a number of variations on SIT, such as efforts to train youth to self-regulate their behavior. These involve teaching children to self-monitor their thoughts and behavior in difficult situations, and to use verbal self-statements as consequences for positive, "I did great that time!" and negative, "I didn't do that well that time; next time, I'll have to try harder" performances. A technique that we have found particularly useful is goal-oriented thinking (Graziano & Mooney, 1982). Using this procedure, children are taught to ask themselves four questions prior to, during, and after a challenging situation: 1) What is my goal for this problem? 2) What can I do about it? 3) How's my plan working? and, 4) How did I do? Goal-oriented thinking is particularly useful in helping children to see how maladaptive some behaviors or thoughts are. An example of such an insightful statement would be, "Thinking about how much I hate math is not helping me to finish this test." The authors have found this technique useful in their own lives, for example, "becoming angry at other drivers does not help me get home any sooner or more easily!"

Another prominent CBT intervention is to train youth in systematic problem-solving strategies. For example, Shure and Spivack (1980) described an interpersonal problem-solving program that trained children to guide their behavior systematically through problem situations by: a) generating a list of behavioral alternatives, b) evaluating each alternative based on its costs and benefits, c) selecting one alternative, d) trying it out, and e) evaluating its impact. A major function of the intervention was to get children to slow down and carefully guide their behavior through challenging situations versus reacting impulsively.

For children who have problems with anxiety and other problems such as motor overactivity, relaxation training is a valuable clinical intervention. Commonly, children are trained in three techniques: 1) Progressive Muscle Relaxation, which involves training in tensing and then relaxing muscles from the feet to the head, and then back to the feet, all the while focusing on the feelings of relaxing muscle groups, 2) Imagery, which involves training in vividly imagining a peaceful and pleasant scene, and 3) Deep Breathing, or training the child to inhale purposefully and slowly, expanding the diaphragm, and then purposefully exhale. Each of these techniques requires a number of demonstrations by the therapist, followed by in-session practice by the child, followed by home assignments to use the techniques, followed by in-session practice again. Once the child has experience with each of these techniques, we recommend that therapists ask him or her for his or her preferences on favored ones. Often, children will choose to use a combined strategy such as deep breathing and imagery at the same time.

We must emphasize that for all of the CBT strategies reviewed, therapists need to provide adequate modeling of skills, have the child practice the skills repeatedly during and in between sessions, and provide encouragement and reinforcement to the child for using the skills. It is also important to train the child's caretakers in the same skills, and to encourage them to provide rewards to the child for demonstration of the skills in situations at home. Clinicians should be aware of the common tendency to provide brief and insufficient training in CBT strategies. This is partly related to the somewhat awkward nature of direct skill training with children (e.g., modeling skills, role-playing). As such, it is "easier" for the therapist to address problems that are presented in the office each week reactively rather than to implement a comprehensive plan to improve the child's skills. Further, such therapy can become monotonous, as skills need to be practiced every week for children to learn them and incorporate them into their behavioral repertoires.

We use the analogy of "cognitive muscles" that before training were "very small and weak," and will only get "bigger and stronger" through repetitive practice in a range of situations. This analogy applies to the learning of these skills by children, but also to the comfort level of the clinician in doing CBT. Importantly, such repetitive and cross-situational practice serves to promote maintenance of the skills over time, and their generalization across challenging situations and tasks (Stokes & Baer, 1977). In the following discussion, we provide more detailed description of CBT strategies, highlighting approaches varying in their relative focus on overt behavior versus cognitive factors. Just as there is diversity in CBT approaches, there is diversity among practitioners of CBT, with some placing relatively greater emphasis on overt behavior, and some placing relatively greater emphasis on cognitive factors.

Representative Techniques and Case Studies

Parent Training Programs   Since the first parent training program was published (Hawkins, Peterson, Schweid, & Bijou, 1966), hundreds of research articles have attested to its efficacy. Parent training involves systematically teaching parents techniques that shape and maintain developmentally appropriate behavior, particularly compliance with parental directives in their children. These programs usually include therapist explanation and modeling, followed by parent practice with therapist feedback. Techniques for toddler-through latency-age children include appropriate presentation of commands, praise for compliance, reprimands for noncompliance, time-out for continued noncompliance and intense misbehavior such as aggression, and backup consequences for time-out refusal such as privilege loss. Strategies for parents of adolescents include monitoring whereabouts and activities, setting up point charts, and the use of work chores or removal of privileges as discipline. Often in conjunction with parent training programs, efforts are conducted to improve the communication between children, adolescents, and their parents, and to address problems such as marital disharmony and maternal depression.

Case study.   Brad, a 6-year-old boy, was referred by his pediatrician because of significant behavior problems at home. Structured interviews and standardized rating scales completed by his mother suggested that he met diagnostic criteria for oppositional defiant disorder. His developmental history was within normal limits and intellectual testing indicated functioning in the average range. Functional analysis revealed that when mother imposed commands upon Brad, his stubborn and demanding responses often led his fatigued mother to either repeat commands incessantly or to acquiesce and allow Brad to have his way.

Parent training in child management was elected as the primary course of treatment to address Brad's oppositionality. Over the course of 14, one-hour sessions, a strategy known as the Behavior Management Flow Chart (Danforth, 1995) was taught to the mother. The intervention began with didactic instruction on appropriate developmental expectations and social learning principles relevant to how children learn to misbehave (see Bandura, 1977), emphasizing problems of parental acquiescence when children are openly defiant. Then a number of skills were taught to the mother. The teaching format was explanation and modeling by the therapist, followed by parent practice of trained skills while the therapist presented constructive feedback. The mother's progressive learning of new skills was facilitated by weekly homework assignments on the skill being trained. The mother was taught skills that included how to give effective commands to increase the probability of compliance (e.g., giving simple commands that focus on one clearly labeled behavior), waiting five seconds for compliance without arguing with the child, praising compliance, reprimanding noncompliance, using time-out for continued noncompliance and aggression exhibited by Brad, and implementing stronger discipline for time-out refusal such as no television for the day. The mother was encouraged to use cognitive strategies to self-monitor and track her implementation of the child behavior management program. She was also provided with written materials and a flow chart that corresponded to each step of the training program. Standardized child rating scales completed by the mother each week of therapy revealed that compliance increased and disruptive behavior decreased to developmentally appropriate levels over the course of therapy. There were concomitant improvements in the mother's mood state and rating of her marital relationship.

   Treating Selective Mutism   Children with selective mutism decline to vocalize in certain settings while speaking in a typical fashion in other settings. Often, nonvocal communication in the form of head nods, pointing, and hand waving emerges. The effectiveness of this nonvocal communication impedes the development of language in some contexts, or generally. Selective mutism may also reflect anxiety about speaking in certain situations. Regardless of the etiology, nonvocal communication may be considered a behavioral excess, failure to speak may be considered a behavioral deficit, and both classes of behavior may be targeted in a CBT intervention. If the focus is on nonvocal communication, such communication is explicitly ignored in an effort to eliminate its function, while programs are instituted to praise and reward speech of sufficient volume and appropriate content. Treatment plans rarely include efforts to punish insufficient speech. If the disorder is based on anxiety, a technique called stimulus fading is often utilized. Using this technique, people to whom the child regularly speaks are gradually moved into settings where the child does not speak. These people can be conceived of as stimuli that evoke speech; as speech emerges, the people (e.g., parents, friends) are gradually withdrawn (faded) from the setting.

   Case study.   Danny was a 9-year-old boy referred by school personnel in September for excessively quiet behavior in the classroom. Structured interviews and standardized rating scales completed by the teacher and his mother suggested that he met diagnostic criteria for selective mutism; he spoke normally at home but rarely spoke in school, which was interfering with his academic achievement. Developmental history and intelligence were within normal limits, although there was a paternal history of anxiety disorder. Functional analysis revealed that Danny had developed a wide array of nonverbal gestures and signals that his teachers had positively responded to, and in spite if his reticence, Danny was a popular child whose classmates did a fair amount of speaking for him. Related to these contingencies, Danny had essentially learned that he did not need to speak in school.
   Using a consultative approach at the school, the intervention consisted of a series of meetings with the mother and relevant school personnel. First, the therapist explained how Danny's nonverbal behavior was supported by staff and by peers, and how such nonverbal behavior needed to be replaced by vocalizations. It was decided that teachers would tell Danny that they were not going to respond to his nonvocal gestures, and they formally forbade other children to speak for him. A team meeting served as a forum for staff to determine consistent criteria for sufficient speech volume and content. Verbal praise was ongoing and formal rewards were scheduled to be presented twice each day when Danny's speech met these criteria. Danny spoke in the presence of his mother, so twice a week at the beginning of the program she "visited" Danny in the classroom for a half day. As his speech volume and content improved mother visited progressively less often. After two months of this intervention, Danny's teacher reported that he was raising his hand to participate in class, clearly speaking louder and with appropriate content, laughing aloud in class, and had even presented a report to the class, after which he quickly scurried back to his seat. Follow-up rating scales revealed that withdrawn behavior had decreased to the normal range. In spite of Danny's improvements, to promote maintenance of his gains, the program was continued for the entire school year. At the end of the year, Danny's speech appeared to be at normative levels.

Addressing Children's Fears   Most children at some point in their development experience excessive fear. One of the most common fears in latency-age children is of contracting a serious illness (Ollendick, Matson, & Helsel, 1985). If untreated, this fear may assume phobic proportions and contribute to the development of a generalized anxiety disorder. Specifically, confrontation with illness cues such as someone with a cold, a television commercial for medicine, or dirty silverware leads to avoidance of such cues, and overwhelming fear of encountering them in unanticipated times or places. Eventually, the child may experience ongoing anxiety and distress that consumes much of his or her free time, and precludes involvement with the full range of daily social and academic involvements (Hagopian, Weist, & Ollendick, 1990). CBT interventions can effectively halt the progression of this pattern, and in successful cases, lead to resolution of fearful behavior and anxiety.

Case study.   As presented by Hagopian, Weist, & Ollendick (1990), Randy was an 11-year-old girl who reported severe worries and fears pertaining to her physical health. The symptoms surfaced approximately one year earlier, and had progressed markedly in recent months. She expressed fears of contracting HIV and being poisoned, and became excessively concerned and anxious anytime she found any kind of unusual mark or rash on her skin, believing that it signified severe illness. Any commentary or mention of HIV on television, in the newspaper, or by a friend led to a marked exacerbation in her symptoms. Randy also expressed worries about her father's health and employment status, and her divorced parents' relationship. Structured diagnostic interviewing indicated that she met criteria for a simple phobia (of illness), and for overanxious disorder. On self-report measures, she reported high levels of fears, and general anxiety, with scores on these measures approaching the clinically significant range. On a parent-report behavioral checklist, Randy was rated as presenting very high levels of anxious behavior by her mother.

In this case, CBT involved parallel interventions with Randy and her mother. Randy received training in goal-oriented thinking (Graziano & Mooney, 1982). In response to stimuli provoking her fears and anxiety, Randy's therapist modeled coping self-statements, followed by practice with her to imagined illness cues. Randy was also trained in relaxation skills involving deep breathing and positive imagery. Her mother was trained in the same skills, and prompted to encourage Randy's practice of these skills at home at regular intervals, and especially when confronted with an illness cue. Following nine sessions of such training, a reinforcement program was implemented wherein Randy was rewarded for behavior she displayed at home when confronted with illness cues. For each incident, she earned one point each for calmly reporting the onset of anxiety, using deep breathing techniques, using coping self-statements, recovering from anxiety within five minutes, and quickly resuming her prior activities. Her mother rated Randy's performance during each episode, and averaged her points each day, which then could be exchanged for extra privileges and rewards if she met a cutoff (average of 4).

Based on her daily monitoring of anxious episodes, and weekly completion of self-report measures of fear and anxiety, Randy showed steady and progressive improvements over the course of therapy which lasted 25 weeks. Her improvements were particularly dramatic once the reinforcement contingency was implemented. Further, Randy reported decreased fear, and her mother rated her as less anxious from pre- to post-intervention, with the gains she made maintained at a follow-up assessment 14 months after the termination of treatment.

Treating Traumatized Youth   Traditionally, children who have experienced significant life trauma such as abuse, neglect, rape, and other forms of victimization are treated
with psychodynamic approaches. For example, using such an approach, the child is assisted in revisiting past traumas, describing them in detail to the therapist, and assisted in
expressing emotions related to the trauma (see James, 1991). However, such treatment can
be conceptualized in behavioral terms. Essentially, memories of past trauma(s) represent
conditioned aversive stimuli for the child. Because the process of remembering the trauma
is painful and aversive to the child, he or she may deny or repress the trauma to avoid
the re-experience of pain and emotional distress. This process of denial and repression is
commonly associated with depression (often for reasons that the child cannot identify),
self-concept deficits, and other traumatization symptoms such as avoidance and hypervigilance that do not improve over time. The child is thus in a "catch 22 situation: To deal
with past trauma means considerable emotional distress, to avoid the trauma(s) means the
perpetuation of maladjustment."

CBT strategies can be used to encourage the child to report on past traumas and to
express relevant emotions to the therapist. These strategies include normalization of the
experience of, and emotional reactions to, trauma; development of adaptive methods to
ventilate and control feelings such as anger and depression; and cognitive restructuring
aimed at debunking irrational thoughts that the abuse was the child's fault and that he or
she is now damaged for life, and controlling cognitive reactions to events. Emotional and
anger expression activities in such work serve to desensitize the child to the trauma(s), such
that over time these past incidents lose much of their threatening value. Cognitive restructuring activities directly address depressive and traumatization symptoms, and promote
improvements in self-concept.

Case study.   Kisha was an intelligent, attractive, and socially skilled 17-year-old
young woman, who had recently transferred to an urban school on the East Coast after
spending two years in high school in California. She had experienced considerable life
stress related to her mother's drug addiction, and her father's inconsistent involvement
in her life associated with his military career and subsequent incarceration. Kisha had at
least 10 past placements, at various times, with her mother, father, other relatives, and
friends. In some of her placements, there was active drug and alcohol abuse by adults in
the home, and periods of functional neglect. In this context of extreme familial instability,
life stress, and chronic "mini-traumas" of observing mother use drugs, witnessing domestic violence, and being unsupervised for days at a time, Kisha experienced three severely
traumatic events: being molested at age 10 by a male friend of her mother's, being raped
at age 15 by an unknown male assailant, and undergoing a problematic abortion at age 16.
Diagnostic interviewing indicated that Kisha presented symptoms consistent with major
depression, demonstrated symptoms of Post-traumatic stress disorder, and was having significant problems with her self-concept, as well as life stress associated with being a senior
in high school at a new school in a new geographic location.

Treatment with Kisha began during the assessment process. The therapist encouraged
her to tell her life story, and throughout empathized with the numerous difficult life circumstances and traumas she had confronted. During discussion of past sexual abuse (without
significant details, but ruling out the need for protective services involvement), the therapist emphasized the unfortunate fact that many girls and women have been victimized, and
tried to normalize emotional and psychological reactions. For example, feelings of guilt,

of being damaged, and of being unworthy in dating relationships were presented as normal reactions, but, nonetheless, untrue and needing to be challenged.

In the third session, an exercise to improve her self-concept was initiated. The therapist had Kisha describe herself; the few positive qualities she listed were amplified, and, together, numerous others were generated. In a perspective-taking activity, the therapist encouraged her to imagine herself as another person, and to predict how this person would be functioning. This served to highlight that she was a person deserving of compassion, and underscored the many positive qualities that she possessed in spite of the significant adversity she had encountered. For homework, Kisha was encouraged to think of herself every day in these new, positive terms, and using cognitive restructuring techniques, to actively challenge negative self-depictions. Sessions followed which focused on controlling her reactions to life events related to her report that if her morning went wrong, her "whole day was bad." Kisha was assisted in learning that emotions are controllable, that after events, we often decide how we will feel. This was combined with a goal-oriented thinking strategy (Graziano & Mooney, 1982), which helped her to see that her nonspecific sadness was not helping her situation in any way.

During the fifth and sixth sessions, Kisha reported in detail on past traumas. During these lengthy sessions, she was encouraged to express her emotions, and again it was reinforced that she had done nothing wrong. She was instructed on appropriate anger management techniques, and encouraged to express her anger at home when thinking of past trauma. After nine sessions, Kisha reported that her depression had lifted; she was feeling much better about herself; was more comfortable and assertive in dating relationships; her school performance had improved considerably; she had received an award for a poem she wrote; and she was actively completing college applications. Kisha's case exemplifies the effectiveness of CBT strategies combined with strategies considered more psychodynamic such as focusing on historical factors and emphasizing emotional expression.

These four cases, although different in approach and treatment foci, highlight commonalities in CBT. These include: (a) careful assessment, including diagnostic, self-and parent-report measures, obtained before, during, and following intervention, (b) developing and implementing specific treatment plans to address specific problem areas, (c) the proactive versus reactive nature of such therapy, (d) the involvement of significant others in the child's life in all phases of treatment when indicated, (e) the use of homework and between-session assignments, (f) the active use of strategies to reinforce treatment gains, (g) the appropriateness of CBT for problems that are traditionally treated with more psychodynamic approaches (e.g., selective mutism, traumatization), and (h) the effectiveness of CBT in spite of relatively short treatment durations.

CONCLUSION

The construct of child therapy is changing related to economic factors and increased pressures for accountability. Cognitive-behavioral therapy (CBT) offers considerable advantages in the current environment. Its empirical basis, with its emphasis on systematic and comprehensive assessment, focus on validated and clearly defined treatment targets, and ongoing evaluation of the impact of treatment, promote quality and accountability in services. The fact that CBT can be completed in relatively brief periods is also consistent with major forces (e.g., managed care) operating to shorten mental health interventions.

However, CBT is not a panacea. Studies which have sought to document the effectiveness of CBT compared to other therapeutic approaches (e.g., Miller & Berman, 1983;

Shapiro & Shapiro, 1982) have provided only suggestive evidence that CBT may be mildly more effective for some problems. Clearly, more research is needed on the effectiveness of CBT to address the full range of psychosocial and emotional/behavioral difficulties for youth. In addition, while we suggested an interface for cognitive-behavioral and other therapeutic approaches in one of our case studies (Kisha), more explicit efforts are needed to explore integration of CBT with other psychotherapeutic and psychopharmacological interventions.

We express appreciation to Raquel Arbizia for assistance in reviewing literature for this chapter.

REFERENCES

Bandura, A. (1969). *Principles of behavior modification*. New York: Holt, Rinehart & Winston.

Bandura, A. (1977). *Social learning theory*. Englewood Cliffs, NJ: Prentice Hall.

Beck, A. T. (1967). *Depression: Clinical, experimental, and theoretical aspects*. New York: Hoeber.

Braswell, L., & Kendall, P. C. (1988). Cognitive-behavioral methods with children. In K. C. Dobson (Ed.), *Handbook of cognitive-behavioral therapies*. New York: Guilford Press.

Ellis, A. (1962). *Reason and emotion in psychotherapy*. New York: Lyle Stuart.

Danforth, J. S. (1995, August). Recent advances in behavior therapy for oppositional ADHD children. Paper presented at the annual convention of the American Psychological Association, New York.

Dattilio, F. M., & Freeman, A. (1992). Introduction to cognitive therapy. In A. Freeman & F. M. Dattilio (Eds.), *Comprehensive casebook of cognitive therapy*. New York: Plenum Press.

Graziano, A. M., & Mooney, K. C. (1982). Behavioral treatment of 'night fears' in children: Maintenance of improvement at 2-1/2 to 3-1/2-year follow-up. *Journal of Clinical and Child Psychology, 50*, 598–599.

Hagopian, L. P., Weist, M. D., & Ollendick, T. H. (1990). Cognitive-behavior therapy with an 11-year-old girl fearful of AIDS infection, other diseases, and poisoning: A case study. *Journal of Anxiety Disorders, 4*, 257–265.

Hart, K. J., & Morgan, J. R. (1993). Cognitive-behavioral procedures with children: Historical context and current status. In A. J. Finch, W. M. Nelson, & E. S. Ott (Eds.), *Cognitive-behavioral procedures with children and adolescents: A practical guide*. Boston: Allyn and Bacon.

Hawkins, R. P., Peterson, R. F., Schweid, E., & Bijou, S. W. (1966). Behavior therapy in the home: Amelioration of problem parent-child relations with the parent in a therapeutic role. *Journal of Experimental Child Psychology, 4*, 99–107.

Jones, M.C. (1924). A laboratory study of fear: The case of Peter. *Pedagogical Seminary, 31*, 308–315.

Meichenbaum, D., & Goodman, J. (1971). Training impulsive children to talk to themselves: A means of developing self-control. *Journal of Abnormal Child Psychology, 77*, 115–126.

Miller, R. C., & Berman, J. S. (1983). The efficacy of cognitive behavior therapies: A quantitative review of research evidence. *Psychological Bulletin, 94*, 39–53.

Ollendick, T. H., Matson, J. L., & Helsel, W. J. (1985). Fears in children and adolescents: Normative data. *Behaviour Research and Therapy, 23*, 465–467.

Ross, A. O. (1981). *Child behavior therapy: Principles, procedures and empirical basis*. New York: John Wiley & Sons.

Shapiro, D. A., & Shapiro, D. (1982). Meta-analysis of comparative therapy outcome studies: A replication and refinement. *Psychological Bulletin, 92*, 581–604.

Shure, M. B., & Spivack, G. (1978). Interpersonal problem solving in young children: A cognitive approach to prevention. *American Journal of Community Psychology, 10*, 341–356.

Skinner, B. F. (1938). *The behavior of organisms: An experimental analysis*. New York: Appleton-Century-Crofts.

Stokes, T. F., & Baer, D. M. (1977). An implicit technology of generalization. *Journal of Applied Behavior Analysis, 10*, 349–367.

Weist, M.D., Ollendick, T.H., & Finney, J. (1991). Toward the empirical validation of treatment targets in children. *Clinical Psychology Review, 11*, 515–538.

Chapter 19

Individual Psychotherapy and the Use of Play with Children

Lance D. Clawson, M.D.

INTRODUCTION

Fantasy play most always takes on a significant role within individual psychotherapy with children. Its function or importance in any particular instance is dependent on the age and developmental capacities of the child in question. Early in the evolution of psychoanalysis and then, subsequently, psychodynamically oriented psychotherapy, adapting the theory and technique of individual work with adults to the emotional and cognitive abilities of children was a challenging and important step. This "adaptation" was the incorporation of the use of play into the consultation room. George Moran (1987), summarized the developmental aspects of play by describing it as "crucial for the child's acquisition of the capacity to differentiate 'me' and 'not-me' experiences, self and object representations, and fantasy and reality." Fantasy play is therefore critical to the intrapsychic and interpersonal development of children. It "offers opportunities to gratify wishes and work through conflicts which are not permitted gratification in reality." Understood in this way, play has become the necessary vehicle which allows therapists to engage children in the therapeutic process, and gain access to their inner world of delights, fears, and conflicts.

Play Therapy may take many forms and utilizes a number of various play and interpretive techniques. Some forms can be useful with certain types of children, for example, certain games or approaches may be used with specific types of psychopathology, or the play may be varied to fit with a particular therapist's approach and philosophy of treatment.

This chapter reviews psychodynamically oriented individual therapy in the ambulatory setting, and the use of play in this form of treatment. Play can and has been used widely as a therapeutic tool in individual cognitive and behavioral therapies, group, and family therapies, to mention a few, the descriptions of which are beyond the scope of this chapter.

HISTORICAL NOTES

Although Sigmund Freud was the first to apply the theories and techniques of psychoanalysis to treat a child through correspondence with the patient's father in the case of "Little Hans" (Freud, 1909), the first psychoanalyst to formally describe the use of play in the psychotherapeutic process was Hermine von Hug-Hellmuth. Von Hug-Hellmuth, a child analyst, described the use of play in work with children as young as 6 years old, considering it helpful to elicit material for the analysis. She did not develop a technique for analyzing children, per se, but was the first to formally use play as an adjunct to working with children (von Hug-Hellmuth, 1921).

Melanie Klein developed play with children into an actual therapeutic process, first describing it in 1919. In working with her child analysands, Klein used a variety of toys and human figures, and broadly interpreted the themes, transferences, conflicts, and issues which arose in the play sessions. Klein saw play as similar to the "free association" which adult work heavily relied on, and so made active use of play material, while practicing along traditional psychoanalytic lines by minimizing outside contact with "contaminants" such as parents, teachers, and the like (Klein, 1932).

Anna Freud, by 1927, had developed her own concepts regarding the use of play in child analysis. She considered children to be different enough from adults to necessitate a more drastic departure from traditional "adult" psychoanalytic technique. Freud was more willing to take into account a child's need for preparation and education about the process of therapy, focused less on "depth" interpretations, and was more willing to intervene in the outside world if the situation dictated (Group for the Advancement of Psychiatry, 1982). Both Melanie Klein's and Anna Freud's texts of child psychoanalysis were significant historical markers, and were indicative of how the use of play as a central modality in child psychoanalysis had become broadly accepted throughout the professional community by the end of World War II.

As play became synonymous with child psychoanalysis, child therapists began to explore the use of play in therapies with more limited goals, along with modifications of traditional therapeutic technique and philosophy. Notable contributions to this effort were Levy's (1939) strategy to achieve therapeutic effects through the cathartic aspects of play which he called "release therapy." He postulated that needs and conflicts could be re-experienced through play, and if the play material captured the salient emotional states of the child, it would, in and of itself, resolve emotional conflict and trauma. Allen (1942) first articulated the therapeutic importance of the relationship between the child and therapist which was initiated and sustained through the process of play. He emphasized that insight and interpretation were not the only important factors which positively affected the outcome in child psychotherapy. It was the relationship with the therapist which he felt was the major contributor to therapeutic success.

As play therapy clearly began evolving outside the bounds of traditional psychoanalysis with children, Virginia Axiline (1947) published her seminal text on play therapy. Axiline was influenced by the concepts of Carl Rodgers' "client-centered therapy," and utilized reflection back to the child of those emotional states, wishes, or conflicts which arose in the play. In keeping with a more Rogerian approach, and diverging from traditional psychoanalysis, she did not attempt to "interpret" any of the "unconscious" roots of what was manifest in the play. Her work was significant in that her ideas were somewhat less theoretical compared to traditional psychoanalytic thought, and focused more exclusively on what the child was presenting in the play in the "here and now."

Winnicott (1953) proposed the idea of the "transitional space" which furthered the understanding of the therapeutic as well as developmental functions of play. In this "intermediate area," experiences of external reality and the inner world of affect and need were theorized to coalesce. Inanimate objects or phenomena (e.g.,. a song, a cuddly blanket, a stuffed toy) could be imbued with the gratifying properties of an internally generated wish. Winnicott wrote that this ability allows the child to create a "transitional object" or soothing companion to ward off the fears and frustrations of a sometimes harsh reality. The transitional object can then be "played" with within the "transitional space," as the child attempts to master the unmet or frustrated need. This conceptualization was important as it further defined play as a amalgam of a child's inner world and external reality, and a place (both literally and figuratively) where the therapist could intersect with the patient's psyche.

Throughout the 1950s and beyond, child therapists like Winnicott and a number of others independently developed their ideas about the function of play in normal development and in the therapeutic setting. The basic consensus, and the foundation of our current understanding of what play represents, was that it was a means for children to modulate and master emotions (such as anxiety) in incremental quantities, and that unconscious impulses could be acted out through play and worked through without ever reaching full awareness, making it the prime therapeutic modality in work with children (Coppolillo, 1996; Moran, 1987).

THERAPEUTIC ACTION

The question, What are the active therapeutic ingredients in play therapy? remains controversial. For many years, attaining "insight" was considered paramount, yet the common experience of clinicians who work with children (and adults as well) is that insight per se is not an essential ingredient for positive therapeutic outcomes (Neubauer, 1987). Simple catharsis of past trauma and conflict have met with a similar demise as to its central importance in child therapy. Mayes and Cohen (1993) stated that "the very act of playing carries much of the therapeutic work aimed toward facilitating their return to developmentally appropriate and adaptive psychic functioning." Psychotherapy researchers have observed that many of the common aspects of therapeutic interventions are the salient factors which bring about change. Elements such as a supportive and empathetic therapist, the power of suggestion, and a positive relationship in the therapy are common among the various types of "therapies." These "common aspects" of psychotherapy have been more powerful in explaining the variance in treatment outcomes than the formal "technique" that any particular type of therapy espouses (Luborsky, Singer, & Luborsky, 1975).

In line with the observations of comparative psychotherapy research, the "active ingredients" which many authors have felt bring about the desired changes in psychotherapy are not necessarily the particular therapeutic technique, but certainly are closely related to the process of psychotherapy. These active ingredients are the experience with the psychotherapist as a strong, emotionally modulated model for identification, intimate exchange with an empathetic and accepting adult, a setting that allows the child to experience strong affects in a protected environment encouraging verbal and symbolic mastery versus acting out, and the opportunity to establish a relationship with the therapist which is then created in a new light as compared to being patterned on intense and conflicted prior relationships (Cohen & Solnit, 1993). These "nontechnical" factors, accompanied by therapeutic techniques such as interpretation within the play scenario, reflection and labeling of emotional states, the reenactment of past trauma and emotional conflict through displacement into the play, problem solving, and so on become intertwined into the process of the therapy.

Maximizing these "nontechnical" elements in any therapy relies heavily on the therapist's personality and individual characteristics. The Group for the Advancement of Psychiatry (1982) summarized these important factors to be:

- the ability to inspire confidence in the patient and parents
- the quality of therapeutic "zeal" or enthusiasm
- the ability to tolerate the inherent ambiguity of the therapeutic situation
- flexibility to experiment with action and attitude so as not to become "stuck" in the "technique"of the work
- warmth and empathy
- self-knowledge and self-acceptance so as not to contaminate the work with his or her own issues and projections
- awareness of one's limited perspective in any given situation
- the capacity for adult gratifications to avoid relying on conducting therapy to fulfill personal needs, and,
- the avoidance of an anti-parent and anti-sibling bias.

These qualities are most likely the most challenging aspects of conducting child play therapy, as they require much of the therapist which may be "personality-driven" or "unconscious" in nature, and counter to those unconscious and preconscious forces which brought the individual into the practice of child psychotherapy in the first place.

It is also apparent that the anticipated changes with which a child first enters psychotherapy may be, to varying degrees, the result of normal development. For example, a young child engaging in primary process thinking and play in therapeutic sessions, would be expected, as part of normal development, to increase the use of verbalization and secondary process thinking over time. This normally reflects a maturing central nervous system as well as representing benefits from the therapeutic process. In this way, all the processes which facilitate normal development will also enhance the goals of psychotherapy (Lewis, 1996).

INDICATIONS FOR THE USE OF PLAY THERAPY

Most child therapists feel fortunate when a single form of treatment will suffice for a given child. The roots of a child's presenting complaints may stem from many sources such as family dysfunction, loss, trauma, genetic vulnerability, and/or subtle neuropsychiatric deficits in attention, learning, and social capacities to mention only a few. This implies that play therapy will many times be only one part of a comprehensive treatment plan which might involve school programming, medication, pediatric intervention, family therapy, group therapy, and other activities. Lewis (1996) stated that such a comprehensive treatment plan evolves out of an in-depth understanding of the child which starts with a diagnosis from the *Diagnostic and Statistical Manual of Mental Disorders (DSM-IV)* (American Psychiatric Association [APA], 1994) but goes beyond the categorical assessment of *DSM* and provides a comprehensive developmental formulation.

Building on much of the "formulative" work of psychodynamic, cognitive, and behavioral therapy, Strayhorn (1988) operationalized, in an atheoretical fashion, the process of evaluating and determining the needs of child patients. He has created a "Skills X Methods" matrix which aligns a child's social/emotional skills deficits on the "Y" axis, and the methods of influencing or creating change in these specific problem areas along the "X" axis. Developing such a grid does indeed develop out of an in-depth understanding of the individual child and his or her strengths and weaknesses, and forms a useful way of planning the multidimensional approach to comprehensive therapeutic intervention as third-party payers demand greater and greater specificity in treatment plans.

Seeing only the child in dynamically oriented play therapy is appropriate when a child's presenting complaint can confidently be considered intrapsychic, and no other factor which may be changed, treated, or modified is present. Otherwise, individual play therapy becomes part of the larger treatment plan. The therapy itself is utilized to address the needs of the child with regard to emotional support, a safe haven for exploration and mastery of strong emotions, traumas, and conflicts, improved reality testing of present and past relationships and events, development of a positive self concept, and developing the use of verbalization over acting out. By speaking within the displacement by utilizing dolls, figures, animals, drawing, and other measures the overpowering emotions can be expressed and manipulated within the play, leading to a growing sense of mastery and resolution (Conn, 1989).

Although play is used exclusively mostly with preschool and young school-age children, play as an element of therapy can be and often is used in older school-age children and young adolescents. In fact, despite the proven efficacy of cognitive-behavior therapy, such interventions have had difficulty adapting to the developmental needs and limitations of young children, and only begin to show outcomes similar to the adult literature when addressing the adolescent population (Spence, 1994). Almost by definition, "cognitive" implies the use of sophisticated cognitions and cognitive defenses as an important element of change. Such abilities are often beyond the preschool and young school-age child, and are often beyond children with developmental delays or significant histories of trauma and neglect.

Play, as a therapeutic venue, suffers no such limitation. In its application, one of the greatest advantages that the use of play in child therapy has is that it is part of normal childhood experience. Play promotes cognitive and emotional growth in the course of normal development. It can therefore be utilized with children as early as infancy and as late as a patient may need to utilize it in the service of maturation and growth (for instance, even younger adolescent patients may have great difficulty engaging in therapy as a purely verbal exercise, yet jump at the opportunity to "play" with the therapist). As a central component of child development it can be effectively used with children who may suffer language, hearing, or physical handicaps. It may address specific symptoms such as separation anxiety, encopresis, and aggression, or for children who may have fallen off the pathway of normal development for reasons of abuse, neglect, trauma, loss, or physical illness to name a few. Its appropriateness to any given situation is only limited by the creativity of the therapist and the willingness of the patient and family.

GOALS AND THE LENGTH OF TREATMENT

The goals of psychodynamically oriented individual play therapy with children are usually either focal (limited) or broad (far-reaching). Generally, the expressed purpose for which a child enters therapy is for symptom reduction, the promotion of normal development (often within the social/interpersonal realm), the fostering of autonomy and self-reliance, or for a change in a real life setting such as how the child gets along/performs at home and school. These global endpoints can present as fairly simple issues or may be multifactorial and complex problems.

Therapy which engages fairly limited goals tends to create a more focused and more time-limited process as compared to the far-reaching goals of modifying coping styles, ingrained patterns of behavior, and character traits which are maladaptive. Limited goals of treatment might center attention on the alleviation of symptoms such as adjustment difficulties, depression, anxiety, or encopresis. The "limited" or more focal nature of a treatment is dependent on numerous factors which pertain to the specific patient at hand. Factors such as the inherent resiliency of the child; the presence or absence of long-standing, maladaptive behavioral patterns; severe trauma, abuse, and neglect; and the ability of the child's family to support the child's emotional growth and individuation must all be taken into account when planning a focal play therapy intervention. An overabundance of the life circumstance and developmental factors listed previously often make time-limited play therapy more complex and difficult, as there is often an inadequate caretaking environment, deviant character development, and multiple symptoms to address in too short of a time.

In brief forms of play therapy, children are selected based on their displaying a limited number of symptoms, the presence of a supportive home environment with motivated and involved parents, a lack of excessive neurological dysfunction (e.g., ADHD or PDD), the capacity to use fantasy and symbols, and a lack of problems involving attachment/basic trust (e.g., abuse, neglect), or what might be conceptualized as mostly the "opposite" to those factors previously mentioned (Racusin, 1994). There is sufficient data to conclude that a majority of patients in psychodynamic psychotherapy actually receive brief treatment (less than 26 sessions) (Howard, Davidson, O'Mahoney, Orlinsky, & Brown, 1989), a statistic that has been, in the past, applied to limit total allowed sessions by many third-party payers. The art to brief play therapy then is the careful selection of patients, setting of appropriate and limited goals, and remaining focused on those goals without experiencing "therapeutic creep" as the therapist allows the suggestions, clarifications, psychoeducation, and interpretive interventions to stray from the original purpose of the treatment.

Play therapy which addresses the multiple symptoms and problems of children who may be neurologically compromised, have suffered significant neglect and/or trauma, and whose families range from unsupportive to toxic often require more far-reaching goals (in addition to involving the family in therapeutic work) and time-intensive therapy. These interventions certainly rely on many of the contributing (non-technical) therapeutic factors listed previously, which in turn rely heavily on the relationship to the individual therapist and the therapist himself or herself.

The evidence supporting the efficacy of psychodynamically oriented play therapy has been mounting in recent years, even as compared to other forms of treatment (e.g., purely behavior therapy). The evidence is also strong in supporting more intensive and longer-term play interventions for children who do not respond, or who clearly are inappropriate for shorter-term treatments. For instance, Fonagy and Target (1994) demonstrated the feasibility of studying, and the efficacy of treating, children with disruptive behavior disorders. Mann and McDermott (1983) reviewed their own work, and that of previous studies, which state that in the population of traumatized and abused children, those who remain in therapy at least one year gain lasting benefits in the areas of behavioral symptom control, social relationships, school performance and self-esteem.

THE PROCESS OF PLAY THERAPY

Play is both an adjunct to, and a vehicle for, communication between child and therapist which reveals to the therapist glimpses of the child's inner life, such as misconceptions about the world, fears, misinformation, wishes, anxieties, conflicts, and anger. In the context of play, human interaction and emotion may be demonstrated fairly directly, such as through doll play. At other times the therapist must look for the "theme" of the play; those repeating elements of emotion, memory, action, and interpersonal relatedness contained within the form and content of the play material. Elucidating the themes, and then bringing them to the awareness of the child through observation, play action, clarification, and direct and displaced interpretation is the major technical scheme of play therapy, and normally occurs in the "middle" phase of treatment (see following discussion). These themes may represent past trauma, distortion, conflicts, fears, transference, and the like, and are therefore the "grist" of the process of working though and mastery for the child patient.

The ability of the therapist to detect the child's play themes, and select which to address, and in what way, at the appropriately timed moments is of utmost importance, and has been addressed thoroughly by previous authors (Sandler, Kennedy, & Tyson, 1980). The therapist's ability to regress within the play session, yet remain observing as to the themes the child presents without becoming mired in his or her own inner conflicts, is paramount. It has only been in recent years that techniques for studying the thematic content of children's play has come under more systematic scrutiny (Marans, Mayes, Cicchetti, Dahl, Marans, & Cohen, 1991), so that more systematic ways of approaching theme development within play therapy can be established.

Generally, psychotherapy with children is conceptualized to occur in three major phases or stages. Most authors have generally divided these into the initial phase, where the "treatment alliance" and treatment preparation/education transpires. Here, the hope for and the expectation of help is a key factor in getting therapy started, along with understanding and gratifying the child patient's overt and latent needs to some extent to allow the child to begin to experience the therapist as "helpful," and lower the natural resistance to revealing oneself to a stranger. The child is often taught about the ground rules and "what we do" in therapy during this period as well. This initial phase is often more prolonged in working with children because many young patients may not perceive a need for treatment in the same way their families or schools might.

The middle phase comes next, and it is where the bulk of the therapeutic work takes place, such as interpreting the play through elucidating themes, and analyzing the transference/countertransference issues which occur in the process of "working through" the child's intrapsychic issues. It is here where the goals, or central issues, or skill deficits are addressed repeatedly over time.

Finally, the termination phase is the ending period of the work where the results of the therapy are "tested" to see if they have taken hold under the stress of ending of the relationship with the therapist. Issues which relate directly to the ending of the relationship with the therapist are addressed so to maximize the ability of the patient to "carry" with himself or herself the therapeutic gains of the work, and master the feelings of dependency which have arisen in the course of the treatment. Termination depends to a great extent on the therapist's, child's, and family's agreement that an acceptable balance of mastery over certain presenting problems and a satisfactory adjustment to others has been accomplished. The patient and family are charged with the task of "taking it on the road" and utilizing the skills learned in therapy to master new challenges as they arise.

Variations on this traditional three-stage schema have generally added clarity to the understanding of the process of psychotherapy with children. An excellent formulation of the phases of psychotherapy was described by The Committee on Child Psychiatry within the Group for the Advancement of Psychiatry (1982) which, because of its more "operationalized" nature, fits well with the "Skills X Method" grid approach (Strayhorn, 1988) mentioned earlier. Here the process includes five stages, the first (establishing a working relationship/treatment alliance) and last (termination) being identical to the three-phase scheme. It is the middle phase, referred to previously, that is more deliberately broken down into its component parts. These intermediate phases are (situated between the working alliance and termination phases): analysis of the problem and its cause, an explanation of the problem, and establishing and implementing the formula for change. When "analyzing the problem and its cause," the child's life experience is examined within the context of the play and through direct inquiry. In the instance of dynamically oriented play therapy (although this schema applies to all forms of child therapy) a cause is searched for, and may be seen within the themes of the play. The child's willingness to explore potential "causes" of the current presenting problems, either through displacement within the play, or more directly, is an important next step.

Flowing out of the search for a cause is then "an explanation of the problem." In play therapy, the explanation phase is somewhat more protracted as compared to behavior therapy which often posits causes early and briefly in the work. This phase is educative and learning-based with linking of strong affective states to the "explanation." Here, the "explanation" of the problem may be completely executed over and over within the play process as the therapist fits the "explanation" to the play scenario at hand and the strong emotions associated with it. Here is where the "corrective emotional experience" is thought to occur, as the past traumas and conflicts are reenacted, relabeled, understood, and mastered within the play, with the "ego" or "modulating" support of the therapist (Carek, 1990).

The last phase of the "middle section" of treatment is "establishing and implementing the formula for change." Here the focus is more on behavioral adaptation, and may successfully be enacted more directly in exchanges with the child if the previous foundation of play therapy has led to more "personalization" of the material. In this phase, theoretical orientation is thought to wane as the therapist's understanding of the child expands and making changes in behavior and symptoms increases in focus. Solutions for change may be explored within the displacement of play, in the realm of guided fantasy, in composition of stories, or in intervening with the child's family and/or school environments. Here is where the original goals of the treatment are most actively sought in a flexible way.

THE ENVIRONMENT

The foundation to any therapeutic intervention is the creation of a proper "holding environment" which allows the child and therapist to immerse themselves together in play (Coppolillo, 1987). Establishing such an environment requires that the therapist have the ability to engage the child at his or her developmental level, that the physical space is comfortable, free of distraction, and safe, that certain ground rules exist which maintain the safety of the environment, and that confidentiality is clearly communicated by the privacy of the setting. Donovan and McIntyre (1990) clearly delineated a number of "ground rules" when creating this therapeutic environment. Such basics as "no adults" in the play therapy room; all communications in therapy are confidential (except cases of potential harm which are in question); toys remain in the therapy room and go back in their proper place at the end of each session; toys contained within the play therapy room are in general "generic" and sturdy, so as not to limit the fantasy play of the child or interfere with enthusiastic use; play room equipment should be "uninviting" with regard to aggressive acting out or hostility; and harming self, others, or objects is never permitted. Disrobing is also forbidden, and anything created by the child (e.g., block constructions) is disassembled at the end of each session.

Some may find this approach rigid, and certainly all therapists have breached these basic tenets, if not disregarded them all together in the name of therapeutic flexibility and utility. Yet, it is important for any child therapist to consider the meaning of repeated trangression of these basic ground rules. What could such ground rule violations imply about the patient and the possible countertransference issues, as well as the "safety" and "ego supporting" structure that are of central importance in conducting this type of work. Addressing the myriad uncomfortable and difficult moments in play therapy such as when a child threatens to run away or steals from your office, ending a session with an unwilling participant, or birthday and holiday gift giving and receiving is generally beyond the limitations of this chapter, yet has been well addressed in child therapy by such authors as Sandler, Kennedy, and Tyson (1980), and Gabel, Oster, and Pfeffer (1988) in their guides to working with children.

ADAPTATIONS AND USES OF INDIVIDUAL PLAY

What transpires in the actual "play" during therapy is often a combination of what the child brings to the situation developmentally and psychologically, and the therapeutic style of the psychotherapist (which often is reflected in how the play room is supplied with toys). Play may be very unstructured, using materials such as sand and water as espoused by Anna Freud, or as regimented as engaging in a "therapeutic" board game frequently seen in therapists' offices. Most "modern" play rooms contain variations on dolls, puppets, blocks, or other materials for building, a doll house or its equivalent for "home" play, and drawing materials. Beyond these basics, most therapists supply the play room according to taste, although the constant search for new toys and new gratifications for one's child patients by an ever-increasing warehouse of toys should be understood more as a need within the therapist to gratify the patient versus a primary need of children to have only the latest in toy hardware.

The importance of the use of art materials in play therapy cannot be overemphasized, and there is a rich history with regard to the use of art in child psychotherapy. As in most forms of play, children may represent many conscious and unconscious ideas through drawing and art which may then be open for understanding and interpretation. Art therapy per se is a field in its own right, yet as with all types of play, expression through art materials is generally quite helpful in the context of psychotherapy if a child is drawn to this type of expression.

There have been many specific forms of play prescribed for general and specific therapeutic uses. There are innumerable examples such as the "squiggle game" (Winnicott, 1965), Lego therapy (Altman & Esber, 1995), hide-and-seek (Frankiel, 1993), writing as the therapeutic means (Demb, 1993), the use of "cooperative games" (Bay-Hinitz, Peterson, & Quilitch, 1994), medical play as preparation for surgery (Ziegler & Prior, 1994), the mutual storytelling technique for Oedipal problems (Gardner, 1983), the use of clay (Feldman, Villanueva, Lanne, & Devroede, 1993), or various forms of "dramatic play." These examples and many others have all been used in the service of psychotherapy. Computers are the newest addition to the play armamentarium, as writing, cooperative games, educational material, or simply acting as a buffer to the intensity of therapy all lend themselves to this form of play. These "variations" on the approach to play are rarely contradictory to the goals of therapy, and can be quite useful to the play therapist as they offer new approaches to old problems, and can be of considerable help in devising a plan of intervention with a child who may challenge the therapist for a variety of reasons. The following are examples of play therapy process which illustrate many of the preceding points.

Examples of Play Therapy Process

Case #1   Susan was an 8-year-old girl who presented with occasional encopresis, oppositional behavior at home and school, and poor peer relationships. She had been in the care of her concerned and supportive father and stepmother for three years since being removed from her mother's home for allegations of neglect. Susan was a very verbal girl, yet had little demonstrable insight into the causes of her problems. In the therapy two scenarios rapidly established themselves in series. The first involved doll play in a doll house where a very loud and angry mother continually disparaged and punished her children. The emotional intensity of the play often resulted in the patient rebuffing the therapist for comments as to how the children must feel at the hands of such a mother, and she would often fall to the floor at the end of such an interaction giddy and disorganized, unable to continue.

After a time Susan began the teacher game, making herself the teacher and the therapist the "student." The student, despite his best efforts, could never be assured of the teacher's reaction to his work, as the teacher personified an erratic and hypercritical task master. As this material was interpreted repeatedly over several months, the patient would at times lose control and attack the therapist, attempting to scratch him, which required physical restraint and letting the patient know that the sessions were to be safe, and feelings could be spoken of or played out, without real harm coming to anyone. The intensity of the teacher game lessened over time as the "teacher" became more tolerant and encouraging within the play, eventually branching out into mutual activities with the patient becoming a "benevolent" tutor while engaging in play cooking and writing stories together with happy endings of family togetherness. This process paralleled Susan's gradual improvement in peer relations, cooperation with authority figures, and real enjoyment of her present family and younger half-sibling. After one year, nearing the time of termination because of a family move, she was alternately directly speaking of and playing about her feelings of loyalty conflict, worrying that a summer visit to her biological mother, who had reentered her life, might threaten her relationship with her present family.

Case #2   James was a 7-year-old boy who originally presented with the complaint of encopresis and a non-progressive neuromuscular disorder. He was initially diagnosed, in the course of evaluation, with a gender identity disorder. The treatment involved both conjoint family and intensive individual work as until noted in the evaluation his cross dressing and obsessive doll play had been generally unnoticed. Both of his parents were emotionally engrossed in issues of their own childhood sexual abuse. Therapy covered many forms of play over a three-year period. James' initial play would always involve a Barbie doll as the omnipotent player in a house of other figures whom she would attack, kick, and destroy after only brief periods of nonaggressive interaction. He articulated within the play the sense of Barbie's all-powerful beauty and strength, and her disdain for the lower soldiers

and dolls. This scenario was played out often over time, and with clarification and interpretation of the fascinating and terrifying power attributed to girls, the play evolved into
more direct interaction and talking

James' encopresis resolved and was successfully managed though the interpretation
of his feelings of anger when his mother would unpredictably demean him (the success
was also a result of his mother's gradual understanding of this dynamic as well). His intense identification with female stereotypes lessened, although the male world of rough and
tumble play was never available to him because of his disability. He often brought in items
he had worked on in school, looking for the admiration of the therapist, and would often
create art projects and wish to decorate the office. His wish to be ever-present in the office
was interpreted along with his concern that the therapist spent time with other children as
well. An erotic transference accompanied by intense anxiety eventually emerged. The patient became quite focused on love for the therapist and the therapist keeping him in mind
when outside the sessions. These issues were gradually placed into words though summarization and interpretation, and well as assisting him in understanding the meaning of his
defense of the erotic feelings through highly regimented and repetitive, yet disorganized,
paper cutting and taping.

Case #3   Tim was presented at age 5 after innumerable surgical procedures and traumas since his diagnosis of Hirshprung's disease shortly after birth. He was initially described as unhappy, with poor self- esteem, and would battle his parents over self-hygiene
because he had never gained fecal continence. How to handle this was a frequent point
of conflict with his parents. His play evolved slowly over an extended course of therapy.
Initially he drew "ghosts" and "mazes" which could not be escaped from. He was verbally
aggressive as the treatment alliance grew, cursing at and threatening to "poo poo" on the
therapist's shoes.

He steadfastly engaged in "wars" between toy soldiers over an extended period. He
always ensured his side victory. The war play was interpreted over time as an expression
of hostile feelings and a need to feel invulnerable, with limited success. His play evolved
into competitive games such as soccer and basketball, pitting himself against the therapist.
His competitiveness and need to win and "feel" victorious and in control were clarified
and interpreted. Tim had a particular fascination with "disembowelment" and would re-
count vividly the latest horror film he had seen, often referring to grisly scenes over a
period of weeks. Summary interpretations were possible eventually, linking his behavior
and play within the session to past feelings of helplessness, rage, pain, fear, a feeling of
defectiveness, and the defense against them. His resistance to becoming responsible for
his own bowel hygiene was also interpreted, within the transference, because control and
aggression were significant themes in relation to his parents as well as within the treatment.

Case #4   Sam was first presented at age 5 for excessive emotional lability, a seeming absence of social skills, and questions about proper school programming as he was
observed to be exceptionally bright. He was eventually diagnosed with a "genius" IQ,
ADHD, and Asperger's disorder. The focus of the therapy was the actual building of play
and interactional skills through games, as well as beginning to use his considerable intellect
to "problem solve" social issues which he had no intrinsic grasp of. Much of the play and
problem solving with Sam began with, and remained focused on, mutual activities which
did not overwhelm him with anxiety. The computer, its manipulation, and playing simple
card games or chess were ideal as the interpersonal intensity was modulated enough for

him to tolerate the direct interaction. Poignant observations and issues were often dealt with during the simultaneous playing of a computer game, as well as the developing of a close interpersonal relationship with the therapist so that issues such as social convention, separation, and awareness of the feelings of the others could all be addressed within the therapeutic relationship.

CONCLUSION

Individual psychotherapy with children and the use of play as the main mode of therapeutic intervention has been shown over the past 70 years to be a reliable and effective means of treating the many emotional and behavioral disorders presenting to the therapist's office. A thorough understanding of the child and his or her environment, and developing a focal or far-reaching set of goals along with the plan of interventions are the starting point for all treatment. From this beginning, therapist and patient set out on a mutual exploration of a child's inner conflicts and fears, while providing the very real support and understanding that such a therapeutic relationship entails. The flexibility, wish to help, and persona of the therapist is as important as the accuracy and timing of the interpretations of the child's play. Much work still lies ahead for play therapists to continue to operationalize and individualize those elements of the work that bring about the desired changes in a caring and efficient way.

REFERENCES

Allen, F. H. (1942). *Psychotherapy with children*. New York: Norton.

Altman, A., & Esber, J. (1995). Lego therapy. *Journal of Psychosocial Nursing and Mental Health Services, 33*, 48–49.

American Psychiatric Association (APA). (1994). *Diagnostic and statistical manual of mental disorders* (4th ed.) (*DSM-IV*). Washington, DC: the Association.

Axiline, V. (1947). *Play therapy*. Boston: Houghton Mifflin.

Bay-Hinitz, A. K., Peterson, R. F., & Quilitch, H. R. (1994). Cooperative games: A way to modify aggressive and cooperative behaviors in young children. *Journal of Applied Behavior Analysis, 27*, 435–446.

Carek, D. J. (1990). Affect in psychodynamic psychotherapy. *American Journal of Psychotherapy, 44*, 274–282.

Cohen, P. M., & Solnit, A. J. (1993). Play and therapeutic action. *The Psychoanalytic Study of the Child, 48*, 49–63.

Conn, J. H. (1989). Play interview therapy: Its history, theory and practice—A fifty year retrospective account. *Child Psychiatry and Human Development, 20*, 3–13.

Coppolillo, H. P. (1987). *Psychodynamic psychotherapy of children*. Madison, CT: International Universities Press.

Coppolillo, H. P. (1996). The use of play in psychodynamic psychotherapy: In M. Lewis (Ed.), *Child and adolescent psychiatry: A comprehensive textbook* (2nd ed.) (pp. 801–815). Baltimore: Williams & Wilkins.

Demb, J. M. (1993). The written word in psychotherapy with a latency girl. *Journal of the American Academy of Child and Adolescent Psychiatry, 32*, 1028–1031.

Donovan, D., & McIntyre, D. (1990). *Healing the hurt child: A developmental-contextual approach*. New York: Norton Publishers.

Feldman, P. C., Villanueva, S., Lanne, V., & Devroede, G. (1993). Use of play with clay to treat children with intractable encorpresis. *Journal of Pediatrics, 122*, 483–488.

Fonagy, P., & Target, M. (1994). The efficacy of psychoanalysis for children with disruptive disorders. *Journal of the American Academy of Child and Adolescent Psychiatry, 33*, 45–55.

Frankeil, R. V. (1993). Hide-and-seek in the playroom: On object loss and transference in child treatment. *Psychoanalytic Review, 80*, 341–359.

Freud, S. (1909/1968). Analysis of a phobia in a five-year-old boy. In S. Freud, The *sexual enlightenment of children* (pp. 47–183). New York: Collier Books.

Gabel, S., Oster, G., & Pfeffer, C. R. (1988). *Difficult moments in child psychotherapy*. Northvale, NJ: Jason Aronson.

Gardner, R. A. (1983). Treating Oedipal problems with the mutual storytelling technique. In C. Schaefer & K. O'Connor (Eds.), *Handbook of play therapy* (pp. 355–368). New York: John Wiley & Sons.

Group for the Advancement of Psychiatry, Committee on Child Psychiatry. (1982). *The process of child therapy*. New York: Brunner/Mazel.

Howard, K. I., Davidson, C. V., O'Mahoney, M. T., Orlinsky, D. E., & Brown, K. P. (1989). Patterns of psychotherapy utilization. *American Journal of Psychiatry, 146*, 775–778.

Klein, M. (1932). *The psychoanalysis of children*. London: Hogarth Press.

Lewis, M. (1996). Intensive individual psychodynamic psychotherapy: The therapeutic relationship and the technique of interpretation. In M. Lewis (Ed.), *Child and adolescent psychiatry: A comprehensive textbook* (2nd ed.) (pp. 802–809). Baltimore: Williams & Wilkins.

Levy, D. (1939). Release therapy. *American Journal of Orthopsychiatry, 9*, 713–736.

Luborsky, L., Singer, B., & Luborsky, L. (1975) Comparative studies of psychotherapies: Is it true that 'Everyone has won and all must have prizes?' *Archives of General Psychiatry, 32*, 995–1008.

Mann, B. & McDermott, J. F., Jr. (1983). Play therapy for victims of child abuse and neglect. In C. Schaefer & K. O'Connor (Eds.), *Handbook of play therapy*. New York: Wiley & Sons, pp. 283–307.

Marans, S., Mayes, L., Cicchetti, D., Dahl, K., Marans, W., & Cohen, D. J. (1991). The child-psychoanalytic play interview: A technique for studying thematic content. *Journal of the American Psychoanalytic Association, 39*, 1015–1036.

Mayes, L. C. & Cohen, D.J. (1993). Playing and therapeutic action in child analysis. *International Journal of Psychoanalysis, 74*, 1235–1244.

Moran, G. S. (1987). Some functions of play and playfulness: A developmental perspective. *The Psychoanalytic Study of the Child, 42*, 11–29.

Neubauer, P. B. (1987). The many meanings of play: Introduction. *The Psychoanalytic Study of the Child, 42*, 3–9.

Racusin, R. (1994). Brief psychodynamic psychotherapy with mono-symptomatic children. Lecture presented at the 1994 Annual Meeting of the American Academy of Child and Adolescent Psychiatry, New York.

Sandler, J., Kennedy, H., & Tyson, R. (1980). *The technique of child psychoanalysis*. Cambridge, MA: Harvard University Press.

Spence, S. H. (1994). Cognitive therapy with children and adolescents: From theory to practice. *Journal of Child Psychology and Psychiatry, 35*, 1191–1228.

Strayhorn, J. M. (1988). *The competent child: An approach to psychotherapy and preventive mental health*. New York: The Guilford Press.

Von Hug-Hellmuth, H. (1921). On the technique of child analysis. *International Journal of Psychoanalysis, 2*, 287–305.

Winnicott, D. W. (1953). Transitional objects and transitional phenomena. *International Journal of Psychoanalysis, 24*, 89–97.

Winnicott, D. W. (1965). *The maturational process and the facilitating environment*. New York: International Universities Press.

Ziegler, D. B., & Prior, M. M. (1994). Preparation for surgery and adjustment to hospitalization. *Nursing Clinics of North America, 29*, 655–669.

Chapter 20

Individual Psychotherapy with Adolescents

Richard M. Sarles, M.D.

Adolescence is one of the most critical growth phases in the human life cycle. Puberty, the physical stage of development, ushers in profound changes in the body habitus, primarily through the acquisition of secondary sex characteristics. Hormonal and endocrine changes along with maturation of the cerebral cortex all contribute to significant personal, social, physical, sexual, and cognitive development of the teenager.

Although the period of adolescence was once considered to manifest an almost universal "sturm und drang" phenomenon, more contemporary studies indicate that only 15 percent of adolescents demonstrate significant psychopathology (Offer, 1992). However, epidemiological surveys indicate that adolescence represents a time of life during which the onset or accentuation of many psychiatric disorders occurs, including schizophrenia, major depression, adolescent suicide, bipolar disorder, obsessive compulsive disorder, and substance abuse disorder, for example. Therefore, ambulatory mental health child and adolescent psychiatry services are faced with a significant population of adolescents who may require the full range of mental health services, including individual psychotherapy.

There are several essential elements in individual psychotherapy with adolescents. First and foremost is the therapist's interest and desire to work with this particular age group. Why certain professionals are drawn to this age group remains a question; what is not in question is that working with adolescents is usually fascinating and often frustrating, always creative and frequently confusing (Sarles, 1994).

Providing psychotherapy with adolescents seems almost counterproductive considering the normal developmental tasks of adolescence such as identity formation, and autonomy and independence acquired through the separation-individuation process. Why, we could ask, would an adolescent want to sit and talk with an adult from whom the adolescent is working so hard to differentiate? It is characteristic of adolescents to develop their own music, styles, vocabulary, and causes, for example, to rebel against parental and adult values in order to carve out an identity of their own through the separation-individuation process. What is often overlooked in this developmental process is that while most adolescents plunge headlong toward independence there lurks an intense insecurity within many regarding the uncertainty and the unpredictable nature of that sought for independence. It is within this context that psychotherapy with adolescents has the greatest opportunity to work. Few adolescents will admit to this concept but many look toward grandparents, teachers, coaches, and even a therapist as a special friend to guide them on their way to adulthood.

All therapies rely upon a working alliance between the therapist and the patient. The beginning of the alliance starts with an initial assessment of the patient. Many adults seek treatment on their own or at the suggestion of loved ones, employers, or friends. Most adolescents do not seek treatment on their own but usually through a request or requirement of parents, school, or the juvenile justice system. Although there are many approaches to the diagnostic assessment process, one approach to facilitate a working alliance with the adolescent is to see the adolescent initially, alone, to "get his or her side of the story" to develop the history and obtain his or her understanding of the reasons for referral. The rationale for the approach is explained to the adolescent and the parent in terms of the therapist obtaining a fresh, unbiased, personal view and opinion by hearing all sides of the story.

The second visit with the parents is accompanied by information such as written materials from the school, psychological tests, previous evaluations. The therapeutic alliance must also extend to the parents; without their input and support, therapy cannot work and the adolescent's progress to healthy development will be thwarted. Naturally, only the parents or parental figures can help the clinician understand the patient's developmental history, including strengths and weaknesses. The process of having the parents list the strengths and weaknesses of their adolescent acknowledges strengths which the therapist can build upon and weaknesses to be addressed in therapy. Even if the adolescent has been fully evaluated or has been in therapy previously and is receiving medication, a fresh view helps establish the therapist's interest in the current problem and the current status of the patient. In addition, a clinician usually gets to know a patient best when personally involved in the diagnostic or evaluation process.

In the third sum-up visit, the adolescent is seen once again, first alone. A summary of the parents' views and concerns is given, including perceived strengths and weaknesses and a summary of written materials such as psychological tests and so on. To reinforce the alliance with the patient, findings and recommendations are discussed. The adolescent learns how the problem is conceptualized by the therapist, as highlighted by presenting symptoms, developmental difficulties, and other factors, codifying the diagnosis by reading DSM-IV diagnostic criteria for each potential diagnostic issue. A brief formulation of the problem in a biopsychosocial format should also be presented to the adolescent patient at this time. This diagnostic formulation is followed by treatment recommendations, including medications and psychotherapy as needed. When indicated, weekly psychotherapy sessions of 45 minutes for a minimum of six months with re-evaluation and renegotiation at six months (dependent, of course, on managed care allocation of the number of sessions) is recommended. The adolescent's response to the diagnostic formulation and treatment recommendation is sought, with the therapist never entering into an argument but only reinforcing the duty as a clinician to give an honest opinion. This presentation to the adolescent is followed with a repeat presentation for the parents with the adolescent present. A discussion of epidemiological data, prevalence figures, and prognosis is always included. The parents and the adolescent are encouraged to discuss the findings and recommendations as a family and to call if they wish to work with the therapist

To minimize dependency pulls on the adolescent, it should be emphasized that it is not a question of whether or when the adolescent needs treatment but with whom. The adolescent and the family can then be offered the option of a referral should the adolescent and/or family desire a therapist of the opposite sex, a younger therapist, or someone closer to their home, for example.

THE PSYCHOTHERAPEUTIC PROCESS

The basic principles of all individual psychotherapy—privacy, freedom of distraction, adherence to time structure, empathy, mutual respect of safety issues, and confidentiality— all apply to the psychotherapy with adolescents. Confidentiality issues should be discussed early, explaining to the adolescent that confidentiality is a critical factor to facilitate the patients' trust in the therapeutic relationship. It is important to emphasize that confidentiality is meant for the benefit of the patient: therefore, any issues which arise in therapy that could be detrimental or harmful to the patient transcend confidentiality. Examples can help emphasize the point, such as, "If you were to harm (or attempt to kill) yourself or others this would not be good for anyone and I would be obliged to inform someone, the parents or the intended victim and the police." In matters of drugs, alcohol, and unprotected sex it is important to note with the adolescent patient that these behaviors are self-destructive and potentially fatal but the therapist would be willing to work with the adolescent on these issues to help him or her alter these dangerous behaviors without informing the parents as long as progress is made in therapy.

Another issue unique to the psychotherapeutic encounter with children and adolescents is the relationship with parents and confidentiality. Parents must be part of the process; parents who are concerned enough about their children to invest the time, energy, and money to help their adolescent should be given as much help as possible by the therapist. How to support the parents' efforts while maintaining patient confidentiality and transference-countertransference issues is critical. In general it is helpful to accept parent calls or requests to talk during an appointment as long as the adolescent is informed and made aware of the issues. A balanced approach is to acknowledge the parents' concern and the therapist goal to help both patient and parents to achieve normal development. It is helpful to inform the adolescent that the therapist will "stick up" for the adolescent's position, if possible, but will also side with the parents if their requests are reasonable.

Conversely, there are differences in the psychotherapeutic approach with adolescents. Generally, the therapist has to take a much more active and interactive role. In contrast to working with adults where silence by the therapist usually generates anxiety in the patient, resulting in verbal output, silence with adolescents also generates anxiety but this anxiety often results in greater silence, resistance, and a negative therapeutic encounter. Psychotherapists working with adolescents must also be willing to be more self-revealing; adolescents tend not to do well with the "tabula rosa" or blank screen often utilized to facilitate transference with adult patients. Most questions by an adolescent patient should be answered by asking him or her, first, why he or she asks, second, what he or she would guess the answer might be, and then, eventually, answering as appropriate.

The therapist must be prepared and willing to offer advice to the adolescent patient. However, as is true of all therapies (and, in fact, life), timing is crucial. To avoid early advice-giving it is generally best to try to understand what the question, the conflict, and the meaning of the question or behavior are. It is helpful early in therapy to acknowledge that the therapist needs to know the patient better, otherwise it would be presumptuous to give premature advice. It is wise to ask the adolescent to avoid any major decisions or moves and even curtail or contain certain behaviors until both the therapist and patient can better understand the issues and create an agreed upon "game plan."

Helping the adolescent discover healthier, more adaptive problem-solving strategies by looking at options, even acknowledging the maladaptive options, can be a major step in alliance formation and successful therapy. The position, which is openly expressed with the adolescent, is that he or she is always ultimately responsible for his or her behaviors and is able, in reality, to accept or reject anything discussed in therapy, including medication. Assuming this position addresses the adolescent's drive toward separation-individuation and autonomy but subtly provides guidance and direction. This technique enables the therapist to serve as a parent but not *the* parent, a very important distinction. The therapist who inadvertently and certainly inadvisably transgresses the transference-countertransference line of the therapeutic relationship will create significant difficulties with possible regression and acting out by the adolescent. In most cases the adolescent does not need or want another parent but can use and welcome an adult "special friend" to help him or her negotiate the way through adolescence.

In the initial stages of psychotherapy it is advisable to attempt to explain to the adolescent patient what the therapeutic encounter will entail. Most adult patients have little understanding of how "talking" with a therapist can help, and "working through" issues is a jargon term unique to the mental health field. Adolescents have even more trouble understanding what psychotherapy is, let alone how it works. One explanation of psychotherapy for the adolescent is that it is similar to a jigsaw puzzle; a puzzle as to why the adolescent is having the trouble he or she is having, a puzzle as to how it occurred, and a puzzle as to how the problem can best be addressed. The early stages (visits) of therapy can be described to the adolescent as spent turning over the pieces of the puzzle to begin grouping colors together and picking out flat-sided pieces to construct a frame within which to work. The adolescent's task, he or she is told, is to bring in material (the pieces) to the therapy, the conjoint work of therapist and patient is to toil together framing, sorting, and synthesizing, utilizing the experience and skills of the therapist in puzzle (problem) solving. This metaphor of the puzzle defines a true working relationship of the patient and therapist in solving the problem; it also avoids the potential transference problem of the adolescent labeling the therapist as a "know-it-all," insinuating the therapist knows what's best for the patient just like the parent.

Psychotherapy can be conceptualized as a learning experience, the balance of the learning weighted for the patient; yet all therapists generally acknowledge how much they have learned from their patients. There is often a thin line between teaching and learning in psychotherapy but with adolescents there must be a very clear distinction between teaching and preaching. Preaching usually indicates that the therapist, in the countertransference, has transgressed the role of serving as a parent and lapses into becoming the parent. The therapist should create this learning environment by constantly seeking information from the adolescent about contemporary life in high school, and current music trends and attitudes in his or her school and with peers regarding drugs, alcohol, and sexual behavior. The therapist needs to be cautious, however, to avoid trying to "seduce" the adolescent by adopting the adolescent's language, styles, or mannerisms. The therapist must always maintain a positive, optimistic attitude toward the adolescent's struggles.

One method to employ teaching in psychotherapy is to utilize a third-person technique, with the therapist commenting on normal adolescent developmental tasks—for example, the therapist might say "it's fairly common for 15-year-old teenagers to find their parents' rules and regulations as silly or stupid at best." "In general, this is not altogether a bad thing for teenagers since it helps them establish their own ideas and values as they begin to carve out who they are in life."

Using nonpsychiatric sayings is also helpful for the patient in understanding the conflicts inherent in life. For example, "you're caught between a rock and a hard place" and "there are no easy solutions and everything in life is a trade-off" so "you have to give something up to get something." Such sayings are meant to help the adolescent self-reflect, to develop an observing ego, and to teach him or her to talk himself or herself through difficult issues and emotions.

CONCLUSION

Psychotherapy with adolescents is a process. In general, there are no quick fixes, even in the contemporary world of psychopharmacology and managed care. In the biopsychosocial model of etiology, pathogenesis, and treatment the psychotherapeutic process supplies the required treatment, structure, and support for the patient. The therapeutic alliance is critical with the adolescent, yet the therapist must always be mindful of the need for a working alliance with the parents or primary caretaker. Adolescents by the very nature of their developmental stages frequently provoke countertransference feelings in the therapist. Recognizing and dealing with these issues is the essence of psychotherapy with adolescents.

REFERENCES

Offer, D., & Schonert-Reichl, K. A. (1992). Debunking the myths of adolescence. *Journal of the American Academy of Child and Adolescent Psychiatry, 31*, 1003–1014.

Sarles, R. M. (1994). Transference-Countertransference issues with adolescents: Personal reflections. *American Journal of Psychotherapy, 48*, 1, 64–74.

Chapter 21

Behavior Therapy with Children and Adolescents

Sheridan Phillips, Ph.D.

Behavior therapy has grown from its status as a revolutionary "upstart" in the late 1960s to the most common form of treatment used with children and adolescents (Powers & Rickard, 1992). In part, this has been prompted by the very nature of behavior therapy. Although often mistakenly perceived as a collection of techniques, the essence of behavior therapy is an experimental approach to human behavior (Goldfried & Davison, 1994). The use of operational knowledge is fundamental to understanding and altering behavior, whether overt or covert (e.g., thoughts and physical sensations). Behavior therapists operationalize abstractions such as depression or anxiety via concrete descriptions of behavior or physiological measurement. Therapeutic change involves the search for and manipulation of the strongest controlling variables, with the patient's behavior assumed to be lawful. Each clinical case is thus essentially a mini-experiment. Data collection is central to developing and testing the therapist's working hypothesis and judging the success of treatment, and the patient is often involved in recording his or her actions and in planning and evaluating therapeutic interventions. The behavioral approach to therapy is thus inherently compatible with evaluating the efficacy of therapy, and it is not surprising that most outcome research has focused on behavioral and cognitive-behavioral interventions. The documented efficacy of behavior therapy has obviously played a major role in its widespread acceptance.

The recent prominence of cost containment in health care has highlighted another aspect of behavior therapy, its relative brevity. The goal of behavioral intervention has always been to identify and alter problematic behavior as specifically and efficiently as possible. Well before the advent of limitations on length of treatment, it was generally a matter of pride with behavior therapists to effect treatment in as few sessions as feasible. While some patients will require a lengthy course of behavior therapy, many can be helped by relatively brief intervention, typically three to six months' duration with follow-up checks to assess maintenance of change. This focus on efficiency enhances the appeal of behavior therapy in the current health care climate where cost is of paramount concern and an estimated 11 million to 14 million American children are in need of treatment for significant developmental or emotional problems (Kazdin, 1994).

BEHAVIORAL ASSESSMENT AND CASE CONCEPTUALIZATION

Advances in behavioral assessment have produced a host of standardized measures (Mash & Terdal, 1988). These range from overall measures of functioning, such as the Child Behavior Checklist, to in-depth measures of specific problem areas, such as the Revised Fear Survey Schedule, and vary from self-report to systematic observation of children's play. Such standardized instruments are valuable for screening purposes as well as for clinical evaluation. However, the key component of assessment remains the functional analysis of a patient's behavior, and the resulting behavioral formulation (Goldfried & Davison, 1994).

As with all assessment, the functional analysis is based on self-report of history and current behavior, and reports of others such as parents and teachers, observation of patient and family, school or court records, and standardized assessment instruments. The behavior therapist may also arrange to observe the child at school or home, or in a setting such as a day treatment program.

Initially, behavioral analysis used a stimulus-response approach, with the goal of determining those stimuli that provoked a specific reaction. The consequences of that reaction were also assessed (e.g., was the child reinforced, punished, or ignored?). In the mid-1970s, behavior therapists began to incorporate the role of cognition and other "person variables" such as autonomic reactivity/arousability as well as overt behavior. These were viewed as organismic variables (specific to that organism) and the functional analysis was conceptualized as SORC (identifying the relevant stimulus, organismic variables, response, and consequences).

Stimuli can be external and overt, or covert such as a physical sensation or thought. Stimuli can also be perceived differently by different individuals because they are filtered through that person's expectations (organismic factors). Similarly, responses can consist of overt or covert behavior such as self statements. The behavior therapist thus attends to such questions as the patient's expectations of himself or herself and others, how events are labeled, and the nature of self statements.

In conceptualizing a case, the behavior therapist considers the patient's problem in the context of his or her history, identifies variables that control the problem behavior, and develops a hypothesis from the functional analysis of the data to serve as a guide during therapy. Operational knowledge and data collection are central to developing and testing the working hypothesis. The clarity and accuracy of the behavioral formulation are crucial in effecting successful treatment because the requisite intervention is readily apparent given the specific formulation, in the same manner that the design of a study emerges naturally once the research question has been clearly formulated. For example, one goal of assessment is to determine whether the patient lacks appropriate skills (a behavioral deficit) or whether these skills have been learned but are only evidenced in some circumstances (an inhibition). In the former case, therapy would focus on skill acquisition; in the latter, interventions would be directed at reducing the inhibition.

Behavioral analysis and individual case formulation were major strengths of behavior therapy in the 1970s and early 1980s. Goldfried and Davison (1994) suggested that the prominence of manualized treatment for specific *DSM* disorders has currently eclipsed this crucial aspect of clinical behavior therapy. Although it is necessary to develop standardized treatment packages that may be evaluated to document efficacy, clinical application often requires modification and/or extension to tailor intervention to an individual case. Practicing clinicians are well aware that two individuals may present with the same *DSM* profile and yet be quite different people with different life circumstances, requiring different approaches to intervention. "Top Gun" was established to address fighter pilots' over-reliance on computers by focusing on instinctual and creative dogfighting. In the same manner, behavior therapists need to develop their clinical instincts and case conceptualization skills to make flexible and creative decisions with individual patients. To benefit from the advantages of both approaches to assessment, Hersen and Last (1989) recommended a two-tiered approach, where psychiatric diagnosis represents the first tier. For the second tier, behavioral analysis would identify specific targets for intervention with specific techniques.

THEORETICAL UNDERPINNINGS OF BEHAVIOR THERAPY

It is crucial to understand the theoretical principles on which intervention is based. Therapists may find themselves inventing new procedures which are logically indicated by the patient's needs but which have not been reported in the literature. Manualized treatment packages may be appropriately applied with some patients with little adaptation. Possibly their main value, however, is to provide therapists with ideas and techniques for individualized intervention.

Behavioral intervention is based on empirically derived principles and models, largely from research in psychology. Many are learning models: classical and operant conditioning, observational learning or modeling, information processing, problem solving, and development of self-control. However, any empirically based principle is fair game for application to clinical practice. For example, one area of social psychology research focuses on the process of attitude formation and change, providing information that is clearly relevant to clinical intervention. With children and adolescents, findings from research on cognitive, social, and moral development are also applicable to treatment.

Classical Conditioning

Certain stimuli (e.g., electric shock) appear physiologically programmed to elicit a response (e.g., pain) in animals and humans. The classical conditioning model describes these as the unconditioned stimulus (UCS) and unconditioned response (UCR) because no specific learning experiences are required to produce a UCR in response to an UCS. If an originally neutral stimulus is presented contiguously with the UCS, the organism detects this pairing and it becomes a conditioned stimulus (CS) that then elicits a conditioned response (CR) of fear or anxiety that antedates the UCS and is considered to be an anticipation of the fearful event. Laboratory experiments with animals and humans have generated laws of classical conditioning that address acquisition, generalization, and extinction of the CR and aspects of the CS such as intensity and timing.

Classical conditioning principles have been employed to devise behavioral interventions such as the urine alarm (or bell-and-pad) treatment for enuresis, although it should be noted that intervention often employs other procedures in addition (Houts, Berman, & Abramson, 1994). The classical conditioning model was also the basis for Wolpe's systematic desensitization procedure (Wolpe, 1995). This uses the concept of reciprocal inhibition, where evoking one response inhibits the production of other responses, particularly those that are functionally opposed to the one being evoked. Wolpe used responses such as

eating or relaxation and paired them with originally fear-arousing stimuli. At a low level
of fear, he found that it was possible to produce the incompatible response which then reciprocally inhibited the fear, weakening it further. Using a progressive hierarchy of low-to
high-intensity examples of the feared stimulus, Wolpe employed such counterconditioning
to produce a relaxation response which reciprocally inhibited the anxiety response, eventually enabling a patient to confront previously fearful situations without maladaptive anxiety. While theorists currently debate whether systematic desensitization truly represents
classical conditioning versus other forms of learning, there is no doubt that it is effective
both with children and adults (Powers & Rickard, 1992).

The relaxation response required for counterconditioning is produced by relaxation
training (sometimes assisted by biofeedback) (Powers & Rickard, 1992). Because this is
typically conducted in the therapy setting, generalization of the relaxation response is enhanced by (a) differential relaxation, where the patient learns to relax those muscle groups
not involved in performing an activity, and (b) cue-controlled relaxation, where the patient
learns to evoke relaxation by using a cue word such as "calm." While such training has been
used successfully with children, it has received relatively little attention and therapists often
assume erroneously that desensitization is not appropriate for children and younger adolescents. Given its potential utility, desensitization is an intervention that clearly warrants
further investigation, particularly to identify specific modifications for different developmental levels.

Operant Conditioning

Reflecting back to the comprehensive SORC model of human behavior, classical conditioning focuses primarily on the stimulus component. In contrast, operant conditioning
primarily addresses the response and its consequences. The most basic application of operant learning principles is the analysis and manipulation of contingencies that exist in an
individual's environment. These are essentially if-then statements such as, If Mary produces behavior A, what happens to her as a consequence?. One possibility is that nothing happens; her behavior has no effect on the environment. This constitutes extinction;
when this absence of consequence is experienced repeatedly, the frequency of behavior A
decreases over time and eventually is no longer emitted. Extinction is used to eliminate
undesired behavior (e.g., ignoring tantrums). It also explains such phenomena as "learned
helplessness," where animals or people learn by repeated experience that nothing they do is
consistently related to what happens to them and they thus have no influence on or control
over their environment; in other words, they learn actively to become passive because they
are helpless. (Note the applicability to child maltreatment.)

Alternatively, a person's behavior can produce consequences. Contingent upon production of behavior A, the individual may experience positive reinforcement (a pleasurable
stimulus or event), punishment (an aversive result), omission/response cost/time-out from
positive reinforcement (the removal of an ongoing pleasurable event such as turning off the
television), or negative reinforcement (the cessation of an ongoing aversive event such as
escaping from humiliation in the classroom or playground).

Numerous laws of operant learning have been used in designing clinical intervention.
Some describe the frequency with which the contingency is applied (e.g., schedule of reinforcement) and the resultant effect on behavior (e.g., after a behavior has been established,
intermittent delivery of reinforcement will make the behavior more resistant to extinction than will continuous reinforcement). Another example is differential reinforcement

of other behavior, an alternative to punishment when the goal is to decrease production of undesirable behavior A (i.e., reinforce a child when he does anything other than A). Overcorrection (or massed practice) refers to a process in which the child is repeatedly prompted to engage in multiple instances of a target behavior in order to effect habit reversal (e.g., alter tics) (Ammerman & Hersen, 1995), eliminate undesired behavior (e.g., fire setting) (Kolko & Kazdin, 1992), or learn new behavior (e.g., toilet training) (Azrin & Foxx, 1976).

Other useful laws describe stimulus control (e.g., under what circumstances the contingency will be applied versus when it will not) and stimulus generalization (e.g., extending training conducted in session to real-world settings). Another example is fading, where prompts initially used to guide behavior are systematically reduced and eventually eliminated. Shaping is used to develop complex behaviors, that cannot be produced initially, by reinforcing successively closer approximations to the target behavior. Complex sequences of behavior can be learned by systematically chaining behaviors. As with contingencies, all operant principles can be useful both to analyze and understand the evolution and maintenance of maladaptive behavior and also to alter it.

Most operant-based interventions employ the application of contingencies. (Note that this is not always a straightforward process; novices often make errors in analyzing and designing contingencies, and selecting optimal levels of reinforcement, such as food versus praise, and appropriate reinforcers.) With very young children, the therapist works primarily with parents to alter the contingencies they employ at home so as to increase desired behavior and reduce undesired behavior. With school-age children and adolescents, the therapist increasingly involves the child as well as parents and/or teachers. Explicit contingency contracting is often used, where parents and child agree to participate in a planned program where specific contingencies are applied to target behavior. Although parents almost always have some involvement in treatment, it is common to include individual sessions with the older child or adolescent if this is appropriate for treatment goals. For example, an adolescent may be experiencing independence struggles at home with parents, and also some difficulty with peer relationships. The therapist could meet weekly with the parents and teenager to address family interactions, and weekly with the teenager alone to work on peer interactions.

Parent training has been used extensively to treat a host of clinical problems, ranging from anxiety disorders to eating disorders and pediatric pain (Powers & Rickard, 1992; Kazdin, 1994; Hersen, 1989). The most detailed, comprehensive, and evaluated parent training program is that developed by Forehand (Forehand & Long, 1988) for children with disruptive behavior and conduct problems. A body of research compiled over 20 years has generated specific training programs addressed to younger versus older children, training aids such as therapist and parent manuals and videotapes, and documentation of generalization to other settings, effects on siblings, social validity, and comparative effectiveness with other forms of intervention.

Operant procedures have also been used extensively in other settings such as residential programs (Ammerman & Hersen, 1995) and the classroom (O'Leary & O'Leary, 1980). Intervention in schools has primarily focused on teacher training in contingency management, but procedures have also been developed to address issues specific to the classroom. These include the use of loud versus soft reprimands, the effects of an individual program on classmates, the Turtle Technique for self-control in the classroom, group contingencies, and the use of older children and peers as change agents (O'Leary & O'Leary, 1980). While the focus is on behavior change at school, intervention with individual children often also involves parents who can be very useful in providing back-up reinforcement at home for achieving behavioral goals at school.

The application of specific contingencies is typically employed to increase the frequency of desired behavior that already exists in the child's behavioral repertoire. If academic or social skills are deficient, operant procedures are also used (in conjunction with other procedures) in skill training. For example, improving interpersonal skills might include teaching children how to make requests of others, respond to comments, give and receive praise, and approach others to enter into a group activity (Kazdin, 1994; O'Leary & O'Leary, 1980). Operant procedures are also commonly used in conjunction with other procedures such as modeling, behavior rehearsal, problem solving, self-evaluation, and self-control to provide comprehensive intervention.

Preparing parents, teachers, and children for operant-based intervention involves at least as much clinical skill as does designing the specific intervention procedures. Seasoned behavior therapists spend considerable time with parents, children, and teachers in preparation and planning prior to intervention, and coordination and feedback once it has begun. Failure to do so often results in failure of the program. Addressing parents' and teachers' objections and concerns should occur throughout assessment and treatment planning because successful behavioral intervention often involves at least as much attitude and behavior change for relevant adults as it does for the child.

Initial expectations of parents and teachers can be problematic. Parents often do not anticipate the amount of effort that will be required of them. In addition to providing a rationale, the therapist should be careful to structure parental contributions that are feasible and maximize success, and generate record sheets or calendars in session with parents rather than sending them home to devise these on their own. Teachers generally are aware of time demands, and are often concerned about this and other appropriate issues such as how to incorporate this program smoothly into other activities and the potential impact of it on other classmates. A teacher will appreciate the therapist demonstrating respect for his or her time by minimizing the effort required via preparing forms that are printed on unusual-colored paper (distinguishing these from hundreds of white pieces of paper that he or she processes) and require him or her to write as little as possible.

Parents sometimes have expectations for their child's behavior that are inappropriate for his or her developmental level and require modification during treatment planning. Also, both parents and teachers often have unrealistic expectations for the extent and rate of change that will result early in intervention. The therapist's challenge is to identify initial targets for change that are both an acceptable first step and also virtually guarantee success, encouraging all concerned to continue with the next steps in treatment.

Some parents are uncomfortable with the whole issue of "controlling" and manipulating their child's behavior. The therapist will need to provide information about motivation and human behavior, noting examples of how their own behavior is influenced at home, at work, and in other social situations. It may be helpful to provide reading material that addresses these and other relevant issues; Research Press (in Champaign, Illinois) publishes numerous books designed for parents, teachers, and children (e.g., *Putting Up with Parents*).

Parents and teachers often evidence a preference for aversive control, and are reluctant to "bribe" children, especially for doing things that they ought to be doing anyway. O'Leary, Poulos, and Devine (1972) encouraged therapists to note that the dictionary defines a bribe as offering an inducement to do something wrong, in contrast to the clinical use of reinforcement, and to provide examples of reinforcement and its effects in the parents' own lives. I have found it useful to conduct "empathy training" with parents and teachers by asking them to describe the affective result of situations relevant to them when reinforcement is inadequate. For example, Mr. B works at a job and is paid for this (hence reinforced) and ought to produce the best work that he can. How would he feel, however, if no one ever thanked him for putting forth a special effort or praised a product of particularly high quality? Similarly, Mrs. B is a homemaker and it is her responsibility to provide good, nutritious meals (potentially three times a day) for her family. How would she feel about doing so if her family merely consumed the food and no one ever said, "That new casserole you tried is terrific" or "Wow, we're having steak!" or "Thanks for making my favorite, Mom."

Another common challenge to the behavior therapist is a parent's or teacher's statement that "We tried that behavior modification stuff, and it didn't work." Actually, this is helpful because nothing provides more useful information than a detailed description of behavioral intervention that failed. In eliciting a description, the therapist can acknowledge that it is not as easy as it sounds and that their well-intentioned effort may have lacked the skill required to maximize its effectiveness.

Finally, adults may need assistance in learning how to reinforce children. Specific, systematic praise for targeted behavior often feels particularly artificial and ungenuine, and yet it is important in effecting behavioral intervention and also in assisting children to identify their special assets and strengths (in contrast to general statements such as "I love you" or "You're a great kid"). Praise can be altered from more stilted feedback (e.g., "Thank you for helping me with that") to statements that feel more comfortable and genuine but clearly convey the same message (e.g., "Boy, you sure are handy to have around"). Assessing the parent's typical mode of communication enables the therapist to provide creative examples of alternative messages that employ the same style or format. For example, a parent may obliquely convey criticism by comparing her child with Mrs. Jones' daughter (a paragon of virtue), describing Miss Jones' actions and accomplishments and concluding with "Why can't you be more like that?" In contrast, the parent could describe Mrs. Smith's daughter and her errant behavior, concluding with "Am I ever glad that you're more responsible than that!"

Two-Factor Learning

Mowrer's two-factor theory was constructed to address situations in which two different learning processes (classical conditioning and operant/instrumental learning) are involved (O'Donohue & Krasner, 1995). Although the theory has been applied to such problems as vaginismus and substance abuse, its primary clinical application has focused on phobias and compulsions (O'Donohue & Krasner, 1995). Mowrer hypothesized that the first phase of learning occurs via classical conditioning when an originally neutral stimulus (the CS) has been paired with an aversive or noxious stimulus (UCS) such that the CS has come to elicit a conditioned fear response (CR) that has motivational properties. This fear motivates operational responding which, if it is successful in reducing the fear, is reinforced by the fear reduction (hence operant conditioning occurs).

From the clinical perspective, two-factor theory explains maladaptive behavior (e.g., repetitive counting) that results from an attempt to deal with learned fear, and which persists even when it appears to serve no purpose. It also explains "vicious circle" behavior such as that of a college football player who fears failing and losing his eligibility, drinks excessively to alleviate his fear, which negatively impacts on his academic performance and increases his fear, which in turn increases his drinking; such behavior is both self-defeating and yet self-perpetuating. Finally, the theory clarifies the basis of maladaptive behavior which persists indefinitely even when the originally feared situation has been altered such that the original stimulus for pain and fear no longer exists: if the fear-reducing behavior involves avoidance of the originally fear-producing situation (e.g., agoraphobia), an individual will never have the opportunity to re-encounter the situation and learn new responses to it. The advantage of this conceptualization of anxiety disorders is that it makes available all the known laws of classical and operant conditioning when designing interventions.

Two-factor theory implies that therapeutic intervention should include prolonged exposure to the feared stimulus coupled with escape prevention. Implosion or flooding has been employed, in conjunction with response prevention, with adults with anxiety and/or obsessive-compulsive disorders (OCD); the procedure involves prolonged exposure in vivo or imaginally to the most intensely feared stimulus (Emmelkamp, 1994). In general, exposure appears to be the most crucial component of treatment, with in vivo being superior to imaginal exposure, and prolonged being superior to brief exposure. Preventing escape is not vital for phobic patients but response prevention is important for OCD patients. Graduated exposure is as effective as flooding albeit considerably lengthier. Treatment can be conducted effectively in groups and via self-help programs. Beneficial effects have generally been maintained at four-year follow-up although patients vary in amount of improvement.

Remarkably few controlled studies have been conducted with children and adolescents, considering the prevalence of phobias in childhood and the typical age of onset for agoraphobia in late adolescence or early adulthood. Case studies and imperfect group studies have generally employed graded exposure, possibly because implosive techniques are nerve-racking for the therapist (Reed, Carter, & Miller, 1992) and unpalatable to parents. However, with funding issues prompting an ever-increasing search for more efficient interventions, this appears to be an area that warrants further exploration. It is noteworthy that one imperfect study of school phobia reported dramatic effects of in vivo flooding (Reed, Carter, & Miller, 1992).

Modeling, Role Playing, and Behavior Rehearsal

The learning that occurs in classical and operant conditioning involves direct personal interaction with one's environment. In contrast, we also learn by observing others, noting how they behave and what happens to them. Such learning influences our own actions and attitudes despite the absence of any direct personal experience. Bandura's study of observational learning generated many useful applications to clinical intervention (Powers & Rickard, 1992). Bandura delineated two important factors: characteristics of the model being observed that will make observers more likely to attend to the model's behavior and learn how to produce it, and consequences to the model as a result of engaging in the behavior. For example, a child might observe Model A engaging in behavior A and thereby learn to produce it (doing so when specifically prompted) but not engage in the behavior spontaneously even if Model A was reinforced because the child perceives himself to be so different from Model A that he or she anticipates that behavior A would not meet with reinforcement for him or her. Alternatively, Model B might be perceived as very similar to him or her, but the child may still not produce behavior B (even though he or she learned it) because he or she observed that Model B was punished for behavior B.

Modeling procedures have been used to reduce fears in children, ranging from specific phobias to anxiety about dental and surgical procedures (Powers & Rickard, 1992). When studies have compared them, a coping model (initially fearful, then gradually coping better) has been superior to a competent model (evidencing no fear from the outset). Modeling has also been an invaluable component of skill training programs, where the therapist and other children model the desired behavior as well as prompt the patient to engage in behavior rehearsal (Goldfried & Davison, 1994; Kendall, 1991). Role-playing is incorporated as well in many behavioral procedures as part of facilitating the patient's participation in new behavior patterns. At least as important, however, is the opportunity offered by role-playing to enable the patient to put himself or herself in the place of other people and experience being on the receiving end of his or her own problematic behaviors, as they are produced by the therapist role-playing him or her.

Cognition

By the mid-1970s, behavior therapists had begun to delineate the organismic variables in the SORC model, focusing on such issues as the patient's expectations of himself or herself and others, how events are labeled, and the nature of self-statements. Basic research in cognitive psychology provided principles of information processing, problem solving, attribution, and self-control that were applied clinically. In cognitive-behavioral intervention, the same empirical approach and many of the same procedures (e.g., reinforcement) used to modify overt behavior are used to identify and alter covert behaviors (cognitions) such as irrational beliefs.

BEHAVIOR THERAPY AND OTHER APPROACHES

While still functioning conceptually as behavior therapists, many clinicians have incorporated techniques from other orientations such as play therapy and gestalt therapy (Goldfried & Davison, 1994; Phillips & Weist, 1997). Others have blended concepts from traditionally different approaches. For example, Robin and Foster (1989) have developed an integrated approach to negotiating parent-adolescent conflict that combines aspects of behavior therapy (behavioral contracting, reinforcement, modeling, skill training, and rehearsal), cognitive behavior therapy (addressing irrational beliefs and expectations), and systems therapy (placing intervention in the context of the family system). This blending of approaches incorporates specific family-related concepts with an empirical approach to analyzing and altering maladaptive behaviors, both overt and covert. Finally, behavior therapy has been used in combination with pharmacotherapy and produced major advances in treatment in several areas of adult psychopathology (Hersen, 1989). Considerably less research to date has focused on combined interventions with children and adolescents, but findings regarding such treatment of ADHD suggest that combined treatment may substantially improve outcome for this and other psychiatric disorders (Barkley, 1990; Phillips & Soffer, 1996).

OTHER APPLICATIONS

Behavioral principles have been used extensively in nonclinical settings in industry and education. More recently, child behavior therapists have developed interventions with pediatric patients to assist with a wide range of medical disorders (Hersen, 1989). In addition, behavioral programs have been employed in primary prevention efforts to reduce problems such as accidents, cigarette smoking, and antisocial behavior (Hersen, 1989).

COMMON ISSUES

The Novice Behavior Therapist

To the newcomer to behavior therapy, particularly one who reads about interventions and techniques in an "overview" chapter, its application sounds simple. It is not. In their effort to bridge the gap between written descriptions of behavior therapy and what occurs in practice, Goldfried and Davison (1994) described the "therapeutic underground" that underlies clinical practice. When clinical reality reveals that behavior therapy is not so straightforward, the novice (as well as seasoned therapists) will wonder: Why don't my patients keep good records? Am I the only one who has trouble getting them to do their homework? Why don't these proven techniques always work for me? Why won't these parents/teachers do something that is obviously so sensible?

The requisites for training in behavior therapy are no different from those in any other orientation. In addition to course work and reading, it is vital to be supervised by a specialized behavior therapist.

Where Should I Begin?

Because an isolated problem rarely presents in clinical practice, therapy usually must address multiple and interrelated presenting problems. A common question is which of these to select first for intervention. In the abstract, one would ideally select a relatively minor and isolated problem as the initial target for intervention because it would be less affect-laden and less complex, hence amenable to fairly rapid resolution. This positive experience with an effort to change would reinforce the patient and increase his or her motivation to work on more difficult areas. Such theoretical considerations, however, are quickly superseded by more vital clinical ones. If one of the presenting problems is causing considerable distress or interfering significantly with the patient's functioning, or threatening major disruption soon if not addressed (e.g., the patient will be expelled from school), this problem would assume a high priority for treatment.

Another consideration is whether there is a functional relationship between problems. For example, a teenager might present with depression and feelings of worthlessness, and also with academic underachievement. If the depression appeared substantially a function of not achieving important academic goals, improving his or her study skills would be a logical first intervention, specifically addressing one problem and serving as a first step to alleviating another. On the other hand, if the patient's grades were excellent prior to the onset of depression, it would not be appropriate to focus on academic skill-building.

Finally, the most vital consideration is that of the patient's own preferences. Goldfried and Davison (1994) have commented that it is remarkable how many therapists fail to consider the patient's desires when planning treatment. Both the therapeutic relationship and the patient's participation in therapy are enhanced when the goals and plans for treatment are endorsed by both therapist and patient (Garfield, 1994). There will certainly be times when the therapist does not agree with the patient's choice of targets for change, and he or she must give his professional recommendation to alter the targets or the sequence in which problems are targeted for intervention. However, therapy is unlikely to proceed well (if at all) unless the therapist thoroughly explains the rationale for this alteration and the patient truly agrees with the resultant treatment plan.

Resistance

Resistance to therapy can occur at several points along the road to behavior change. First, the referring agent (e.g., pediatrician or teacher) may find that the child and/or parents flatly deny that the problem exists or that they need assistance in resolving it. Second, the child or parents may appear to accept the referral recommendation, but somehow never manage to appear in the therapist's office. Third, they may present for treatment but evidence reluctance to engage fully in therapy. Fourth, during the course of treatment, patients or parents may re-evidence reluctance to accept the therapist's recommendations regarding specific activities designed to produce behavior and/or attitude change.

The first two types of resistance represent referral failures and are discussed elsewhere (Phillips, Sarles, Friedman, & Boggs, 1997; Phillips, 1997); this section focuses on reluctance to accept the therapist's recommendations. When children and parents are resistant to the need for assistance, it is helpful to "normalize" the situation. It is interesting that reluctance to use professional assistance is not evident in most other areas of life. Plumbers, accountants, dentists, and lawyers are employed routinely without extensive soul-searching. In contrast, even mild deficiencies in interpersonal or parenting skills are often viewed as evidence of personal abnormality. Here, behavior therapists have an advantage in espousing a behavioral/learning view of personality, noting that one is not born with such skills, that all skills in life are acquired quasi-randomly, and that most individuals possess a collection of stronger and weaker skills in different areas.

Group intervention that focuses on "normal" parenting problems or "normal" issues for adolescents is more likely to appeal to resistant parents and teenagers than is individual intervention. Resistance in less urgent cases can be lessened by recommending participation in groups for normal teenage problems or targeted groups such as Alateen. Groups that include normal children can be highly therapeutic. In fact, one large-scale study that evaluated various interventions for antisocial youth reported the greatest improvement for those treated in "mixed" groups including both referred and nonreferred (normal) teenagers (Feldman, Caplinger, & Wodarski, 1983). Such a mixture provides several models and enables teenagers to learn from one another. Participants also learn that all teenagers have some kind of problem, which makes it less threatening to acknowledge their own. Another advantage of group intervention is increased familiarity with the group leader. As children and parents come to believe that this therapist can truly assist them, they become increasingly willing to consider individual or family treatment.

Once patients and families have accepted the fact that a problem exists and that they can benefit from professional help, a major source of resistance in therapy is the human inclination to resist being controlled or influenced by others. While individuals vary along the submissive-controlling dimension, it is clearly advisable that all patients and their families participate actively in goal-setting and treatment planning. Patients ultimately have the control in the therapy setting; children can refuse to talk to the therapist and parents can stop bringing their children to treatment. It thus is sensible to acknowledge the patient's power and promote an active partnership in effecting change.

Initial treatment planning necessitates clear determination of goals, the patient's expectations regarding the therapeutic process, and the likelihood that he or she can change. It is crucial that both strategy (goals) and tactics (intervention procedures) are mutually agreeable to the therapist and the patient/family as this enhances the probability that patients will remain in treatment (Garfield, 1994). This process culminates in a therapeutic contract which addresses what is expected of the therapist and of the patient. Behavior therapists often put the contract in writing, with copies for all involved. It is also common to set a limited time period for the initial contract (e.g., six sessions), after which the therapist and patient will stop and evaluate the progress of treatment, with the expectation that some behavior and attitude change will be achieved by that time. In addition, it may be necessary to reformulate goals and plans at other points in therapy, either because the therapist has reconceptualized the problem or because the child and/or family has presented additional problems that they would like to address.

Another important source of resistance is the amount of work involved in changing behavior. The need for complex and often multifaceted change can feel overwhelming to a patient and family at the beginning of treatment. Behavior therapy generally addresses such problems via the development of graduated tasks. By focusing on first one problem area and then another, and by developing hierarchies to deal successfully with easier situations before moving on to more difficult ones, the change process is broken up into components which appear more feasible. Progressing through this series of positive corrective experiences promotes the cyclical process of attitude and behavior change that comprises therapy. In addition to a gradual increase in behavior change, the patient's success at change gradually persuades him or her that he or she is able to change undesirable aspects of his or her life. It is this change in perceived "self-efficacy" that Bandura (1986) hypothesized to underlie all successful therapy.

Resistance to behavioral intervention on the part of parents or teachers sometimes represents anger that has developed over time with a difficult child. Such negative affect may be particularly evident in reluctance to praise or reward the child, or difficulty in describing anything positive about him or her. In such cases, one of the first goals of therapy will be caretaker attitude change, directing his or her attention to the child's assets, strengths, and positive behavior. This can be facilitated by also assisting the child to learn to reinforce positive actions by parents and/or teachers. Caretakers need reinforcement too, and are inclined to take a more positive view of a child who does so. In one classic study, teachers significantly increased their positive interaction, and decreased negative interaction, with children who received no intervention other than training in reinforcing teacher behavior (Graubard, Rosenberg & Miller, 1980).

Family Issues and Resources

Research in child psychopathology has increased our sophistication regarding concurrent presentation of problems by both child and parent(s). The respective effects of parental modeling and genetic transmission are not yet specified, but it is clear that we should be alert to the presence of similar disorders in parents of children who present with anxiety or mood disorders, or with ADHD. The resulting clinical question is whether the child can be treated effectively in isolation or whether intervention would be most successful if the child and parent were treated in tandem. If the parent refuses treatment, an alternative would be to increase the child's interactions with other adults who do not model a similar disorder.

Another issue is how to provide reinforcers for contingency management in a family with very limited financial resources. It is possible to find many reinforcers that do not need to be purchased. Many of the most potent reinforcers represent activities or privileges, such as being able to choose which television show will be watched by the family. In one instance, a family had a tradition of going to an inexpensive restaurant (e.g., Denny's or Pizza Hut or Popeye's Chicken) for dinner on Fridays; I found that being able to choose where to go was one of the most powerful reinforcers for the children. In another family, the favorite reinforcer of a 5-year-old was to help his mother make dessert. Not only was this useful in treatment, but its identification surprised and delighted his mother, who had no idea how much he enjoyed this activity.

Some families are impoverished in parenting resources. Parents may have debilitating problems of their own and be unable or unwilling to participate actively in treatment. In such instances it may be possible to enlist an older sibling to conduct the home-based aspects of treatment. Even fairly young children can be helpful as change agents. Fifth-graders have proved to be effective behavior managers with first-graders (Surratt, Ulrich, & Hawkins, 1969), and peers have been employed successfully in several efforts to increase prosocial behavior (O'Leary & O'Leary, 1980; Fantuzzo et al., 1988). In one study of withdrawn, maltreated preschool children, the peer intervention increased social responding and subsequent school adjustment significantly more than did adult intervention (Fantuzzo et al., 1988).

When parents are unwilling or unable to assist with treatment, a second option is to search for another adult whom the child likes (e.g., relative, neighbor, teacher's aide), enhance the child's affiliation with him or her, and involve him or her in treatment. If no such relationship exists, it may be possible to place the child in circumstances where beneficial relationships may evolve (e.g., with a coach in a neighborhood center). An example is the case of a 13-year-old ("T") being treated in our pediatric ward for a bullet wound through her lung that resulted from her unsuccessful suicide attempt. Her parents adamantly refused to participate in treatment although they were pressured into allowing T to come regularly for therapy. We observed that T returned repeatedly to the adolescent medicine ward, where she charmed the nurses who allowed her to assist with a variety of tasks. We arranged for her to become a candy-striper at a hospital near her home, where she was "adopted" by several staff members, one of whom actively participated in T's treatment.

THE THERAPEUTIC RELATIONSHIP

The behavior therapy literature seldom specifically addresses the therapist-patient relationship whereas the "therapeutic underground" clearly acknowledges that a positive alliance is necessary (though not sufficient) for effecting change. Goldfried and Davison (1994) noted that the therapeutic relationship provides a sample of the patient's interaction with others and is also important in preparing the patient for change. They emphasize that the therapist may be tough-minded and yet tenderhearted in interaction with patients. In fact, the few studies that have evaluated the therapeutic alliance effected by behavior therapists suggest that important therapist characteristics are similar to those found in other orientations: empathy, warmth, genuineness, and respect (Beutler, Machado, & Neufeldt, 1994).

Although qualities of the relationship may be similar, the type of relationship may not be identical in different psychotherapies (Beutler, Machado, & Neufeldt, 1994). In behavior therapy, the therapist-patient relationship can comprise the primary medium for the therapeutic work, or at least some of it. However, it is generally viewed as being most powerful as a catalyst to bring about change outside the therapy setting in the patient's daily life. Goldfried and Davison (1994) suggested that it is unduly limiting to decide in advance whether to focus on within-or between-session change. As with most behavioral intervention, this decision should be based on the individual behavioral analysis, and the focus of change may well shift when in different phases of intervention with the same case.

Goldfried and Davison (1994) also make an interesting analogy between the therapeutic alliance and anesthesia during surgery:

> Not only is anesthesia essential for surgery to take place, but once administered, it must be continually monitored. If at any time during the surgery there appear to be problems with the anesthesia, then it becomes the central focus. We would suggest that an ongoing monitoring of the three components of the therapeutic alliance—the interpersonal bond between therapist and client, and their agreement on both the therapeutic goals and intervention procedures—is essential in dealing with client resistance and noncompliance. (p. 288).

ETHICAL CONSIDERATIONS

Therapists of any orientation who work with children confront the same major ethical challenge that has been discussed prominently regarding behavior therapy: because therapy is generally initiated by adults, and not the child, to what extent are the goals for the child's treatment determined by others? I would suggest that there are two major reasons why this concern is more salient for behavior therapy. First, the determination of targets for change is so explicit that it highlights the issue of goal selection. Second, behavioral intervention often works.

A classic paper, "Be Still, Be Quiet, Be Docile" (Winett & Winkler, 1972), challenged behavior therapists to consider whether teachers' (and parents') goals are in the best interest of the child. Ongoing discussion of the issue of conformity versus individuality has continued in the literature; the imperfect resolution is that each therapist must exercise his or her professional judgment in setting goals for individual cases. This sometimes represents a complex juggling act to define therapeutic goals that are endorsed by the patient, therapist, family, and others such as teachers. Especially with older children and adolescents, it may be necessary to redefine the goal as "getting the teachers off your back," or even begin with a different target for change (e.g., peer relationships) that represents a pressing concern of the patient's, in order to engage the patient in a genuine therapeutic partnership. A major consideration must be the consequences of waiting to address the presenting problem (Will the child be expelled? Will the family withdraw from treatment?). If the presenting goals need substantial alteration to proceed effectively with treatment, it is vital to explain the rationale thoroughly to relevant adults and ensure that they genuinely accept the change.

Another consideration that confronts all child therapists is the problem of providing special treatment (and privileges) for the child in therapy, in contrast to other siblings in the family. While attempting to bring about needed behavior change in the "problem child," the therapist does not want to exclude recognition of the already extant positive behavior of siblings who are functioning well. One must proceed cautiously in reinforcing siblings so as not to disrupt behavior that is being maintained by natural reinforcers. However, it is important to address the issue and avoid decreased attention and recognition of siblings' accomplishments as a consequence of increased attention being focused on the child in treatment.

One circumstance unique to behavior therapy is the use of group contingencies, where all members of a group (e.g., all siblings, all children in a classroom) are reinforced contingent upon their collective behavior (e.g., absence of fighting or tattling, completion of a specific task). Group contingencies are very efficient and peer pressure can be extremely effective in producing behavior change. O'Leary and O'Leary (1980) pointed out that peers often influence children to engage in undesirable behavior, with considerable success, and mobilizing such influence toward desirable ends is an appealing use of its potential. One must be careful, however, to (a) target behavior that can be produced by all members of the group to avoid scapegoating the "laggards," and (b) monitor the group to ensure that children are influencing their peers in nondestructive ways.

CONCLUSION

The behavioral literature abounds with criticism of behavior therapy as we know it. Kazdin (1996) pointed out that the field has progressed considerably by improving the quantity and quality of studies evaluating efficacy, that consistent effects are found for treated versus control children, and that effect sizes parallel those found with adults. However, the extent of research with children and adolescents still lags considerably behind that conducted with adults, there are still relatively few controlled studies comparing different modalities of treatment (e.g., behavioral versus client-centered) and/or different techniques within treatment, and behavior therapy has not always been found to produce superior effects, although significant differences, when found, generally favor behavioral and cognitive-behavioral treatment. It is true that there are extensive methodological problems and challenges involved in conducting high-quality outcome research (Kazdin, 1994; Phillips & Weist, 1997). However, there is a clear need to expand the range of treatments studied, research questions asked, and clinical populations and types of problems, and to address long-term treatment effectiveness (Kazdin, 1994; Ammerman & Hersen, 1995).

Most theorists would agree that behavior therapy has become more sophisticated and useful by including cognitive factors, incorporating concepts and techniques from other orientations, considering the importance of diagnosis, and combining behavioral and pharmacological treatment. Yet all of these advances increase the methodological complexity of assessing the effectiveness of specific treatment and its most appropriate applications. The last source of additional complication is the need to pay more detailed attention to developmental factors (Hersen, 1989).

Although not abandoning a commitment to efficiency, behavior therapists have increasingly acknowledged that certain problems are not amenable to a "quick fix," (Goldfried & Davison, 1994; Kazdin, 1994; Hersen, 1989). Expectations for treatment "success" need to be adapted to the child's personal and family resources. Highly recalcitrant problems such as antisocial behavior will require extensive and lengthy intervention that includes relapse prevention, extended follow-up, and booster sessions. Some problems (e.g., ADHD) may best fit a chronic disease model (Barkley, 1990). In reflecting on some 30 years of clinical experience, Goldfried and Davison (1994) encouraged therapists to acknowledge to themselves, and to their patients, that there are realistic limits to what can be changed and that it is a disservice to expect that one can totally overcome biological constraints and the influence of past experiences. Accepting realistic expectations for behavior therapy itself may ultimately represent the maturation of the field.

REFERENCES

Ammerman, R. T., & Hersen, M. (1995). *Handbook of child behavior therapy in the psychiatric setting.* New York: John Wiley & Sons.

Azrin, N. H., & Foxx, R. M. (1976). *Toilet training in less than a day.* New York: Pocket Books.

Bandura, A. (1986). *Social foundations of thought and action: A social cognitive theory.* Englewood Cliffs, NJ: Prentice-Hall.

Barkley, R. A. (1990). *Attention deficit hyperactivity disorder: A handbook for diagnosis and treatment*. New York: Guilford Press.

Beutler, L. E., Machado, P. P. P., & Neufeldt, S. A. (1994). Therapist variables. In A. E. Bergin & S. L. Garfield (Eds.), *Handbook of psychotherapy and behavior change* (4th ed.) (pp. 229–269). New York: John Wiley & Sons.

Emmelkamp, P. M. G. (1994). Behavior therapy with adults. In A. E. Bergin & S. L. Garfield (Eds.), *Handbook of psychotherapy and behavior change* (4th ed.) (pp. 379–427). New York: John Wiley & Sons.

Fantuzzo, J. W., Jurecic, L., Stovall, A., Hightower, A. D., Goins, C., & Schactel, D. (1988). Effects of adult and peer social initiations on the social behavior of withdrawn, maltreated preschool children. *Journal of Consulting and Clinical Psychology, 56*, 34–39.

Feldman, R. A., Caplinger, T. E., & Wodarski, J. S. (1983). *The St. Louis conundrum: The effective treatment of antisocial youths*. Englewood Cliffs, NJ: Prentice-Hall.

Forehand, R., & Long, N. (1988). Outpatient treatment of the acting-out child: Procedures, long-term follow-up data, and clinical problems. *Advances in Behavior Research and Therapy, 10*, 129–177.

Garfield, S. L. (1994). Research on client variables in psychotherapy. In A. E. Bergin & S. L. Garfield (Eds.), *Handbook of psychotherapy and behavior change* (4th ed.) (pp. 190–228). New York: John Wiley & Sons..

Goldfried, M. R., & Davison, G. C. (1994). *Clinical behavior therapy* (expanded ed.). New York: John Wiley & Sons.

Graubard, P. S., Rosenberg, H., & Miller, M. B. (1980). Student applications of behavior modification to teachers and environments, or ecological approaches to social deviancy. In K. D. O'Leary & S. G. O'Leary (Eds.), *Classroom management: The successful use of behavior modification* (2nd ed.) (pp. 235–250). New York: Pergamon.

Hersen, M. (Ed). (1989). *Innovations in child behavior therapy*. New York: Springer.

Hersen, M., & Last, C. G. (1989). Psychiatric diagnosis and behavioral assessment in children. In C. G. Last & M. Hersen (Eds.), *Handbook of child psychiatric diagnosis*. New York: John Wiley & Sons.

Houts, A. C., Berman, J. S., & Abramson, H. (1993). The effectiveness of psychological and pharmacological treatments for nocturnal enuresis. *Journal of Consulting and Clinical Psychology*.

Kazdin, A. E. (1994). Psychotherapy for children and adolescents. In A. E. Bergin & S. L. Garfield (Eds.), *Handbook of psychotherapy and behavior change* (4th ed.) (pp. 543–594). New York: John Wiley & Sons.

Kazdin, A. (1996). Developing effective treatment for children and adolescents. In E. D. Hibbs & P. S. Jensen (Eds.), *Psychosocial treatments for child and adolescent disorders: Empirically based strategies for clinical practice* (pp. 9–18). Washington, DC: American Psychological Association.

Kendall., P. C. (Ed). (1991). *Child and adolescent therapy: Cognitive-Behavioral procedures*. New York: Guilford Press.

Kolko, D. J., & Kazdin, A. E. (1992). The emergence and recurrence of child firesetting: A one-year prospective study. *Journal of Abnormal Child Psychology, 20*, 17–28.

Mash, E. J., & Terdal, L. G. (Eds). (1988). *Behavioral assessment of childhood disorders* (2nd ed.). New York: Guilford Press.

O'Donohue, W., & Krasner, L. (Eds.) (1995). *Theories of behavior therapy: Exploring behavior change*. Washington, DC: American Psychological Association.

O'Leary, K. D., & O'Leary, S. G. (Eds.). (1980) . *Classroom management, the successful use of behavior modification* (2nd ed.). New York: Pergamon.

O'Leary, K. D., Poulos, R. W., & Devine, V. T. (1972). Tangible reinforcers: Bonuses or bribes. *Journal of Consulting and Clinical Psychology, 38*, 1–8.

Phillips, S. (1997). Compliance with medical regimens. In J. D. Noshpitz (Ed.-in-Chief) (vol. 3), *Handbook of child and adolescent psychiatry*. New York: John Wiley & Sons, Inc.

Phillips, S., Sarles, R. M., Friedman, S. B., & Boggs, J. E. (1997). Consultation and referral for behavioral and developmental problems. In R. A. Hoekelman, S. B. Friedman, N. M. Nelson, H. M. Seidel, & M. L. Weitzman. (Eds.), *Primary pediatric care* (3rd ed.) (pp. 772–776). St. Louis: C. V. Mosby.

Phillips, S., & Soffer, S. L. (1996). Recent advances regarding attention deficit-hyperactivity disorder in adolescence. *Current Opinion in Pediatrics, 8*, 310–318.

Phillips, S., & Weist, M. D. (1997). In R. A. Hoekelman, S. B. Friedman, N. M. Nelson, H. M. Seidel, & M. L. Weitzman.(Eds.), *Primary pediatric care* (3rd ed.) (pp. 761–771). St. Louis: C. V. Mosby,

Powers, S. W., & Rickard, H. C. (1992). Behavior therapy with children. In C. E. Walker & M. C. Roberts (Eds.), *Handbook of clinical child psychology* (2nd ed.) (pp. 749–763). New York: John Wiley & Sons.

Reed, L. J., Carter, B. D., & Miller, L. C. (1992). Fear and anxiety in children. In C. E. Walker & M. C. Roberts (Eds.), *Handbook of clinical child psychology* (2nd ed.) (pp.237–260). New York: John Wiley & Sons.

Robin, A., & Foster, S. L. (1989). *Negotiating parent-adolescent conflict: A behavioral-family systems approach.* New York: Guilford Press.

Surratt, P. R., Ulrich, R. E., & Hawkins, R. P. (1969). An elementary student as a behavioral engineer. *Journal of Applied Behavioral Analysis, 2,* 85–92.

Winett, R. A., & Winkler, R. C. (1972). Current behavior modification in the classroom: Be still, be quiet, be docile. *Journal of Applied Behavior Analysis, 5,* 499–504.

Wolpe, J. (1995). Reciprocal inhibition: Major agent of behavior change. In W. O'Donohue & L. Krasner (Eds.). *Theories of Behavior Change: Exploring Behavior Change.* Washington, DC: American Psychological Association, pp. 23–57.

Chapter 22

Group Psychotherapy with Children and Adolescents: Key Issues

Eric P. van Schoor, Ph.D., Kristen Schmidt, Ph.D., and
Harinder S. Ghuman, M.D.

HISTORICAL BACKGROUND AND SOCIAL CONTEXT

The origins of child group psychotherapy may be traced to Alfred Adler's work in Vienna, Austria, and the development of the Child Guidance movement. In the United States, Aichorn and Redl pioneered a psychoanalytic approach to group therapy with adolescents. Helen Durkin, working in 1937 at the Brooklyn Child Guidance Center, applied John Levy's "Relationship Therapy" to a children's play therapy group. This method involved interpretation of how children played, engaged with each other, and related to the therapist in dealing with their conflicts. Slavson (1950), established "group play psychotherapy" with preschool children, "activity-interview group psychotherapy" with latency children, and "interview group psychotherapy" with adolescents and adults. Slavson considered Activity Group Therapy and Analytic Group Therapy two basic approaches in his group work. The former he applied to group work with latency-age children where "free play and unrestricted acting out without restraint or interpretation are the sole treatment process." Here the emphasis is on the expression of fantasies and drives through play and action. The latter he employed for all types of therapy groups whether activity or verbally oriented, for children or adults, when transference and interpretation are used to bring about insight. (For a more detailed history of child group psychotherapy, see Slavson's (1943), "An Introduction to Group Psychotherapy."

RATIONALE

Groups are fundamental to child and adolescent developmental processes. From kindergarten throughout their school years children are immersed in groups. Peer group relationships are used to validate feelings and develop social skills. Children and adolescents often feel isolated and emotionally alone, and group support helps to unburden them. In a therapy group, children can experience being loved, trusted, and encouraged. They may also feel valued for just being themselves and gain a basic sense of security, safety, and trust, perhaps for the first time. Peer groups also serve to facilitate a transition from relatively constricted family life to a wider network of social relationships with others and the community at large. Developmental tasks such as seeking independence and autonomy (separation-individuation), gaining a sense of identity, discovering sexual relationships, and generally assuming more of the responsibility of early adult roles may be usefully shared and experimented with in a peer group forum. A positive group experience is socially important in our increasingly fragmented, economically pressured, and alienated society. Group members bring their school, church, and community life involvement into treatment. Sharing this wider social matrix in turn develops a good sense of reality testing and community values for the young person.

With the thrust of deinstitutionalization there has been an increasing emphasis on outpatient treatments. Socioeconomic changes, increasing substance abuse, the collapse of intact family life, increasing teenage pregnancies, to mention a few factors— all have placed intense demands on ambulatory services. This is especially pertinent to many inner-city children who are born to drug-addicted mothers and have suffered organic brain damage with concomitant developmental delays. Increasing numbers of children with learning difficulties and limited social skills are seen in inner-city clinics.

There is also much evidence of severe physical neglect, sexual abuse, physical violence, and emotional trauma. Many of these children experience uncontained, chaotic family and community life, and are often significantly undersocialized, lacking basic interpersonal and social skills. Frequently they present serious antisocial behaviors, including violence toward others, destructiveness, and disregard for authority figures. In the past, many of these children would have been treated in inpatient facilities for extended periods of time, but economic pressures now demand only brief inpatient interventions. Outpatient group therapy with its economic viability and psychosocial therapeutic potential, is therefore an important treatment modality for helping dysfunctional young people.

However, outpatient therapy groups are intrinsically more difficult to establish than groups in inpatient or residential settings where captive patient groups are defined by the social milieu. Irrespective of the theoretical orientation, key issues which the outpatient group therapist inevitably struggles with include: (a) the initial pre-group context and processes, including assessment, selection issues, and determination of treatment goals; (b) establishing the group and difficulties associated with boundaries; and, (c) maintenance and termination issues.

In this chapter, we explore certain key issues for establishing and conducting groups with children and adolescents in a range of ambulatory settings. It is not a "how to" approach, but an attempt to provide clinicians with a framework of fundamental issues that need to be addressed when conducting groups in various outpatient settings. How at ease the therapist(s) feel in a group setting, and the level of training and experience in groups, will have a significant bearing on outcome. We broadly address dynamic and administrative issues concerned with group establishment, process, structure, and termination.

MODELS AND TREATMENT FOCUS

A variety of theoretical models of psychotherapy may be drawn from when developing a focus and structure for group psychotherapy with children and adolescents. In effect, a continuum of approaches to group treatment is employed, ranging from relatively unstructured supportive or psychodynamic play groups to highly structured didactic or cognitive-behaviorally oriented groups. Taking into account the developmental levels and presenting problems, practical constraints, and therapeutic goals, a wide range of group treatment approaches can be developed (see Table 1).

Wherever a group falls along the continuum of models of psychotherapy, considerable freedom exists when selecting a treatment focus for the group. Often, the focus of a group is determined from a description of the children, as well as the composition and quality of their social, physical, and emotional environments. A review of the literature reveals a wide range of applications for group therapy with children, including "inner-city children with aggressive behavior," (Eargle, Guerra, & Tolan, 1994), "survivors of sexual abuse" (Silovsky & Hembree-Kigin, 1994), "parentally bereaved children" (Lohnes & Kalter, 1994), and "children of fathers with PTSD" (Jacobsen, Sweeney, & Racusin, 1993). Many other groups have been established based on the (a) identified focus of treatment, such as social skills training or problem-solving therapy; (b) enhancement of intimate friendships; and, (c) self-esteem, where the participants are then matched to the group based on common needs or deficits.

CONTEXT AND STRUCTURE

Pre-Group Considerations

Initially, the aim and purpose of the group must be established. Depending on the goal of the group, there may be a need to respond to specific presenting problems, and to screen selectively referrals for suitability. For example, in an outpatient clinic, a group may be focused on problems of unresolved grief, impulse control, sexual abuse, substance abuse, improving self-esteem, or developing social skills. In a school setting, specific school-related issues such as violation of school rules, truancy, fighting and anger management, difficulty in relating to peers in class, and disrespectful behavior toward teachers may be of primary concern.

In working with children and adolescents, a developmental perspective must always be kept in mind. Kraft (1983) emphasized that, "traits of developmental stages influenced the growth of group psychotherapy techniques more than perhaps any other factor." Child mental health work is fundamentally a contextualized discipline: It embraces a historical, social, and family perspective. It locates the child or adolescent within this wider context in trying to understand emotional and psychological growth. This may be contrasted with decontextualized practices such as clinical descriptions and classifications such as *DSM*, which promulgates a system devoid of historic, developmental family systems.

Group Composition

Group composition refers to the mixture and balance of group member characteristics such as age, sex, level of emotional functioning, diagnosis, and verbal skills. It is recommended that a balance be obtained between verbal and less verbal, and withdrawn and assertive patients in a group. More than two passive, nonverbal members in a group of six to eight may significantly stifle the group process. On the other hand, more than two assertive, demanding members may overwhelm the less active ones. The more structured and focused the group approach, the more latitude is available in accepting a wider range of emotional functioning. Conversely, with a more unstructured approach, the group composition becomes much more critical, particularly in balancing levels of pathology.

Table 1 Group Models and Defining Features

	Psychodynamic	Ego-supportive	Interpersonal	Cognitive-behavioral	Educational
Focus	Genetic interpretation of current dysfunction and definition of group members' emerging object relations.	Therapy as a relational experience to support patients in the use of ego functions for controlling and organizing their behavior adaptively. Often focused around specific life stressors/events.	Identification of problems associated with the onset of symptoms and improvement in the quality of interpersonal functioning. Addresses developmental issues (e.g., peer pressure, separation from parents, development of intimate relationships, etc.).	Modification of maladaptive belief systems and behaviors; homework-based assessment and skills-building assignments.	Provision of accurate information relevant to identified problem area or to development, maintenance, and treatment of symptoms (e.g., cancer or diabetes patients, substance abuse, children with learning disabilities).
Time Frame	Unlimited, usually long-term	Varied dependent upon patients needs/wants	Usually brief, time-limited (e.g., 12–16 weeks)	Brief, time limited (e.g., 12–16 weeks)	Brief, time limited (e.g., 6–10 weeks)
Patient Composition	Individuals with minimal or manageable regressive behaviors. More highly developed cognitive and verbal skills. Adolescents need motivation for treatment and capacity for observing ego.	Children prone to more severe acting out, with unstable defenses and poor observing ego.	Individuals with prominent interpersonal difficulties, poor social adjustment (e.g., depressed adolescents).	Individuals with homogeneous problem or social skills deficits, depression, problem-solving deficits, anger management needs).	Individuals with homogeneous problem or identified knowledge deficit relevant to symptom presentation (e.g., affective education, substance abuse education).

Table 1 (Continued)

	Psychodynamic	Ego-supportive	Interpersonal	Cognitive-behavioral	Educational
Dynamics/Process	Activity, play, and fantasy. Therapist works interpretations into play themes. With adolescents, development of insight and working through of transference reactions.	Ego training in action. Non-interpretive, here-and-now focus with emphasis on reality testing.	Development of an understanding of the interpersonal context in which symptoms occur with focus on interpersonal problems associated with the onset of symptoms. Group process provides in vivo therapeutic experiences.	Maladaptive thoughts and behaviors are identified by other group members; social dynamics of group and group feedback help to bring core issues to forefront for individual patients. Role-playing, exposure, cognitive restructuring exercises.	Primarily educationally oriented, but patient's own experiences and reactions
	Minimal. Open-ended group play and/or discussion.	Moderate with emphasis on maintaining secure boundaries within the groups.	Focus is maintained on one or two problem-areas in patients' current interpersonal functioning.	Highly structured. Therapists are active and directive to meet specific treatment goals.	

This issue was highlighted in a long-standing group for early adolescent boys many of whom were described as "peer-rejected and intellectually defended." When a new member joined the group, the boys were engaged in drawing pictures and sharing what had happened to them during the week. The new member who had been acutely depressed revealed that he had experienced thoughts of suicide. This immediately became quite anxiety-provoking and overwhelming to the other members, who adamantly maintained they had never had such thoughts or feelings. The group leader was concerned with not alienating the new member by focusing too much on his suicidal ideation, but the leader needed to address this issue and the other group members' anxiety about such self-destructive ideas. The group leader dealt with this situation by processing with the group as a whole the possibility of having self-destructive thoughts, attempting to normalize this, but also respecting their fears and defenses against such dangerous destructive thoughts. Thus, the new group member did not feel stigmatized as being the only one with such thoughts. The other members were also able to gain access to their more repressed depressive feelings about being rejected and how emotionally despairing they might also feel.

The aim and goals of the group will also determine the structure and duration of the group, for example, whether the group is "closed" and time-limited or "open" with a longer time span. In a day hospital setting or school, an open group may be more viable, with new members joining as others terminate and depart, and the group slowly develops a history and culture. Such a structure is more organic and fluid, rather than goal-oriented, as the children participating bring their specific needs and issues to the group.

Age and Sex

Generally, it is expedient to keep preschool children, latency-age children, and adolescents in separate groups, as each major age group presents different developmental and psychosocial needs. Working in a school setting with latency children, Corey (1977) found it most productive to have groups with three to five children of the same sex and age. This optimum composition helps the therapist relate to individual children, avoid slipping into a disciplinary role, and minimizes the children's need to compete for the therapist's attention. It also enables the therapist to focus on group dynamics.

Preschool groups are usually structured around activities such as artwork, puppet theater, and other facilitative play activities. As in individual psychotherapy, children may use such play activities to enact aggressive impulses and emotional conflicts they may be experiencing at home. In play group therapy with children, Ginnot (1961) aimed to change the individual child's intrapsychic structure through group relationships which involved catharsis, reality testing, sublimation, and insight. The process of identification, in particular, enabled the child to identify him or herself with others and the therapist. Ginnot did not, however, consider group dynamic processes, focusing instead exclusively on the individual child.

Latency-Age and Pubescent Groups   Latency-age and pubescent groups have evolved from Slavson's early work on "activity-interview" groups, employing interview techniques, exploration of fantasies, group play, and other communications (Frank, 1983). This approach aims at modifying behavioral, emotional, and intrapsychic difficulties through the application of traditional methods of play therapy with the catalytic effect of a peer group. The method relies on the use of basic dynamics of analytic psychotherapy including transference, sublimation, catharsis, reality testing, and insight. Slavson and Schiffer emphasized that to use this method effectively with latency children, "these dynamics must be modified and scaled down to suit their ages" (Slavson & Schiffer, 1975, p. 298). Activity group therapy has been found particularly helpful for the treatment of children with mild character and neurotic disorders (Coolidge & Grunebaum, 1964). Scheidlinger (1960) developed a modified version to treat more severely disturbed children presenting inadequate impulse control, confused identity, poor reality testing, and poor peer relations (see also Scheidlinger & Rauch, 1972).

Latency-age groups focus on the child's developing relationships with peers, teachers, community groups, and sublimated activities. The process of sublimation is essentially the rechanneling and modification of aggressive and sexual instinctual impulses into ac- culturated, socially valued activity. To a large extent, this is achieved through the wider sociocultural environment the child is born into. It is generally agreed that the function of group psychotherapy during this developmental period is to direct and organize drives into socially acceptable behavior patterns. The child gains coping strategies and begins to master social situations involving more control over impulses.

Adolescent Groups   Adolescents are treated in a wide range of outpatient settings including clinics, schools, day hospitals, and community club settings. The setting itself will strongly influence the total group process. Slavson's interview group psychotherapy approach and various modifications have been widely used with adolescents. Slavson's original group interview method with adolescents involved one-on-one psychodynamic exploration, with therapist and patient, in the presence of peers with similar problems. He saw this as providing mutual support and enabling group members to bring forward latent and repressed feelings: "The therapist helps each member to allay anxieties, gain insight..., and develop more wholesome attitudes towards parents, mates, siblings, and the world in general" (Slavson, 1950, p. 13).

A significant history of psychopathy, severe conduct disorder, drug addiction, and/or psychosis are diagnoses which usually contraindicate inclusion in psychodynamic groups and require further special considerations. Some therapists prefer to separate younger ado- lescents from older adolescents. Kraft (1983) pointed out that, "depressed adolescents need to be evaluated extremely carefully, for this presenting picture may be a facade for extensive substance abuse and for a brooding, preoccupied schizophrenic configuration" (p. 230). An assessment of adolescent suicide attempts and borderline personality features also needs to be considered carefully. Traditional diagnostic categories may not, however, sufficiently serve to guide group selection. In this regard, Sugar (1981) developed "adoles- cent peer group psychotherapy" with teenagers who have "poor-to-moderate reality sense and reality testing, with rigid or unstable defenses and a poor observing ego" (p.119).

Group Setting   The organization, institution, or agency responsible for policies and practices will inevitably impose a context which needs to be taken into account in estab- lishing any group. Organizations and agencies outside the work setting may also have an impact, (e.g., courts, juvenile services, and social services), and this boundary with the outside world must always be kept in mind. Whitaker (1985) noted, "The nature of that boundary, who belongs inside it and outside it, and who decides when persons stay inside it and move outside it, has a substantial influence on how one can go about conducting work with groups" (p. 102).

Farrell (1984) noted that outpatient groups in a clinic setting often encounter "more suspicion and hostility than any other form of treatment" as unconscious rivalries and envy are evoked regarding different treatment approaches. The functioning of a group inevitably makes demands on colleagues to cooperate if the group is to proceed effectively. Conducting a group in any outpatient setting will have an impact on that setting, either creating problems or revealing certain existing policies and practices which may require amendment if the group is to succeed. If an organizational view exists that groups are secondary to individual psychotherapy, or simply a cost-effective way of dealing with patients, then group psychotherapy may never be valued as a significant treatment modality in its own right.

Co-Therapist Considerations   The decision to conduct a group alone or with a co-therapist is an important issue which can have a significant effect on outcome. Certain types of groups will require more than one therapist, such as when children in a group spend time in subgroup activities. In adolescent groups, male and female co-therapists offer better opportunity for role modeling (Corder, 1994). Moreover, as noted by Dick, Lesser, and Whiteside (1980), co-therapy can provide a greater opportunity for shared problem solving and a mutual support system for the therapists when facing difficult and demanding group processes. Co-therapy also provides continuity in the absence of one of the therapists.

Co-therapy, however, may also compound the already complex process of group leadership and may result in dominance struggles and conflicting theoretical perspectives (see Leadership section). Corder (1994) noted that, "Developing a non-sexist, shared orientation toward group leadership and problem solving may be one of the most critical factors in planning for any group" (p. 18). The co-therapy relationship should be based upon mutual trust and certain precautions taken to ensure effectiveness. These include: (a) planning together from the outset; (b) continued consultation and feedback, before and after each group; and, (c) sharing group experiences. For a further analysis of factors related to the general satisfaction of co-therapy relationships see Paulson, Burroughs, and Gelb (1976), and Corder, Cornwall, and Whiteside (1984) on techniques for increasing effectiveness of the co-therapy relationship in adolescent groups.

Group as Primary or Adjunct Therapy

An important issue to consider is whether the group is to function as a primary treatment modality or as an adjunct to individual psychotherapy. If group treatment is the primary approach, will the group therapist function as case administrator? If individual psychotherapy is the primary mode of treatment, how will overall treatment planning be organized, including collaboration and feedback with the individual therapist? As previously mentioned, this raises key organizational issues which, if not appropriately addressed, can lead to the marginalization of group therapy and the failure of groups to become well established. Group psychotherapy can be effective as an adjunct to individual psychotherapy and in its own right, as a primary therapeutic process. In either case, the overall collaboration and clarification of aims, objectives, and responsibilities needs to be carefully analyzed within the organizational setting.

GROUP DYNAMICS AND PROCESSES

In its most general sense, the term group process refers to the way in which the group deals with communications. More specifically, it implies working through and integrating behavior and emotions through interaction. Foulkes and Anthony (1957) first employed the term "group process" to distinguish it from "group dynamics," the latter referring to the psychodynamics of treatment including resistance, transference, and countertransference. Foulkes stated, "The process which we know from a two-person situation can be seen in full in interaction between two, three, and more persons. They... are interactional processes, not as processes in the isolated individual" (Foulkes & Anthony 1957, p. 28). Group process is seen to develop from action, through interaction, to wider and deeper levels of communication, thus establishing attitudes and relationships in the group. Consideration of group-as-a-whole processes is fundamentally important. Schamess (1992) commented on the historical lack of attention to group-as-a-whole processes in child and adolescent group psychotherapy. He stated, "It seems likely that the traditional conceptualization of therapeutic groups for children as environments in which individuals are treated for specific emotional problems, as well as the historical emphasis on differentiating therapeutic from recreational and educational groups, encourages therapists to undervalue the therapeutic significance of group as a whole phenomena" (p. 353).

Establishing Group Culture

The anthropologist Clifford Geertz (1973), stating Max Weber's view that we create and are "suspended in webs of significance," metaphorically, considered "culture to be those webs" (p. 5). In this sense culture pertains to the network of relations and meanings that connects and supports us. In the group psychotherapy context, we speak of the "group matrix" (Foulkes, 1964). Erikson (1950), in *Childhood and Society*, also emphasized the role of cultural context in ego development, specifically in relation to the growth of "ego identity." Erikson commented, "For the growing child must derive a vitalizing sense of reality from the awareness that his individual way of mastering experience, his ego synthesis, is a successful variant of a group identity...." (quoted by Rachman, 1975).

In considering group culture and the development of group process in child and adolescent groups, Pfeifer (1992) drew attention to two complementary group-as-a-whole processes, namely, "indigenous peer culture" and "therapeutic group culture." The former refers to "the natural organization of meanings created and maintained by a given cohort of children," and the latter "grows from the soil of a positive connection between therapist and members" (Pfeifer, 1992, p. 362).

In our group work with children and adolescents in a multicultural, inner-city social context, we were particularly aware of the complex web of cultural diversity and how this manifests in group interactions. For example, in a group with male and female African American adolescents in a middle school setting the indigenous peer culture manifested in spontaneous "rap" songs in the group. In a particular song a sexually attractive girl, referred to as a "bomb," is demanded to "explode" by the excited males. Several such sessions were permeated by sexual themes (the therapist requiring help with "translation" of the songs by group members), which facilitated the group's exploration of sexuality and sex roles. Here the therapeutic group culture developed from a positive connection between therapist and members, and an acceptance and respect for the indigenous peer culture.

A focus on the "here and now," as emphasized by Foulkes and Anthony (1957), is important in working with adolescents who are often struggling with practical day-to-day concerns. Dealing with historical material must be balanced with a here and now focus which also develops spontaneous group experience.

Leadership

The British child psychiatrist and family therapist Robin Skynner (1969) considered child development as a "series of challenges to master group situations of increasing complexity," this developmental process being a preparation for leadership roles through adaptation to the authority of others. In this sense leadership issues may be considered central to human activity and these manifest in much of the interaction in groups. In psychotherapy groups, the therapist in the capacity of group leader exercises a dual function. First, as the "dynamic administrator," he or she takes full responsibility for the provision and maintenance of the therapeutic setting including props and the space-time structure (where, when, and how long the group meets) around which the group matrix organizes itself. The dynamic administrative function includes the all-important monitoring of the flow of communication into and out of the group (see Boundary Keeping below). In conducting groups with children and adolescents, the dynamic administrative function plays a particularly prominent role as boundary incidents impact strongly on the group process. There is also more action, rapidly changing themes, labile and, at times, volatile moods. Second, the therapist(s) functions in an analytic or task-oriented manner, depending on the goals of the group, but always with a special awareness of the group as a whole and the activity concerning the boundary of the group.

Attention to transference and countertransference phenomena is an essential analytic therapeutic function. Grotjahn (1972) identified three levels of transference in the group situation: (1) direct transference to the therapist by individual members; (2) transference relationships developing between members; and, (3) transference to the group as a pre-Oedipal mother. Grotjahn highlighted the significance of the latter dynamic and stated, "This... transference relationship is of decisive importance in groups of adolescents since the central conflict of adolescence takes place between the need for dependency and the drive for individuation and identity" (Grotjahn, 1972, p.173).

Boundary Keeping and Limit Setting

Boundary keeping and limit setting are significant aspects of the role of the group therapist working with children and adolescents. Behr (1988), writing about analytic group therapy, characterized adolescence as a "boundary state which demarcates childhood from young adulthood." With latency children and adolescents, the group boundary is immediately scrutinized and tested. Groups are convened by the adult-authority-figure therapist usually at the time when the child's life and development is under considerable stress. Immature defenses are often operative and include splitting, denial, and projective identification. Moreover, there are confusing changes in the adolescent"s own physical bodily boundaries and subsequent self-image distortions may occur (Behr, 1988).

Adolescents' preoccupation with the group boundary, that is, those conditions (rules, limits, and structural aspects) which define and form the group, appears in several ways: (a) breaching the space-time boundary; (b) action and verbalization boundary; and, (c) teasing and testing the therapist's boundary. The interruption of the space-time frame by "dropping in and out" of the group is ubiquitous in child and adolescent groups. Often, the child wants to use the bathroom, retrieve a schoolbag, drink a soda, or eat something. Such activities need to be monitored and minimized, and the underlying anxieties addressed. Attending sporadically, arriving late, or needing to leave early are also common boundary problems. It is not uncommon for group members to arrive very early or to be reluctant to leave at the stated time. When group members become emotionally invested in the group they also tend to treat other areas of the group setting as an extension of the group, such as the waiting area. Activities in these areas also need to be monitored, as acting out in these areas may occur and needs to be redirected (acted in) to the formal group setting. The therapist(s) need to bring these pre-and post-group exchanges back into the sessions of the group.

An example of the need for such boundary keeping arose in a latency-age boys group: During one of the meetings two group members played "tag." They were unable to settle down at the end of the session, chasing each other into the waiting room, where they proceeded to wrestle on the floor. The parent of one of the boys angrily shouted at the other boy, "Where's your mother? I can't believe she lets you act this way...." (this comment was especially hurtful because this patient's problems centered around his mother's drug use and neglect of him) and stormed out of the clinic, saying she would not let her son return to the group if the other boy also attended. In group the following week, members processed the issue and it was decided that the boy would talk to his mother and let her know that he and his peer had worked out a way to get along in the group. Other group members expressed their discomfort with this situation and one began to arrive late for sessions stating that he did not want to come to the group. It was incumbent upon the therapist to deal with this boundary issue without violating the patient's confidentiality, and to inform this parent that it was not acceptable for her to voice her concerns to this boy in this manner.

The perennial problem of erratic attendance in outpatient settings may be minimized by establishing time-limited groups, up to 10 weekly sessions rather than an open-ended group. A time-limited group allows members an opportunity to work toward completion, to terminate properly, and to gain a sense of achievement. It is useful to establish 10-week block groups throughout the school year, running three 10-week block groups annually. The time span of the sessions should also be regulated depending on the composition of the group. Young children and more immature adolescents can usually only sustain one hour sessions. Groups with older adolescents can run for one-and-a-quarter to one-and-a-half hours. The particular time frame must of course be kept constant for the entire block of sessions.

Action and Verbalization Boundary   In conducting groups with children and adolescents, the ongoing dialectic between regressed behavior and more mature, adult-like communications demands much flexibility from the therapist(s). The aim is how to maintain a structure which is both containing and limit-setting. In preparation for joining the group we clearly state a number of "rules." There is to be no hitting, kicking, slapping, or other such intrusion or violation of body space. It is expected that group members not interfere with any property in the room, remain within the group room for the session, and not attend intoxicated. Despite these injunctions, the high level of activity and reactivity in child and adolescent groups, at times, demands that the therapist say "No!" or "Stop" to establish control, reorganize the group, and direct attention to the therapeutic task.

Such sharp interventions must also be coupled with an attempt to understand individual anxieties and the group-as-a-whole's psychological preoccupation: In a preadolescent male therapy group boundary issues were preeminent. Group members who shared horrific histories of physical and sexual abuse as well as exposure to violence, struggled to manage their own anxieties by deflecting attention to other members' issues. During one particularly charged and unsettled session, one member triggered a traumatic memory in another by forming his hand in the shape of a gun, aiming at his peer, and pretending to shoot him. The therapists intervened in a direct manner, demanding that this highly stress-inducing behavior stop. The group, however, fragmented into a manic defense state, members agitatedly leaving their seats, moving around the room and roaring with laughter, while their peer lay frozen in terror on the floor. Members' defensive behavior was characterized by omnipotence and denial.

The psychic pain of their peer appeared emotionally too unbearable for the other group members who feared that they may also be psychically annihilated. In their attempt at omnipotent mastery of the object, they fantasized that their peer will not only be prevented from further psychological injury to himself, but as a group they will not be a danger to one another. That is to say, that they will not resort to further persecutory attacks. Through boundary management and containment, the therapists enabled the group to reestablish a safe therapeutic space and to slowly begin to process this manic episode. It took many sessions to begin to regain trust and security in the group and enable members to experience the emotional pain of their traumas and resulting depressive feelings.

The important issues of trust and confidentiality must also be addressed. The clear expectation is stated that anything talked about in the group is not to be spoken about elsewhere. This is particularly important where children attend the same school and have close contact in the same neighborhood. Ghuman and Wilmoth (1993) emphasized that, "It is the therapist's duty to evaluate issues of trust as they surface and to explore and discuss methods of enhancing or regaining trust in a time-effective manner" (p. 57). Distrust may arise when members avoid personal disclosure because of feeling fearful of others' reactions.

Teasing and Testing the Therapist's Boundary   The therapist may face quite blunt and intrusive interrogation about a range of personal issues such as sex life, childhood, and marital and parental status. How the therapist(s) deal(s) with these personal inquiries will impact upon the development of the therapeutic culture of the group. A balance should be struck between enhancing and modeling self-disclosure and openness but without transgressing moral and ethical standards. Teasing is an ambivalent playful communication signaling both a wish for intimacy and, at the same time, the need to maintain some distance. It can be benign, affectionate, and gentle or assume aggressive and sadistic qualities. Here again, the therapist(s) must balance playful interaction with a censoring response to overt bullying and sadomasochistic interchanges. Teasing can also become a defense against experiencing painful emotions.

This activity may also operate on the group-as-a-whole level when a particular member becomes scapegoated and represents unbearable vulnerability for the whole group. For example: In an inner-city middle school-based group, four relatively bright Caucasian males struggled with racial tensions, issues of respect and acceptance, and fears of being verbally and physically attacked by peers. In the initial phase of treatment the boys, all friends on "the outside," came to scapegoat the weakest group member much in the same way they were themselves scapegoated as a group in the larger school setting. Resolution of this group dynamic and how it mirrored events for them in the school was necessary before the group could move forward toward more intimate and meaningful interactions.

PHASES OF DEVELOPMENT AND TERMINATION

Behr (1988) pointed out that adolescent groups tend to develop either very quickly or slowly. He suggested that the therapist(s) moderate the pace when too fast, slowing it down, "so that the group is not flooded with material in manic style" (p.128). This especially needs to be borne in mind in time-limited groups where there may be a pressure to work at an accelerated pace. On the other hand, if the pace is too slow, the therapist(s) may provide momentum by stimulating communication using "warm-up" techniques or by stimulating fantasy thinking.

The early sessions of groups with children and adolescents are frequently character-ized by high levels of anxiety, with giggling, restlessness, and overall difficulty in focusing on the task of the group. In these initial sessions the members tend to be egocentric and have difficulty responding to the needs of others. In her work with adolescents in structured psychotherapy groups, Corder (1994) addressed this problem and identified certain general tasks for the group leader: (a) to facilitate interaction by modeling behaviors or structured techniques such as arranging roles; (b) to monitor and regulate the group's anxiety level; © to modify the group's verbal behavior to develop security and protect the self-esteem of individuals; and, (d) to encourage the examination of verbal content and group process behavior to develop insight.

The middle phase begins with the development of group cohesion, trust, and mean-ingful intimacy between members. There is a shift toward mutual exchange of opinion and ideas, sharing of experiences, support, and challenging confrontations. The group as a whole is more coherent and provides a structure to integrate and help work through con-flict and trauma. The group provides a safe containing therapeutic environment in which the child or adolescent can repeatedly experience and attempt to resolve his or her conflicts in different ways until sufficient understanding and mastery is gained. The group member-ship provides opportunities to compensate for developmental deficits and neurotic conflict as the group moves toward greater understanding and maturation. The therapist needs to respond to the various phases of the group, being more supportive and nurturant in the early dependent stage, and more open, playful, confrontative, and challenging when group cohesion and confidence is established.

Toward the later phase alliances among members will deepen. Members may take more initiative, making suggestions and experimenting with different roles. Toward the end, anxieties may again surge and regression occur with fears of separation and broken attachments. Preparation and rehearsal of the leave-taking rituals are important terminating experiences that enable members to practice and integrate the emotions related to future endings in life.

CONCLUSION

Outpatient group psychotherapy with children and adolescents embraces a wide range of approaches adaptable to a variety of settings and presenting problems. Groups are an im-portant medium through which to treat children and adolescents experiencing developmen-tal and psychosocial problems. Issues relating to establishing a group, such as selection and composition, are discussed. The need to maintain a developmental perspective with chil-dren and adolescents in the group setting is considered a guiding principal throughout. Setting conditions, co-therapy, and organizational collaboration are also highlighted in es-tablishing a successful group. The group therapists are seen as having a dynamic adminis-trative and therapeutic role. Boundary keeping and limit setting are primary considerations in developing a safe, contained therapeutic environment with children and adolescents. Attention to group-as-a-whole dynamics as well as individual communications is empha-sized. Phases of development and the termination process, and how they can be modulated to maximize the therapeutic potential of the group, are discussed.

ENDNOTES

1 Following the first World War, Adler introduced educational guidance and parental training groups in Vienna. His basic premise is that we are first and foremost social beings, and he aimed to understand individual psychopathology through the person's relationship to primary groups. The emotionally ill person is considered not to be fully adjusted to the groups in which he or she lives (Rattner, 1983).

2 Slavson adopted a rather stilted, if not contradictory, position. He basically dismissed group-as-a-whole dynamics and stated, "By and large it is an error to speak of the group as an entity in therapy. It is always the individual and not the group as such that remains the center of the therapeutic attention" (Slavson, 1943).

3 Klein believed that, "this mechanism of denial originates in that very early phase in which the underdeveloped ego endeavors to defend itself from the most overpowering and profound anxiety of all, namely, its dread of internalized persecutors and the id.... Klein added that what is quite specific to mania, "is the utilization of the sense of omnipotence for the purpose of controlling and mastering objects" (Klein, 1935, p. 277).

REFERENCES

Behr, H. (1988). Group analysis with early adolescents: Some clinical issues. *Group Analysis, 21* (2), 119–133.

Coolidge, J. C., & Grunebaum, M. G. (1964). Individual and group therapy of a latency age child. *International Journal of Group Psychotherapy, 14,* 84–96.

Corder, B. F. (1994). *Structured adolescent psychotherapy groups.* Sarasota, FL: Professional Resource Press.

Corder, B. F., Cornwall, T., & Whiteside, R. (1984). Techniques for increasing effectiveness of cotherapy functions in adolescent psychotherapy groups. *International Journal of Group Psychotherapy, 34,* 643–654.

Corey, M. S. (1977). Counseling groups for children. In G. Corey & M. S. Corey, *Groups process and practice* (pp. 149–164). Belmont, CA: Wadsworth Publishing Company.

Dick, R., Lessler, K., & Whiteside, R. (1980). A developmental framework for cotherapy. *International Journal of Group Psychotherapy, 3,* 273–283.

Eargle, A. E., Guerra, N. G., & Tolan, P. H. (1994). Preventing aggression in inner-city children: Small group training to change cognitions, social skills, and behavior. *Journal of Child and Adolescent Group Therapy, 4* (4), 229–242.

Erikson, E. H. (1950). *Childhood and society.* New York: Norton.

Farrell, M. (1984). Group work with children: The significance of setting and context. *Group Analysis, 27* (2), 146–155.

Foulkes, S. H. (1964). *Therapeutic group analysis.* Boston: Allen & Unwin.

Foulkes, S. H., & Anthony, E. J. (1957). *Group psychotherapy: The psychoanalytical approach.* Harmondsworth: Penguin Books.

Franks, M. G. (1983). Modified activity group therapy with ego impoverished children. In E. S. Bucholz & J. M. Mishne (Eds.), *Group interventions with children, adolescents and parents* (pp. 145–155). New York: Jason Aronson.

Geertz, C. (1973). *The interpretation of cultures.* Basic Books.

Ginott, H. G. (1961). *Group psychotherapy with children.* New York: McGraw Hill.

Ghuman, H. S., & Wilmoth, E. E. (1993). Group psychotherapy setting, structure and process. In H. S. Ghuman & R. M. Sarles (Eds.), *Handbook of adolescent inpatient psychiatric treatment* (pp. 52–69). New York: Brunner/Mazel.

Grotjahn, M. (1972). The transference dynamics of the therapeutic group experience. In I. H. Berkovitz (ed.) *Adolescents grow in groups: Experiences in adolescent group psychotherapy* (pp. 173–178). New York: Brunner/Mazel.

Jacobsen, L. K., Sweeney, C. G., & Racusin, G. R. (1993). Group psychotherapy for children of fathers with PTSD: Evidence of psychopathology emerging in the group process. *Journal of Child and Adolescent Group Therapy, 3* (2), 103–120.

Klein, M. (1985). A contribution to the psychogenesis of manic-depressive states. In *Love, guilt and reparation* (pp. 262–289). London: The Hogarth Press. First published 1935, *International Journal of Psychoanalysis, 16,* 145–174.

Kraft, I. A. (1983). Child and adolescent group psychotherapy. In H. I. Kaplin & B. J. Sadock (Eds.), *Comprehensive group psychotherapy* (pp. 223–234). Baltimore: Williams & Wilkins.

Lohnes, K. L., & Kalter, N. (1994). Preventive intervention groups for parentally bereaved children. *American Journal of Orthopsychiatry, 64* (4), 594–603.

Paulson, I., Burroughs, J., & Gelb, C. (1976). Cotherapy: What is the crux of the relationship? *International Journal of Group Psychotherapy, 26,* 213–224.

Pfeifer, G. (1992). Complementary cultures in children's psychotherapy groups: Conflict and convergence in group development. *International Journal of Group Psychotherapy, 42* (3), 357–368.

Rachman, A. (1975). *Identity group psychotherapy with adolescents.* New York: Jason Aronson.

Rattner, J. (1983). *Alfred Adler.* New York: Fredrick Ungar Publishing Co.

Schamess, G. (1992). Reflections on a developing body of group-as-a-whole theory for children's therapy groups: An introduction. *International Journal of Group Psychotherapy, 42* (3), 351–356.

Scheidlinger, S. (1960). Experiential group treatment of severely deprived latency age children. *American Journal of Orthopsychiatry, 30,* 356–368.

Scheidlinger, S., & Rauch, E. (1995). Psychoanalytic group psychotherapy with children and adolescents. In B. Wolman (Ed.), *Handbook of child psychoanalysis* (pp. 364–398). New York: Jason Aronson Inc. (1972).

Silovsky, J. F., & Hembree-Kigin, T. L. (1994). Family and group treatment for sexually abused children: A review. *Journal of Child Sexual Abuse, 3* (3), 1–20.

Skynner, A. C. (1969). A group analytic approach to conjoint family therapy. *Journal of Child Psychology and Allied Disciplines, 10.*

Slavson, S. R. (1943). *Introduction to group psychotherapy.* New York: The Commonwealth Fund.

Slavson, S. R. (1950). *Analytic group psychotherapy with children and adults.* New York: Columbia University Press.

Slavson, S. R., & Schiffer, M. (1975). *Group psychotherapies for children.* New York: International Universities Press.

Sugar, M. (1981). Adolescent peer group psychotherapy. In L. R. Wolberg & M. L. Aronson (Eds.), *Group and family psychotherapy* (pp. 118–128). New York: Brunner/Mazel.

Whitaker, D. S. (1985). *Using groups to help people.* London: Routledge & Kegan Paul.

Chapter 23

Interventions with Parents and Children

John J. Gibbons, Ph.D., L.C.S.W.C.

Interventions with parents and children requires a systems orientation to clinical practice. A systems orientation views the unit for treatment as the person in his or her social context. Since its inception in the 1950s, family therapy has tried to understand the relationship between symptom development and maintenance and social context. The underlying assumption of family therapy is that the self is the product of interactions with significant others. The experience of any social interaction is dependent upon the social context and the meaning created by the self through interaction with others. Meaning is dependent on a person's language, social interaction, and inherent biological vulnerabilities and strengths. Meaning is a social construction of reality that has cultural, cognitive, emotional, and behavioral correlates.

Bateson, Jackson, Haley, and Weakland (1956) hypothesized a relationship between communication patterns of parents and symptom development in children described as the "Double Bind" hypothesis. Murray Bowen and his followers (Friedman, 1985) developed a theory of family functioning stressing an intergenerational approach. His adherents have developed strategies of assessment and therapeutic intervention with core concepts such as fusion, anxiety, and triangles. Jay Haley (1973) went on to develop the Strategic School of Family Therapy based on systems concepts and an intervention strategy similar to the hypnotic model of Milton Erickson.

Minuchin, Montalvo, & Guerney (1967) developed the model of Structural Family Therapy working with a lower social economic class population and later expanded to psychosomatic populations (Minuchin, Rosman, & Baker, 1978). Therapeutic interventions were aimed at restructuring family interaction, often using conflict around homeostatic patterns as the stimulus for change.

There are several offshoots and models of family therapy and intervention including dynamic models (Nichols, 1987), one-person models of intervention (Szapocznik, Kurtine, Foote, Perez-Vidal, & Hervis, 1989), family development (Hill, 1964), parent training models (Weiss & Hechtman, 1993), and various models developed to work with specific populations and problems (Pittman, 1987; Boyd-Franklin, 1989).

All these models contain core concepts that describe the family as a system operating within a larger system, having certain properties that can be observed. These concepts are descriptive and provide the clinician with an interactional, cross-sectional sample of behavior among people that can be generalized over time. These models usually provide techniques for change that include modalities ranging from education to direct and/or indirect interventions, cognitive versus behavioral tasks, and paradoxical versus non-paradoxical prescriptions.

Describing the organizational structure that exists between people limits one to observable behaviors that are social in nature and neglects the intrapersonal aspects of behavior. However, many family theorists have included in their methodology questions that not only track social behavior but also track constructed meanings or the reasoning behind a person's decision to act (Boscolo, Cecchin, Hoffman, & Penn, 1987).

The goal in the assessment and treatment of children and their families is to: (a) identify how the symptoms of one person are related to the changes in the family structure through time: (b) ascertain how people within the system make sense of how the symptoms came to be and are maintained, and (c) develop a plan to interrupt the identified patterns with interventions targeted at the biopsychosocial level. Interestingly enough, Karuso (1992) has shown that psychosocial treatment, independent of modality, affects a person at the biological level.

CONTEXT, FAMILY STRUCTURE, AND SOCIAL INTERACTION

Symptoms in children develop within a biopsychosocial context. A family with a depressed single mother, whom could be described as disengaged or distant, may result in a family organization that allows an older female child to develop behaviors consistent with parentalization, leading to an inverted hierarchy in the family. In such a family the child takes over the parenting of her younger siblings and becomes vulnerable to depression because she learns that others are more important than she. The same family structure may provide the context for a male sibling to find himself making his own decisions regarding going to school at the age of 8 years, anxiously attached to adults and at great risk for future problems.

However, a depressed, angry, controlling mother's behavior may be decreased considerably when her 8-year-old son is placed on Ritalin to control behaviors associated with attention deficit hyperactivity disorder. The point is that symptoms in children develop within a biopsychosocial context. The behaviors of each individual in the system must be assessed within the larger context of the family to understand how symptoms develop. Faulty structure in a family—for example, a depressed, distant mother—may not always lead to symptom development in children. The reverse may be true—that is, symptom development in children may lead to symptom development in a parent or guardian.

THE CLINICAL APPROACH

Thinking about symptom development and maintenance, it is useful to approach a discussion of child problem behaviors with parent(s) from the perspective of how their child's behaviors affect them within a specific context. Such an approach sets the stage for learning about parental responses and helps maintain the therapeutic alliance.

Assessment and Interventions

The clinician's main tool is himself or herself, his or her use of language, and the map or model that guides his or her practice. Therapy and or an evaluation of a child and his or her social context is a conversation between two or more people about a set of behaviors, meanings, and potential outcomes. Language is the medium and the capacity to deal with anxious and difficult interactions dictates the clinician's ability to use his or her tools.

Every assessment is an intervention. The average therapy case, regardless of modality, lasts anywhere from six to eight sessions (Brown-Standridge & Standridge, 1995). Thus, if assessment is conceptualized narrowly, the opportunity to create a therapeutic context and take advantage of the most critical time in the therapy, the first interview endeavor is not acknowledged.

The initial session is not only a rapport-building time but, also, a time to begin clarification of problems, potential goals or outcomes, and understanding the interaction between the child with symptoms and other family members. This process can be defined behaviorally, cognitively, and emotionally. The family therapist remains central during this initial process. The conversation about the presenting symptoms/problems takes place with the therapist asking questions and keeping the dialogue between family members to a minimum. The therapist tracks (Minuchin & Fishman, 1977) each family member's behaviors to the symptom and each person's theory or understanding about the symptom's development and his or her implicit or explicit understanding of his or her role in how the symptom affects him or her and gets played out. In essence, this approach asks parents, siblings, and/or guardians to become observers not only of the child's symptoms but also of their own emotional and behavioral responses to the child with the presenting symptoms. This style of questions, asked from the stance of a curious clinician, allows for the family's emotional/behavioral process to unfold. It offers the family a time to tell their story and it gives the interviewer a baseline of the family's cognitive/emotional and behavioral patterns. People are theory makers and their behaviors usually reflect a reason for acting.

During this initial phase of interviewing family members it is useful to interview subsystems; parents/guardians with and without the child present or siblings alone. It is important to interview adolescents alone. It is important to interview parents and children together unless the parent(s) is overly critical or hostile and cannot be redirected. However, even in the case of an openly hostile parent, a sample of the parent/child interaction is essential.

Generally, one should move at the readiness level of the patient and family, moving at a pace that barely exceeds their comfort level to assure that resistances stay at a minimum. The family's nonverbal communications will cue the therapist as to the pace. If the therapist moves too quickly into material that the patient and family are not ready for the family may (a) not return if they are passive or underorganized; (b) state that they do not understand and not return out of anger; and, (c) keep returning and not change.

The clinician must be aware of the messages he or she sends to the patient and family at the verbal and nonverbal level. Emphasizing strengths as opposed to deficits helps build rapport. Focusing on parent/child interactions suggests to the family that potential interventions may be built along the same lines. An exclusive focus on diagnostic issues may give the family the impression that intervention may focus exclusively on psychopharmacology. However, an overly optimistic clinician with a depressed, angry family may be out of rapport with the family's emotional presentation. Referring to a child as young and immature instead of oppositional defiant suggests to parents that the child needs "to be grown up" by them. Such frames or messages used within a developmental model infer behaviors that promote change and define symptoms and from a social interaction perspective.

The therapist should be aware of all the various systems in the family's life including social services and/or other treatment agencies. In such instances other professionals should be invited to the initial meeting to clarify their roles and outcomes. Such meetings also provide useful information as to personal and treatment history. Frequently, the outcomes of the social service agency and the therapist conflict. It is often necessary to develop mutual goals and enlist the social service worker as a therapeutic agent so as to not create confusion for the family (Colopinto, 1995).

Feedback to family members should use direct and jargon-free language. Diagnostic categories should be related to the initial problems related by the family. Positive aspects of family and individual functioning should be emphasized.

Case A

This case highlights the myriad issues and problems that often exist in inner-city families. It also suggests that the clinician working with this population needs to become acquainted with many theoretical approaches in addition to family systems theory, including child and adult psychopathology as psychopharmacology is often a major intervention. This requires working within a team format. The case also demonstrates that our thinking about potential goals or outcomes must be developed within the story of our patients and accommodate their presentation and readiness.

An emergency call comes in from the secretary that a woman is on the phone in "dire need of emergency care." Upon talking to the woman I learn that her 12-year-old son has just disclosed to her that he had been sexually abused by his cousin over the last year. The usual procedure with respect to calling the police and protective services is gone over with her and appointment scheduled which she readily accepts. Mother is informed that if she does not call the police that I would, but her calling would show her son that she was willing to protect him.

Mother is a 28-year-old, overweight, unemployed African American single parent. She complains that her son not only gets in fights at school and in the neighborhood but also eats her food all the time, including all the sugar or bread in the house. She also finds candy wrappers and empty cookie containers under his bed. Mother also notes that she rarely lets him out since she lives in a bad section of town and does not trust anyone, especially men. Mother notes that she and her son spend a lot of time together and argue constantly with each other. She reports frequently retreating to her room to cry after such arguments.

He is average academically, does poorly with peers, and is very unsure of himself. The boy reports symptoms consistent with post-traumatic stress disorder including intrusive visual imagery and misperceptions in social situations that usually accompany trauma victims. He reports difficulty falling asleep. He reports having a few friends but cannot name anyone he consistently associates with or considers his best friend. In fact he names more enemies than friends. He appears of average intelligence. School reports and Achenbach Behavior Checklists show average grades and behaviors consistent with attention deficits, anxiety, and impulsivity.

The boy expressed anger over the sexual abuse. He demonstrated sadness and great anxiety over having to talk about what happened and public exposure if he had to go to court. He feared everyone in his school would find out what happened. Mother described the boy as alternating between explosive outbursts and withdrawn behavior consistent with van Der Kolk's (1987) biphasic conceptualization as characteristic of post-traumatic stress disorder.

During the first interview Mom noted, "I don't know what to do with him anymore, maybe he will have to move out." The patient's father is not in the picture and inquiries about him bring negative comments from mother. During the first three interviews I make sure that I let mother know how impressed I am with her dedication toward her son by taking him to therapy and trying to understand him and why he is so angry all the time. I also do informal and formal education around issues of anger and sexual abuse in an attempt to help her develop understanding and empathy toward his symptoms and help sensitize her to the type of language and content that will eventually get discussed. I make comments to her about treatment, that her strength is crucial in helping her son talk about what happened to him in therapy and possibly in court.

I work alone with her during the later stages of the interview when I make specific suggestions for treatment. For example, I suggest to her that children who experience sexual abuse are not only angry at the perpetrator but also angry at the person who was supposed to protect them. Hopefully, this approach normalizes his anger once mom accepts his anger as inevitable and necessary. I also tell her that part of his therapy is to learn how to express his anger with words and not actions and that she could help me with this task by allowing him to be angry at her with words. Earlier, I had interviewed them together concerning issues of history and symptoms, identifying a timeline when his behavior deteriorated and the sexual abuse incidents began, introducing the sexual abuse issue though not in specific detail.

It is important initially to work indirectly around charged content to assess the family's comfort level in talking about issues. This stage of talking about what is to be talked about assesses the family's style of emotional communication. Talking about talking is a type of question that focuses on future communication and asks the patient to create hypotheses about his own responses (Penn, 1982) and begins to set the stage for the type of dialogue that the clinician hopes to develop between himself or herself and family members.

Clinically, nonverbal communication often gives the clinician more information about the content under discussion than verbal information. Many sexually abused children live in families where one of the parents has a similar history which may or may not have been diagnosed and treated. Discussion of the present abuse often becomes a trigger event (Gelinas, 1983) for the parents' own histories and symptomatology to develop. Asking a parent to be strong in order to discuss the sexual abuse history of their child may be touching issues never before discussed by the parent. Prior histories of trauma in the child or parent are an important predictor of the child's and parents' ability to process the present issues (Friedrich, 1990). In the fifth interview, I asked mother, alone, for permission to ask "a difficult question, one I believe she is strong enough to handle regarding the information I needed to know about her, to help her son talk about what happened to him and to help him talk about it with her." She denied such a history, however her stated anger toward men left me wondering about some form of trauma history.

Mother agreed to accept her son's anger and noted how guilty she felt. This led to a discussion of disclosure patterns in children and how children act out their anger in play and everyday life (Terr, 1991). I asked her to use her guilt to make herself strong for him. I suggested to her that he will continue to get angry and that her job is to listen and teach him how to be angry with words.

In the first several sessions I used subsystems, going from individually oriented treatment to family therapy to individual parent work. This type of multimodal work (Sheinburg, True, & Fraenke, 1994) demands that the clinician be conscious of boundary issues with respect to the content discussed in the family therapy, respecting the abused patient's requests concerning the type of content that gets discussed in the family therapy. This suggestion becomes more important when sexually abused children are involved or when working with adolescents. Control, fairness, and trust are significant issues for sexually abused children. Giving them a sense of control over the issues that are chosen to explore is crucial. Of course, autonomy being a central theme of adolescence dictates that any content explored with parents (besides self-injurious) be a result of permission given by the adolescent.

In this case we have a severely sexually abused preadolescent (invasive contact of long duration and frequency, with threats around disclosure) in an overly close and mutually protective relationship with his mother. Conflict between them usually was expressed metaphorically through issues such as food, schoolwork, and passive opposition, by coming home late or not following through on chores. Mother's responses were to get angry, yell, and then withdraw. His angry, aggressive behavior is a product of his abuse and his inability to express anger and/or create boundaries with others. The enmeshment offers each a sense of togetherness at the expense of a self. Thus, even though the boy notes that he felt something was wrong while the abuse happened, he did not know how to say no. He also noted the perpetrator threatened to hurt his mother if he told, strengthening the protective relationship and affecting disclosure.

In working with this boy, I was careful to state repeatedly and in various ways that he move at his own pace and comfort. During the seventh session it became apparent that he might have to testify regarding the alleged contact between him and his cousin. I framed his testimony for him as his way of protecting others and showing his cousin that he could take care of himself. He was quite anxious about his testimony which presented an opportunity to have him disclose the event by setting the stage for the hearing by: (a) going over procedures, (b) explaining how the judge would ask questions, and then by assuming the judge's role, I went over his testimony by having him disclose the events. He was able to do so, which set the stage for further discussion of the abuse and his thoughts and feelings about it. He still had great difficulty talking about it but was able eventually to discuss his anger and some of the content with his mom. I was also able to have mom ask him to tell her how angry he was at her which allowed them to expand their normal way of relating.

I suggested to mother that she allow him to visit his maternal grandmother more often in order to provide herself a break and give her son an opportunity to do more things outside the neighborhood. Grandmother introduced him to her church which he began to frequent. Grandmother also enrolled him in a karate course which helped him begin to seek even more time away from home.

This was an anxious time for Mother because the boy did not handle his initial forays into the public very well, returning home late and engaging in fights frequently to protect younger children whom he perceived as being taken advantage of.

Early in treatment I referred him for a psychopharmacological consultation to address symptoms of anxiety and depression which resulted in the prescription of an antidepressant which he stayed on for several months. During the sixth month of treatment I referred him to a adolescent group to address social interaction with peers while still doing individual and family work. He attended the group several times but had difficulty getting to the sessions. Also, at this time, mother returned to work part time which precipitated an increase in symptoms. These symptoms were framed to Mother as the boy's way of learning how to set boundaries for himself and interact with others. He was still hypervigilant and prone to angry outbursts in social situations with peers. In therapy, both in individual and family, we continued to discuss how to express his anger with words and his misperceptions in social situations. I continued to process how he goes about getting what he wants and how his history of abuse affects his ability to trust and feel safe. He showed little insight but was able to begin to increase his relationships with other adults and children his age through his grandmother's church and in school. His overall symptoms decreased over several months and Mother felt that his medicine was no longer necessary. As the boy improved his Mother began full time work. Without the crises of the aggressive symptoms to motivate them and with Mother working full time the family dropped out of treatment. However, since developmental transitions usually precipitate a resurgence of symptoms, especially in cases of sexual abuse, continued treatment was recommended as essential.

Case B

The patient is a 12-year-old biracial American female referred because of truant and disruptive behaviors at school. At referral, the department of social services is involved because of a history of parental physical abuse and frequent runaways. Mother is a Caucasian female currently on methadone maintenance and in treatment for bipolar disorder. Also in the home is the patient's "aunt," a sometime lover of Mother, also on methadone maintenance and much more stable in mood than Mother. Father has not been involved with the girl or family for many years.

This family presents the clinician with a set of relationships in which in many ways the adolescent functions at a higher level than her mother with respect to mood and reality testing. On presentation mother is loud and tangential. She becomes hypercritical, walking around the room, and cannot be redirected. Mother notes that her medicine does not help and becomes very angry at daughter for skipping school and not coming home. Mother and patient escalate easily, yelling at each other with no sense of attachment.

Patient appears sad, angry, and withdrawn. She makes her own decisions regarding going to school and curfew. Sessions are chaotic and mirror the family's interaction. The department of social services tells the clinician that it cannot keep the case open since there is no ongoing abuse and the family is in treatment. They drop the case after a month against our advice. The trainee/clinician working the case reports to me that she cannot control mother and is not sure what our goals/outcomes are with respect to treatment.

In supervision the clinician working the case and myself agree to do several things, among them including aunt in the family therapy if mother permits. Mother and her friend were seen together and the adolescent was in individual therapy. This subsystem approach allowed us to praise mother for allowing her daughter to develop relationships with other people and come to the clinic regularly. The trainee could develop a relationship with the adolescent, help her with her school issues, and slowly develop rapport with mother. The aunt was used to structure mom in session and develop a plan to have mom enroll in the adult ambulatory services; she was subsequently seen in the day hospital.

Mother and aunt called the school and with the clinician's help enrolled the patient in an alternative program for students. The girl developed a relationship with a school counselor and started having success in that arena. The therapy continued in this manner with the patient in individual therapy with family consults as needed. The therapist continued to work with mother and aunt. Contracts for safety were written and the patient was educated as to potential mental illness issues for her mother. Themes of anger and safety were explored. Boundary issues among therapist, adolescent, and parent were crucial toward allowing the therapist to work in this fashion.

Mother became more stable after several weeks in day hospital; however, another shift had occurred with mother's stability. Aunt's role had to be redefined. Mother began to assume more parenting responsibilities. This created more conflict for the adolescent. This case is ongoing but demonstrates the need for intervention and continuity of care at various treatment levels and junctures.

CONCLUSION

Interventions with parents and their children assume that for change to occur the child's social context must have an element of stability in it. This stability is characterized by a nonreactive, problem-solving stance on the part of the child's parent/guardian. This allows for dialogue not only at the developmental level of the child but also with the clinician and parent in a working alliance. The therapist working with children and their families creates a working alliance with parents through his or her rapport with each person as he or she assesses family structure and patterns of coping. Rapport with each family member is a function of how well each member perceives the clinician as understanding their behaviors and interactions.

Interventions can then be achieved in a variety of ways. Interventions at the social and/or cognitive level include a new meaning or frame introduced by the therapist into the family's existing story with respect to problematic interactions. Interventions at the behavioral level ask family members to behave in a different fashion around the problem/symptom. Any intervention takes into account each family member's readiness level which is related to individual developmental issues.

The systemic therapist takes an active stance modified by the history of his or her patient. He or she assumes that change in one family member frequently brings new problems for other members. However, through education and the ability to predict and frame change as positive the family learns new coping skills.

REFERENCES

Bateson, G., Jackson, D., Haley, J., & Weakland, J. (1956). Toward a theory of schizophrenia. *Behavioral Science, 1*, 251–264.

Boscolo, L., Cecchin, G., Hoffman, L., & Penn, P. (1987). *Milan Systemic Family Therapy*. Basic Books.

Boyd-Franklin, N. (1989). *Black families in therapy: a multi-systems approach*. New York: Guilford Press.

Brown-Standridge, M., & Standridge C. (1995). Family therapy for the working poor. Presentation at the American Association for Marriage and Family Therapy. Baltimore, MD.

Colopinto, J. (1995). Dilution to family process in social services: Implications for treatment of neglectful families. *Family Process, 34*.

Friedman E. (1985). *Generation to generation*. New York: Guilford Press.

Friedrich, W. (1990). *Psychotherapy of sexually abused children and their families*. New York: W. W. Norton.

Gelinas, D. (1983). The persisting negative effects of incest. *Psychiatry, 46*, 312–332.

Haley, J. (1973). *Uncommon therapy*. New York: W. W. Norton.

Hill, R.(1964) Methodological issues in family development research. *Family Process, 3*, 186–206.

Karuso, T. (1992). The worst of times, the best of times. *Journal of Psychotherapy Research and Practice, 1* (1), 2–15.

Minuchin, S., & Fishman, C. (1977). *Family therapy techniques*. Cambridge, MA: Harvard Press. Minuchin, S., Montalvo, B., & Guerney, B. (1967). *Families of the slums: An exploration of their structure and treatment*. New York, Basic Books.

Minuchin, S., Rosman, B., & Baker, L. (1978). *Psychosomatic families*. Cambridge, MA: Harvard University Press.

Nichols, M. (1987). *The self in the system*. New York: Brunner/Mazel.

Penn, P. (1982). Circular questioning. *Family Process, 21*.

Pittman F. (1987). *Turning points: Treating families in transition and crisis*. New York: W. W. Norton.

Shienberg, M., True, F., & Fraenkel, P. (1994). Treating the sexually abused child: A recursive multi-modal program. *Family Process 23*, 263–276.

Szapocznik, J., Kurtines W., Foote, T., Perez-Vidal, A., & Hervis, O. (1983) Structural family versus psychodynamic child therapy for problematic Hispanic boys. *Journal of Consulting and Clinical Psychology, 57* (5), 571–578.

Terr, L. (1991). Childhood traumas: An outline and overview. *American Journal of Psychiatry, 148* (1), 10–15.

Van der Kolk, B. (1987). *Post-traumatic stress disorder: Psychological and biological sequelae: clinical insights*. American Psychiatric Press. Washington DC.

Weiss, G., & Hechtman, L. (1993). *Hyperactive children grown up*. New York: Guilford Press.

Part 5

Day Treatment for Children and Adolescents

Chapter 24

Day Hospital: Planning, Staffing, and Administration

Lois T. Flaherty, M.D. and Susan B. Glassman, Ph.D.

INTRODUCTION

Use of the Term "Day Hospital"

The term day hospital denotes a type of service that is intermediate in level of intensity between impatient and outpatient care. It is generally conceived as a less expensive and less restrictive alternative to impatient treatment, yet one that provides many of the same services that are available in the hospital. While the words "day hospital" are often used interchangeably with "partial hospital," a day hospital is a specific type of partial hospital program, in which patients attend for several hours during the day, returning to their homes in the evening. Partial hospitalization, a broader concept, encompasses after school and evening programs, as well as the "inn" for adult patients. This chapter uses both terms to refer to the definition that follows developed for partial hospitalization for children.

American Association for Partial Hospitalization Definition

The Child and Adolescent Special Interest Group of the American Association for Partial Hospitalization (Block et al., 1991) has developed standards for child and adolescent partial hospitalization programs. These standards define a partial hospital program as "a time-limited, ambulatory, active treatment program that offers therapeutically intensive, coordinated, and structured clinical services within a stable therapeutic milieu" (p. 13). Programs must comprise at least six hours per day of which at least 60 percent must be devoted to active treatment. Programs may be either free-standing or attached to hospitals but must have provision for 24-hour coverage for emergencies. A length of stay of 180 days or less is specified, although a national survey of programs showed that many were more long-term than this (Kiser, Culhane, & Hadley, 1995).

BACKGROUND AND HISTORY

Examples of special day programs for children with serious emotional disturbances can be found in the 1940s and earlier, but the widespread development of day hospitalization is a phenomenon of the past decade. In the United States, the 1963 Community Mental Health Centers Construction Act gave a major impetus to partial hospitalization by including it among the five federally mandated services. However, even with the carrot and stick of federal funding (community mental health centers could only receive federal funds if they had these programs), partial hospitalization programs were slow in developing.

Programs for Children and Adolescents

Day programs for children and adolescents existed outside of the mental health arena long before they were developed in connection with psychiatric facilities. These programs developed as a natural response to the needs of children and adolescents with psychiatric disorders. Most such children and adolescents continue to reside with their families, who assume the burdens of providing for their special needs outside of school hours. All children have educational needs, traditionally met by going to school five days a week. Thus, it is understandable that many programs that would in today's world be termed day hospitals were originally developed as educational services. For example, in Baltimore, the Children's Guild, a program for young children with a variety of emotional and behavioral disturbances, and the Linwood Center, a program for autistic children, both began in the 1950s as free-standing programs with no formal affiliation with hospitals or mental health facilities.

An example of another model is the Forbush School at Sheppard-Pratt Hospital, also in the Baltimore area. This program exists in conjunction with the inpatient services at this private psychiatric hospital. It serves children and adolescents currently and formerly hospitalized on the inpatient service as well as those who have never been hospitalized, but have been referred by their surrounding communities. Length of stay in these programs is usually at least a school year, and may extend throughout the child's educational career.

MARKETING AND FUNDING

Numerous reviews have pointed out that partial hospitalization has been underutilized, despite evidence that it is a cost-effective alternative to hospitalization (Hoge, Davidson, Hill, Turner, & Ameli, 1992; Sharfstein, Stoline, & Goldman, 1993). Factors cited in the underutilization of this treatment modality include third-party reimbursement policies and lack of public awareness.

Third-Party Payers

Third-party reimbursement for day hospital treatment is now common, though it developed slowly. It was not until 1987 that services rendered in hospital-based partial hospitalization programs became reimbursable under Medicare; in 1991 this coverage was extended to community mental health centers. CHAMPUS and private insurance companies did not begin to cover these services until 1992. Medicaid mandates benefits for partial hospitalization in association with outpatient treatment programs.

Managed care organizations, seeing the cost savings of partial hospitalization compared to inpatient treatment, have favored the development of these programs; at the same they have effectively defined this form of treatment as acute, short-term care for the management of acutely ill patients (Hoge et al., 1992). Medical necessity criteria for partial hospitalization with which the authors are familiar approach those for hospitalization in making dangerousness to self or others a prerequisite for admission; the only difference between the inpatient criteria and those for partial hospitalization being the degree to which dangerousness is imminent.

Public Funding through Education and Mental Health Systems

Because the educational component is central to programs for children and adolescents, part of the funding for the day hospital often comes through the educational system. This may involve direct grants to programs, or placement in the program of teachers hired by the educational system. For the Baltimore programs described above, funding is through the youngsters' local school systems as well as the state mental health system. Day hospital programs can meet legal mandates for children to be educated in the least restrictive environment and to remain with their families, as they often serve as alternatives to institutional placement.

In contrast to the acute nature of private sector programs, day hospital programs in the public sector are likely to be long term (Kiser, Culhane, & Hadley, 1995). Some experts have noted that public mental health funding for day hospital programs appears to be diminishing as community mental health systems of care increasingly emphasize assertive community treatment and psychosocial rehabilitation; however, these observations apply mainly to programs for adults, not those for children and adolescents (Hoge et. al., 1992).

Marketing Issues

In spite of the similarities between day hospital and inpatient programs in terms of the types of patients who would be appropriate, professionals in a position to make referrals often do not think first of day programs, because inpatient programs are so much more familiar to them. Institutions that have both partial and full inpatient programs have generally marketed their inpatient programs more aggressively because these generate higher revenues. Thus, effective marketing of day hospital programs is essential to increase utilization.

Marketing of the day program is facilitated if the program is part of a larger parent institution that has the resources to have a marketing department. The day hospital can be promoted as part of a continuum of care. The program the authors are familiar with had a full-time staff person who was involved in visiting schools and hospitals, and other community agencies, as well as organizing educational conferences for professionals in the community. The marketing department must have an understanding of how the child and adolescent programs operate to effectively "sell" the program.

STAFFING AND ADMINISTRATIVE STRUCTURE

General Issues

Staffing of partial hospitalization programs resembles that of inpatient units, with the exception that 24-hour nursing coverage is not required, nor are bedrooms for patients. The AAPH Guidelines call for a patient to staff ratio of 3:1, with no more than six patients assigned to one staff member at any time (Block, 1991). This is a somewhat richer staffing pattern than what was found in the subsequent AAPH survey, where respondent facilities averaged approximately 4 to 1 (Kiser et al., 1995). This survey included both long- and short-term programs, however, and it is important to remember that staffing needs are higher in acute care programs.

Overview of Staff Roles and Administrative Structure

Mental health workers or psychiatric technicians provide the hands-on care of the patients under the guidance of educational and mental health professionals. These professionals include social workers and special education teachers. A clinical psychologist and psychiatrist are used primarily for assessments and medication monitoring and staff supervision. The psychiatrist should be sufficiently involved in the day-to-day operation of the program and have sufficient responsibility for treatment planning for individual patients that the title medical director is appropriate. Nurses dispense medications and are utilized to implement infection control and other policies; they may serve as an important link to the parent institution when the latter is a hospital.

Clinical Administration   Ideally, the doctoral level staff members should be involved in clinical administration as well as in providing clinical supervision for staff and some direct services. In the program the authors are familiar with, clinical psychologists served in the role of program directors for the children's and adolescents' programs. Because of the importance of understanding educational issues and dealing with various barriers to learning, psychologists' knowledge of assessment and cognitive functioning is particularly crucial.

Team Structure   Staff are organized by teams rather than by discipline and there is considerable overlap in roles. For example, a substance abuse counselor may also serve as a teacher's aide in the classroom. In most programs there are too few professionals of any one discipline for them to meet regularly as a group.

The various professionals interact both formally and informally. Brief daily meetings take the place of the morning rounds usually held in inpatient units. More formal treatment planning takes place through regularly scheduled team meetings at which the progress of each of the patients is reviewed. These meetings should be held on at least a weekly basis.

Model Staffing Pattern   A typical staffing pattern for a program designed to handle up to 20 children and 20 adolescents in a program with an average length of stay of four weeks would be:

- 1 full-time-equivalent (FTE) clinical psychologist/program administrator
- Doctoral- or Master's-level clinician with training and experience in child and adolescent mental health services

   - Because of the multiplicity of functions for which clinical psychologists are trained, they may be involved in partial hospitalization programs in a variety of roles. A clinical psychologist may serve as a consultant to the staff and perform assessments as indicated; this person may also function in the role of program administrator and/or primary therapist for some patients, just as in an inpatient unit.

- 4 FTE clinicians

    - These are master's level social workers and/or psychologists. Each serves as case manager and primary therapist for an assigned caseload of 10 patients. These professionals provide group, family, and individual therapy and coordinate communication with outside therapists and community agencies other than schools.

- 8 FTE child/adolescent psychiatrist medical director

    - The psychiatrist's responsibilities include diagnostic evaluations, determination of level of care needs, participation in treatment planning, and prescribing and monitoring of medications. The latter function includes informing parents about the risks and benefits of medications and their role in treatment. The psychiatrist attends treatment team meetings at least weekly and reviews and approves treatment plans. The psychiatrist may be involved in family therapy sessions with the child's or adolescent's primary therapist. He or she is responsible for communicating with referring psychiatrists, particularly with those who are continuing to provide outpatient treatment. In an acute care program, patients are seen individually at least weekly; this would mean an average of 8 patient visits/day for a census of 40.

- 2 FTE special education teachers

    - One teacher is assigned to the adolescent program and the other to the child program. The teachers have the responsibility of organizing and implementing the educational program, assessing and making recommendations regarding children's educational needs, and communicating with their home schools. A one-page summary is prepared in conjunction with the youngster's discharge, giving the diagnosis, medications, educational summary, and recommendations.

- 2 FTE nurse

    - A registered nurse is required to dispense any medications that must be given during program hours, as well to have administrative responsibility for maintaining the medication room and for infection control; this person typically will only need to be on-site for morning rounds and program-wide staff meetings and an hour each day in the middle of the day; about .2 FTE is required.

- 6 mental health counselors

    - These staff members function similarly to psychiatric technicians on an inpatient service. They interact directly with the children on a day to day basis. Just as in an inpatient program they are the ones who are relied on to translate the program goals into a concrete reality. How they talk with patients, set limits and give feedback is crucial in whether the patients experience the program as supportive and helpful. While the children are in the classroom, these staff members function as teacher's aides. In group therapy activities they serve as co-therapists or co-leaders, working with the clinician or leading groups by themselves. They will spend time talking with children in time out, and accompany children on trips, bathroom and lunch breaks.

- 1/2 FTE substance abuse counselor

    - This person provides evaluations of patients for whom substance abuse is an acknowledged or suspected problem, and is responsible for organizing and providing specialized substance abuse services for patients in need of them. These services may take the form of a separate substance abuse track within the regular program that involves attendance at separate group meetings, focused on substance abuse, at designated times during the day. The substance abuse counselor attends all team meetings and provides consultation to other staff and input into treatment planning at these meetings.

Other Specialized Staff   Other staff who may be shared with the adult programs include music and art therapists, who typically may provide one to two hours a week of face-to-face service to each program.

Staffing Needs Vary with Program and Patients   The exact staffing needs are dictated by a number of factors, not the least of which is the level of acuity of the program. A program whose average length of stay is short requires additional case managers and additional time to do assessments and the work associated with admissions and discharges. The AAPH survey found the average caseload for a psychiatrist spending 35 hours a week in a program to be approximately 100 patients; for a psychologist working similar hours, the caseload approximated 179 patients. The programs surveyed included many that had lengths of stay of six months or longer; in such programs, patients will be seen much less frequently by doctoral-level professionals. A psychiatrist working 35 hours a week and seeing each patient once a month could, given the same volume of service (eight patient contacts/day) manage a caseload of 140 patients. In practice, a longer length of stay program is likely to utilize a part-time consultant psychiatrist on the order of one day per week.

Flexible Staffing   In a program in which the census varies considerably, the staffing in terms of counselors and case managers/primary therapists may consist of a core group of people who are augmented by temporary staff when the census is higher. Many staff can be shared between the child and adolescent programs, and some can be utilized by adult programs as well, provided they have the expertise to deal with all age groups. This is of course one of the advantages of housing several programs in one facility. If the program is in proximity to an inpatient service, staff can be shared between the two.

PHYSICAL FACILITIES

The facilities required are similar to an inpatient setting, with the major exception of bedrooms. Optimally, there should be a clear separation of the area for children and that for adolescents. It is particularly important for the children's group rooms, activity rooms, time-out room, and staff offices to be in relatively close proximity to each other. This proximity fosters the containment and holding environment functions of the program. It allows staff to be available quickly in case of a crisis. Finally, it prevents the sounds of the youngsters from intruding on the other patients' activities. Some spaces, such as special activity or group rooms, can be scheduled so that they may be used in a shared manner.

Classrooms

Classrooms should be separate for children and for adolescents. These are the rooms where the youngsters spend most of their time. For each program, a classroom large enough to accommodate up to 12 students is needed. Flexible dividers can be used to divide the group during periods of academic work.

Group Therapy Room(s)

These rooms are furnished with chairs and are large enough to accommodate 8 to 10 children or adolescents. Because these rooms are only used part of the day, they can also double as community meeting rooms. It is desirable that they be distinct from the classrooms to reinforce the distinction between therapy and education.

Community Meeting Room

This must be large enough to accommodate all the youngsters in each program (child, adolescent) at one time. Separate community meetings are held for each group.

Time-Out Room

This is a small room with a carpeted floor and two lightweight chairs that can be removed easily. It should be close to the classroom and group therapy rooms. It is important that this room not be used for any other purpose.

Waiting and Reception Area

Similar to one in an outpatient clinic, this is a place for new patients and families to wait to be seen, and for parents and other family members to wait for their appointments with the staff.

Therapy Offices

These should allow for privacy for individual and family sessions; one should be allocated to each clinician.

Educational Staff Offices

This can be a shared area where teachers can complete their paperwork and work on instructional plans. Ideally it should be situated near the classrooms.

Medication Room

This can be a small office with a desk and locked cabinet with medications to be dispensed during the day, as well as any emergency medications, are kept. It should be equipped with a scale, stethoscope, and blood pressure cuffs. A sink is helpful but not essential.

Bathrooms

These need to be large enough for children to occupy as a group during specified times.

Kitchen/Eating Area

In a facility that is shared by several programs, the kitchen is likely to be used primarily for food storage and preparation. Patients may eat in the classrooms, using their desks as tables. In programs in proximity to a hospital, the hospital cafeteria can serve as a dining area, and indeed the use of this area can be a privilege that must be earned.

Recreational Facilities

These should include an outdoor area than can be used in good weather much as a recess area would be in a school. An advantage of being located on the grounds of a hospital is that there are likely to be facilities for recreation, such as a gym. Lacking this, arrangements can be made with community facilities. Our program developed a creative linkage with a nursing home that had a pool; patients also visited with the residents of the home.

Transportation Vehicles

Some way of transporting patients to recreational activities in the community is essential. It will also be necessary at times to transport patients to and from their homes and even parents for appointments. The availability of one or more vans for these purposes has been an essential feature of the programs with which the authors are familiar.

Flexible Use of Space

Flexible use of space can help the program accommodate to fluctuations in numbers of patients. For example, if there is only one group therapy room, and the group is large enough to be split in two, one group may stay in the classroom while the other goes to the group room. If the person who does group therapy is also responsible for some individual and family therapy, his or her office could double as a group room. The classroom may serve as the locus for community meetings, since all patients are involved in both.

RELATIONSHIP TO OUTSIDE AGENCIES

As partial hospitalization occupies a status that is in between the hospital and the community, close relationships with both inpatient and outpatient facilities as well as other community resources are essential. The AAPH survey showed that over half the patients treated were referred by schools or inpatient programs (Kiser et al., 1995). Most children and adolescents need follow-up treatment following discharge from the partial hospitalization program, and many require special educational placements. The following is a description of how interrelationships with outside agencies operate in a typical program.

Schools

Following the admission of a youngster, the home school is contacted and information is requested regarding the youngster's prior school history. Parents are asked to obtain assignments and books so that the child can keep up with what is going on. A general assessment of the child's educational attainment is done during the stay in the program, but this does not involve formal diagnostic testing. At the time of discharge, a letter is written by the teacher in the partial hospitalization program giving the patient's diagnosis, any medications, a brief summary of his or her progress in the program, and recommendations regarding educational needs. Children often have a transition period during which they begin to attend their home school part-time. This may be a half day, usually in the morning, and then return to the partial hospitalization program in the afternoon, or they may go back to the home school two or three days. This transition does not last more than one or two weeks. It is particularly helpful when the presenting problems have included anxiety related to school.

Outside Therapists

The partial hospitalization program does not preclude continuing therapy with an outside therapist. The youngster will still be assigned a primary therapist/case manager in the partial hospitalization program, and that person's responsibility will be to act a liaison between the program and the outside therapist. Similarly, the psychiatrist in the program may function in a like manner with an outside psychiatrist who continues to provide treatment. In the latter case, it is likely that the outside psychiatrist will agree that medication monitoring and management can best be done by an on-site physician who has the opportunity to observe directly responses to medication.

Hospitals and Clinics

In most cases, entry into the partial hospitalization program will have been preceded by an intake interview that provides an opportunity for the child and family to become familiar with the partial hospitalization program. In cases where the partial hospitalization program is part of a facility that includes an inpatient program, it is possible for a transition to occur to the partial program prior to discharge from the hospital. This means that a youngster may begin attending the partial program during the day while still on inpatient status, returning to the inpatient unit after completion of the day's activities in the partial hospital. In acute programs, this transition will be fairly brief, often only one day.

Outpatient Visits   A child and family who have a preexisting relationship with an outpatient clinic or therapist may be encouraged to attend outpatient therapy sessions during the child's sojourn in the day hospital; it is usually possible to structure these visits at the beginning or the end of the day so that they do not seriously disrupt the treatment in the day hospital. In cases where a new referral is being made for outpatient treatment, it is advisable for at least the initial visit to take place prior to discharge. The fact that parents are often already involved in transporting children to the partial hospitalization program makes the expectation that they take children to outpatient visits less difficult to implement than it might otherwise be. The major barrier to such transitions is often third-party billing policies that make it impossible to bill for more than one service on the same day, or to bill for any outpatient services while a patient is in a partial hospitalization program.

CHALLENGES AND NEEDS

Demonstrating Effectiveness

Because partial hospitalization as a mainstream treatment is still a relatively new phenomenon, studies of outcome and effectiveness are not abundant. Most of the studies that have been done concern adults, and these studies do show that partial hospitalization has similar outcomes to inpatient treatment; given the considerably lower cost of partial hospitalization, this is a powerful argument in its favor.

Grizenko and Papineau (1992), taking advantage of the fact that a hospital program was converted into a day treatment program, compared outcomes at discharge in two groups of children; those treated in the day treatment program were compared with another group who had been hospitalized in the same facility in the past. The authors asserted that the two groups were comparable demographically and had equally severe emotional disturbances. They found outcomes were similar, with the cost of day treatment about one-sixth that of inpatient. The reduced cost was partly a result of the fact that length of stay was much shorter in the day program (6.1 months compared to 19.6 months); however, even if one assumes a comparable length of stay the cost would still be about half.

A more recent study by Kiser and colleagues (1996) of 114 patients completing treatment in two different programs showed positive changes after one year in four salient domains: clinical status, level of functioning, utilization of behavioral health services after discharge, and patient/family satisfaction.

ESTABLISHING CONTINUITY BETWEEN LEVELS OF CARE

The effect of curtailed use of inpatient treatment has been to divert into partial hospitalization many patients who would have been hospitalized, and shorter lengths of stay for those who do go into hospitals means more patients are being discharged into partial programs while they are still in the process of becoming stabilized. The ideal, a seamless transition between levels of care, is far from reality even in institutions where the inpatient and partial hospitalization programs are under the same roof. Lack of communication between the programs and unnecessary duplication of assessment and paperwork makes for less than optimal patient care and wastes staff time.

Given the brevity of treatment episodes in all settings in our current era, linkages that can assure continuity of care are crucial. This is, however, difficult to implement, as each facility tends to cling to its own procedures, resulting in not only much duplication of effort but in lack of communication between them. The need for a complete assessment, including a psychiatric evaluation, to be repeated as the patient passes through each level of care, makes for a costly and not always necessary repetition of effort. Records are likely to be separate and do not follow the patient from one program to the next. In part, these procedures are dictated by accreditation requirements for each type of setting; these requirements reflect the realities of an earlier age when patients did not move as rapidly from one level of care to the next. The use of computerized medical records and electronic data transfer could go a long way toward solving these problems. Perhaps the greatest barrier is the tendency on the part of staff to see their own programs as self-contained entities rather than as parts of a continuum. Institutional policies and accreditation standards need to change to allow for the reality of rapid movement between levels of care. The separatist mind-set of staff must be addressed by administrative leadership that encourages and fosters integration.

CONCLUSION

The day hospital for children and adolescents provides multimodal and cost-effective treatment that can offer alternatives to hospitalization and decrease the length of time of hospitalization. An important advantage is that treatment does not disrupt the child's entire life and routine, and skills acquired in the program carry over in the child's "regular" life. The day hospital occupies a vital part of the level of care continuum necessary for the effective treatment of the youngster with serious emotional disturbance.

REFERENCES

Block, B. M., Arney, K., Campbell, D. J., Kiser, L. J., Lefkovitz, P. M., & Speer, S. K. (1991). American Association for Partial Hospitalization Child and Adolescent Special Interest Group: Standards for child and adolescent partial hospitalization programs. *International Journal of Partial Hospitalization*, 7, 13–21.

Grizenko, N., & Papineau, D. (1992). A comparison of the cost-effectiveness of day treatment and residential treatment for children with severe behavior problems. *Canadian Journal of Psychiatry, 37*, 393–400.

Hoge, M. A., Davidson, L., Hill, W. L., Turner, V. E., & Ameli, R. (1992). The promise of partial hospitalization: A reassessment. *Hospital and Community Psychiatry, 43*, 345–354.

Kiser, L. J., Culhane, D. P., & Hadley, T. R. (1995). The current practice of child and adolescent partial hospitalization: Results of a national survey. *Journal of the American Academy of Child and Adolescent Psychiatry, 34*, 1336–1342.

Kiser, L. J., Millsap, P. A., Hickerson, S., Heston, J. D., Nunn, W., Pruitt, D., & Rohr, M. (1996). Results of treatment one year later: Child and adolescent partial hospitalization. *Journal of the American Academy of Child and Adolescent Psychiatry, 35*, 81–90.

Sharfstein, S. S., Stoline, A. M., & Goldman, H. H. (1993). Psychiatric care and health insurance reform. *American Journal of Psychiatry, 150*, 7–18.

Chapter 25

Therapeutic Milieu in a Day Hospital for Children and Adolescents

Susan B. Glassman, Ph.D. and Lois T. Flaherty, M.D.

INTRODUCTION

Partial hospital programs exert their primary therapeutic effect through the milieu they provide. In this respect, they have much in common with that of an inpatient program. Washburn and Conrad (1979) identified "containment, support, structure, involvement, and validation" as essential elements of both types of programs. But there are important differences; these authors suggested that the crucial difference is that inpatient programs can fall back on coercion, but partial hospitalization essentially relies on negotiation. Containment is achieved by sending patients home, as opposed to secluding or restraining them, and goals are negotiated based on patients' wishes.

They view the day hospital as an open system, inherently more egalitarian than the inpatient ward, which they see as prone to mechanistic approaches, the use of a "prescribed medical model," and communication mainly via instructions with a greater potential for abuse of power. They conclude, "Because the partial hospital system is midway in the spectrum between inpatient physical structure and community freedom and complexity, it may be able to offer a greater range of functions to affect the ego than can the intrinsically more confining inpatient status." These authors were describing programs for adults, but their conceptualization may be particularly relevant for adolescents, for whom the enforced dependency of inpatient treatment runs counter to developmentally based strivings for independence. This chapter summarizes the essential features of a therapeutic milieu in programs for children and adolescents.

PATIENT POPULATION AND TREATMENT APPROACHES

Partial hospital programs have been developed for children and adolescents with almost every category of psychiatric disorder, including conduct disorder, autism, psychoses, mental retardation, and others (Lahey & Kupfer, 1979). Those designed for children and adolescents with severe developmental disabilities generally are long-term programs that focus on habilitation; those that serve as an alternative to hospitalization are usually short-term, with a focus on acute care.

Within fairly broad limits, the kinds of patients appropriate for day hospital programs are limited primarily by the skill of the staff. In general, any patient who does not need a locked unit and 24-hour supervision may be considered appropriate. Nevertheless, for a given program, the patient population and its selection is crucial to the effectiveness of the treatment for the individual and the treatment community as a whole. Because of the heavy dependence on group process, patients who are not able to participate meaningfully in group activities will usually not benefit and may have a deleterious effect on the program. Unlike inpatient wards, where such a patient may be allowed to isolate himself or herself for periods of time, this option is not available other than for brief interludes. It is unlikely that there will be sufficient staff to provide one-on-one attention for other than short periods of time, so patients who need this kind of care will not be appropriate.

Difference Between Children's and Adolescents' Programs

The basics of the treatment approaches for children and adolescents are similar in overall structure and planning. However, the staff and program need to be mindful of the different developmental needs of each group when implementing treatment groups and the thera-peutic community. Socialization and communication patterns are two aspects that differ markedly. Both kinds of programs can consist of the same type of staffing and administra-tive structure and may actually borrow staff from one another, but the children's program should have a higher staff-to-patient ratio. Children require assistance in basic function-ing that adolescents do not and this actually becomes part of their treatment. For example, staff involvement and supervision of bathroom breaks is important for young children. In addition, it is important to have flexibility in each program since the community in a day hospital is constantly changing and the community population determines its level of functioning and, in turn, its need for increased or decreased structure and/or supervision.

Limitations of the Day Hospital

Although the day hospital program is intensive and provides the child or adolescent pa-tient consistent supervision and treatment in a therapeutic environment it is not a locked unit and is not capable of handling severe acting-out behaviors that may require extensive interventions such as seclusion and/or frequent physical restraint. Severe aggressiveness, persistent suicidal and/or homicidal ideation, and/or active drug/alcohol abuse will require more containment than is possible in the open environment of a day treatment program.

Some patients may cause too much disruption by virtue of their regressed, inappropri-ate behavior to be tolerated by the milieu, as illustrated by the following example:

Nina, a 15-year-old with multiple foster home placements and a history of psychotic symptoms since the age of 7 years, was admitted to a partial hospital program after a brief hospitalization. Although she had stabilized in the hospital, she appeared very anxious and depressed and reported hearing voices telling her she still needed to be in the hospital. In group therapy later in the day, she began trying to stab herself with a pencil, and was quickly re-hospitalized when she stated she did not feel safe and could not handle going home in the evening.

In the opposite vein, occasionally a child or adolescent is admitted and it becomes apparent after admission that the youngster does not need partial hospitalization. Once in the program, the youngster no longer exhibits the problem behaviors that were the reason for admission. When this occurs, a re-evaluation should take place involving the child and child's family and an appropriate referral should be made; most probably this will involve outpatient therapy. This does not necessarily mean that the initial assessment has been faulty. Instead, in such an eventuality, the day hospital has actually served as an evaluation and assessment tool to determine the level of severity of an individual's disorder and the level of functioning of the child and his or her family. The actual locus of the problem may be in the child's school setting or the community.

TREATMENT, OCCUPATIONAL, AND RECREATIONAL ACTIVITIES

The treatment in a child or adolescent day program is multi-modal, encompassing a variety of approaches. One of the major goals is the formation of a sense of community, which itself is part of the treatment. This is the essential core of what is commonly called the therapeutic milieu. The experience of being a valued member of a community can provide enhanced self-worth, self-understanding, and self-control.

The behavior modification system, which will be explained in detail, may be the single most important treatment modality for children and adolescents in a day hospital. In addition to the daily groups and activities, there are weekly family sessions, psychiatric care, and case management services provided for each child.

Work with families may take the form of parent education, or involve family therapy with goals of restructuring the family system.

Group Interventions

Group activities, including group therapy, form the backbone of the therapeutic program. A typical day program encompasses six hours of active milieu treatment, supplemented by 24-hour crisis services. The day is highly structured and the behavior modification system is constantly in operation. The day is divided into segments of 45 to 50 minutes each. A morning community meeting provides a time for each patient to "check in" and develop goals for that particular day. Group therapy is usually a verbal group, but may be structured differently, especially for younger children. School activities make up the core of the daily routine: each child receives schoolwork from his or her home school, adolescents usually have more school in their daily program.

Allied therapy may include art, music, or bibliotherapy. Adventure-based counseling comprises group activities that provide confidence-building cooperation through outdoor and challenge activities. A "wrap-up" group serves as a "check in" at the end of the day and a preparation to go home for the evening.

Educational Program

The educational component of the day hospital is essential to the overall interventions for the child or adolescent. It enables the child to earn academic credits under the supervision of certified teachers in conjunction with the child's school district and home school. This link between the hospital and the school is extremely valuable. It gives the treatment team useful information and, in turn, the treatment team teacher can provide the school with information so, upon discharge, the school can better meet the needs of the child. The child is helped to keep up with schoolwork and not to fall behind his or her classmates. Further discussion of the educational component of day treatment is provided in the following chapter.

RULES, STRUCTURE, AND DAILY SCHEDULE

Children who come into day treatment often lack internal controls and have difficulty conforming their behavior to the demands of the usual school environment. With a sense of themselves and the world around them that is confused, conflicted, and chaotic, they need a strong external structure to function more effectively, and it is crucial that the day hospital provide this. A schedule that essentially takes up every minute of the child's time in the program is one form of structure. For adolescents, some brief periods of free or unstructured time are appropriate, during which youngsters can socialize or play basketball, as they wish, always with staff supervision. Table 1 shows a sample weekly schedule.

Behavior Management

Another avenue through which this structure can be provided is a behavior management system designed to teach patients to follow basic rules of accepted conduct while developing an increased sense of self-esteem and responsibility. Essentially, this takes the form of a token economy through which tangible rewards are provided for prosocial behavior and completion of academic tasks.

Children move through four levels or phases designed to reward appropriate decisions and behaviors on their part. They earn points daily for appropriate behavior and advance to the next level on the basis of the points earned. As they move from one level to the next, they earn added privileges and responsibilities.

Individual daily point sheets help children monitor their own progress and understand the steps required to master long-range goals. The staff emphasizes that each child is able to make good decisions; the stress is thus placed on thinking as well as acting.

Table 1   Children's Day Hospital Program Level System

Level	Responsibilities	Privileges
1	Earn 70% of points	Snack at end of each day with wrap-up Friday activity
2	Earn 75% of points	Level 1 privileges Free time in class Lunch in cafeteria Extra snack with Friday activity
3	Earn 80% of points Self-rating	Level 1 and 2 privileges Use of Walkman Canteen on Wednesday Can walk to restroom by themselves Can bring craft projects home
4	Earn 90% of points	All privileges from previous levels Canteen twice a week Leadership role in activities Staff choice for additional privileges

The point sheet lists the three basic program rules plus one individual rule. Additionally, all of the patients can earn bonus points if they meet the group goal set for the day. The group goal is established daily in community meeting and usually relates to a prosocial behavior, such as being supportive or accepting feedback. Points are given out during each group activity by whatever staff members are involved with this activity. An example of a point sheet is given in Table 2.

Patients set individual goals for themselves daily in community meeting; each youngster announces his or her goal for the day. The goal is then written on the child's point sheet. Points earned for individual goals affect a patient's level. These points are also recorded daily in a goals chart. A patient must earn a certain percentage of the total goal points to achieve his or her goal for the day (e.g., 70% for level 1, 75% for level 2, 80% for level 3, and 90% for level 4). If a patient achieves his or her goal at a rate determined by staff (e.g., three out of five days, for two consecutive weeks), he or she is eligible to attend a "goals trip."

Level 1—Orientation Level   The patients earn points and learn the fundamentals of the program standards. During this phase, patients must remain with staff at all times. To move beyond this level, they must exhibit appropriate behaviors to meet level criteria ("make their day") for five consecutive days.

Level 2—Program Level   Patients at this level have the opportunity to earn more privileges while exhibiting increased responsibility. Additional privileges may include more "free time," assisting staff during an activity, or walking alone to the bathroom or group room. Children are encouraged to think of their own special privileges they would like to earn; this facilitates self-esteem and empowerment. To move beyond this level,

Table 2   Children's Day Hospital Program Daily Point Sheet

Name:_____   Date:_____

Individual Goal:_____

	Follow directions	Stay on task and participate	Show respect	Individual goal	Total points	Initials
Community Meeting						
School						
Group Therapy						
Lunch						
Psycho-Education Group						
Recreation Therapy						
School						
Wrap-Up						

Earned Goal Today? Yes:___No:___Bonus Points:___

Table 3   Children's Day Hospital Program Weekly Schedule

Date:				
Counselors:				
Staff Out:				
Patients Out:				
New Patients:				
Discharges:				
Charting:				
Van(s):				
Family Meetings:				
Community Issues:				

8:45–9:30	8:45–9:30	8:45–9:30	8:45–9:30	8:45–9:30
Arrival, work at desk	Arrival, work at desk	Arrival, work at desk	Arrival, work at desk	Arrival, work at desk
9:30–10:00	9:30–10:00	9:30–10:00	9:30–10:00	9:30–10:00
Community Meeting	Community Meeting	Community Meeting	Community Meeting	Community Meeting
10:00–10:45	10:00–10:45	10:00–10:45	10:00–10:45	10:00–10:45
School	School	School	School	School
11:00–11:45	11:00–11:45	11:00–11:45	11:00–11:45	11:00–11:45
Group Therapy	Group Therapy	Group Therapy	Group Therapy	Group Therapy
11:45–12:45	11:45–12:45	11:45–12:45	11:45–12:45	11:45–12:45
Medication and Lunch	Medication and Lunch	Medication and Lunch	Medication and Lunch	Medication and Lunch
12:45–1:30	12:45–1:30	12:45–1:30	12:45–1:30	12:45–1:30
Storytelling	Intergenerational Group	Goals Trip or Group Activity	Storytelling	Art Therapy
1:30–2.30	1:30–2.30	1:30–2.30	1:30–2.30	1:30–2.30
Recreational Therapy	Recreational Therapy	Goals Trip or Recreational Therapy	Recreational Therapy	Recreational Therapy
2:30–3:00	2:30–3:00	2:30–3:00	2:30–3:00	2:30–3:00
Wrap-up and Clean Up	Wrap-up and Clean Up	Wrap-up and Clean Up	Wrap-up and Clean Up	Wrap-up and Clean Up

patients must meet level requirements for 10 consecutive days. If a patient does not meet these requirements more than two times in a week, his or her level will be dropped.

Level 3—Advanced Level   Patients are given the responsibility to rate themselves on the point sheet and compare their ratings with the staff member's rating. The staff rating is the final rating; however, bonus points can be earned if the patient is able to "match" the staff rating. This helps them learn to observe and evaluate their own behavior as others do.

To move beyond this level, patients must meet criteria for 15 non-consecutive days. If a patient does not make his or her day more than two times in a week, he or she will start the next week at the beginning for Level 3. If he or she does not make his or her day more than three times in a week, his or her level will be dropped to the next lower level.

Level 4—Self-Management Level   Patients at this level begin to take a leadership role in the program. They have exhibited a sustained period of acting responsibly and making good decisions. Their goals may reflect activities such as helping to orient new children to the program by explaining the rules to them. Rather than points, they receive checks at the end of each activity. If a patient does not meet his or her daily quota of checks more than once in a week, he or she will start the next day at the beginning of Level 4. If he or she does not make his or her day more than two times in a week, his or her level will be dropped to Level 3.

In addition to the level system, staff may choose to develop additional incentives and rewards for exceptional behaviors. Staff can also develop more specific behavior contracts with individual patients.

Work with Families

Family involvement is always a critical component in the treatment of children and adolescents. Without the support and involvement of the family the child's treatment is hampered greatly. Meetings are scheduled with the child and his or her family and the team therapist at least weekly. The nature of the work with the family in a day hospital will vary just as it does in other settings. In some cases an intensive, crisis-oriented family therapy approach is appropriate, with the goal of resolving whatever acute problems led to the current treatment episode. In others, the main goal will be to keep family members informed of the child's progress in the program and assist them in obtaining needed aftercare services. Family therapy frequently involves scheduling appointments outside of regular program hours to accommodate parents' schedules.

Psychiatric Evaluation and Treatment

Psychiatric evaluation and treatment are essential components. The psychiatrist is active in the daily treatment of the child. Psychiatric assessment is done on admission and periodically throughout the episode of treatment. If indicated, psychopharmacological treatment is instituted and monitored. The daily participation of the child in various activities provides an opportunity to observe the effects of medication in vivo in a less restrictive setting than a hospital; this combined with reports from parents of their observations in the home greatly facilitates medication management.

Other Treatment Modalities

The indications for other specific treatment approaches depend on the particular needs of the community and/or individual.

Specialized Groups   Many adolescents come into treatment with drug and alcohol problems. Treatment for these or other comorbid conditions must be incorporated into the program, the daily schedule, and the patient's treatment. Through flexible schedules, various specialized groups can be offered, so that those patients who need them can attend. Examples are groups with a special focus on sexual abuse, girls' and boys' groups, 12-step groups, and play therapy. Adolescents can benefit from various kinds of psycho-education, such as sex education, drug education, stress management, and education about use of leisure time.

Recreational Activities   Recreational activities comprise an important therapeutic modality for children and adolescents. These activities provide them with opportunities to develop appropriate socialization skill, peer interaction skills along with motor development, increased interests, and an appropriate outlet for excessive energy and negative, overwhelming emotions. Adventure-based counseling, although it may require increased planning and funding, is a powerful therapeutic tool that can enhance the treatment of children and adolescents. It promotes self-esteem, group cooperation, and understanding through outdoor activities, including rock climbing, hiking, caving, canoeing, and a ropes course.

Art and Music Therapy   Art and music therapy are also extremely beneficial for these populations. These treatment modalities provide ways for the child to express feelings and work on problems through nonverbal means. Thus, during the time the child spends at the program, a blending of multiple treatment modalities addresses all aspects of the child's being: thinking, feeling, and behavior. Both careful planning of the program in advance and constant adjustment and adaptation on a daily basis are necessary.

MANAGEMENT OF COMMON PROBLEM IN A DAY HOSPITAL

Dealing with Disruptive and Negative Behaviors   The children's program should be equipped to handle behaviors such as temper tantrums and aggression, which frequently are part of the developmental psychopathology of preschool- and grade school-age children. Staff should always work with the child to de-escalate the situation verbally if possible. Attempts should be made to understand the patient's feelings and provide feedback and redirection. Providing choices and suggesting alternative behaviors often avoids power struggles. If the negative behavior continues, there are three levels of intervention to be employed. In order of restrictiveness, these include "cool out," time-out in the quiet room, and physical restraint.

Cool-Out   Cool-out involves going to an isolated area or chair in the classroom. The student is asked to go cool-out to regain control. Once the child is in control, positive feedback is given for this and he or she is encouraged to rejoin the group.

Time-Out: Use of a Quiet Room   Time out in the "quiet room" is imposed if the child refuses the cool out or is not able to stop the disruptive behavior while he or she is still in the room. It is also appropriate if the behavior continues or escalates and in the staff's judgement it is or could become dangerous or highly disruptive to the group (e.g., hitting, throwing chairs, fighting).

The quiet room is a small carpeted room with two chairs that can easily be removed if necessary and a door that can be closed but not locked. Patients are escorted to the quiet room and remain there with continual monitoring by staff. The staff member may stay in the room with the child or sit in a chair immediately outside, depending on whether the child needs to be alone or needs to be able to talk. Efforts are made to help the student gain control of his or her behavior so that he or she can join the group.

There may be instances when a patient's behavior (i.e., actions that pose a danger to himself or herself or others) necessitates passive physical restraint. The object is to help the patient calm down by insuring safety for himself or herself and staff. Once a patient shows adequate calm for a continued period of time judged to be sufficient by staff (no more than 10 minutes) the physical restraint is discontinued, and the patient will continue to be helped to gain control of his or her behavior in order to join the group. It is generally important that the patient be able to "process" the incident in some way, that is, by verbalizing awareness of antecedents and consequences, before returning to the group. Once back in the group, the student is encouraged to express himself or herself either by talking, or through drawing or completing a writing assignment about the incident.

The use of the quiet room is meant to be only on an occasional basis for fairly brief periods of time; on average children are in the room for 10 to 15 minutes. If the usage is occurring on a daily basis or several times a day, a decision must be made as to whether the child is in need of an inpatient setting.

Physical Restraint   Physical restraint is sometimes appropriate and can generally be accomplished fairly easily with young children. With an adolescent the need for it is a more ominous development; physical restraint is impracticable given the staffing and the adolescent should be re-evaluated and referred to an inpatient unit. Although both programs should have a time-out room, the children's time-out room is maintained to provide safety and containment if a child does need to be restrained physically. If a child requires this type of intervention on a continual and consistent basis, he or she will require a re-evaluation to determine the appropriateness for this level of care.

Logistical Problems Unique to the Day Hospital

Transportation   An essential requirement for a day hospital for children and adolescents is that children are transported back and forth to home and to the program daily. This means that one of the more complicated logistical problems is transportation. Fortunately, many of the public school districts do provide transportation for their students to the day hospital; the program must have a mechanism to inform the school district of the admission and discharge date. However, even when the local school district is responsible for transportation, this service will not be available when the schools are closed for holidays or other reasons, even though the hospital is in operation during many of these days.

Transportation is also needed to take the children and adolescents out of the hospital for earned trips and/or adventure counseling outings. Either parents or the day hospital will have to be relied on in these cases, as well as with children whose schools do not provide transportation. The logistics of transportation can involve an extensive staffing and scheduling operation. However, without providing this service the hospital may not be able to offer its services and treatment to potential patients or serve as an area referral source. If not managed properly and scheduled carefully transportation problems can disrupt the program and hamper treatment. Arrangements for each patient need to be in place on the day of admission. Our program employed a full-time staff person to coordinate transportation, in addition to drivers and vans.

Dealing with Medical Problems   Medical problems can come up often in daily operation. These range from injuries to reactions to medication to the usual viral illnesses. Unlike a hospital, a nurse or physician is not on site continually. Decisions about the care of the child then become the responsibility of the mental health counselor who may not be equipped to handle the situation. This is not only a medical problem, but a management and possibly a legal problem; an on-call system is needed for providing medical coverage by phone at all times. An additional nursing problem can occur when the children or adolescents are scheduled for a day trip, such as an adventure-based counseling trip, and the children who receive noontime medication need to receive their medication from the nurse. Procedures must be developed for administering the medication; one solution is to have medications dispensed in the morning in labeled envelopes, giving the labeled medication to a staff person to dispense.

Meals   Providing lunch for the patients in the program can turn into a complicated management problem. If the day hospital has an operating cafeteria this is optimal. However, if the cafeteria is in another building, such as the inpatient building, this involves another transportation issue. Although, this may seem like a minor formality, it can become a major problem, which in turn can effect the operation of the entire program.

Difficulty Enlisting Family Participation in Treatment

A difficult issue that has implications for both the clinical program and administration arises when working with patients' families is problematic. It is appropriate in an acute treatment program that families are involved in meeting with program staff at least once a week. The expectation of weekly or biweekly family sessions is built into some managed care contracts. Even though this expectation is articulated to families, for a variety of reasons, many families are unable to fulfill a commitment to attend family sessions. This not only hampers the child's treatment but has been the basis for disallowal of continued treatment at this level of care by managed-care companies.

In more long-term programs that are publicly funded, the non-involvement of families in treatment has different, but equally problematic, implications. The decision to discharge a child whose parents do not participate in meetings with staff is often a painful one; the child may receive benefit from the program even without parental participation. Fiscal considerations play a role here as well if the program receives funding based on enrollment.

The program must make every effort to be "parent-friendly" and reduce barriers that impede parents' utilization of the help offered to them. In inpatient settings, parents are involved in visiting their children and sessions can be scheduled around visiting hours; in outpatient clinics, parents must transport their children and so their presence is a precondition of the visits. In the day hospital, neither of these necessities holds and it is often fairly difficult to involve parents meaningfully in the treatment. Parents may have negative expectations of treatment staff based on their past experiences and their expectation that they will be blamed for their children's problems. The authors have found that inviting parents to observe their children in the classroom is often responded to positively by parents and may facilitate their developing and alliance with the staff.

Handling Relationships Outside the Program

Day hospital programs cannot control their patients' activities outside the program, after school hours, and weekends, a significant portion of the day. Given the close contact among patients and the intensity of the shared experience that is inherent in the program, it is inevitable that youngsters will develop intense relationships both inside and outside the program. This is especially true with regard to adolescents. While it is futile to try to prohibit such relationships, the program must address them insofar as they have an impact on the patient's mental health and treatment. Generally, such relationships will become a focus of group discussion and can be talked about in a way that helps patients gain a greater understanding of their emotional needs and the ways in which their relationships with each other are growth enhancing or inhibiting. It has been the authors' experience that very intense, exclusive, and exploitative relationships among teenagers are less of a problem in day treatment programs than in inpatient programs, as the preservation of the adolescent's ties with friends in the community acts to dilute the intensity of relationships within the program.

CONCLUSION

Day hospital programs provide an important link between inpatient and outpatient psychiatric treatment for children and adolescents. This link has become even more significant because managed care companies are trying to curtail costs of inpatient treatment. The major therapeutic effect of the day hospital is through the milieu which provides various treatment activities in a safe and structured environment. Behavior management techniques, limit setting, time out in the quiet room, and physical and chemical restraints help in providing optimal structure and safety for the milieu.

REFERENCES

Lahey, B. B., & Kupfer, D. L. (1979). Partial hospitalization programs for children and adolescents. In R. F. Luber, *Partial hospitalization: A current perspective*. New York: Plenum Press. pp. 73–90.
Washburn, S., & Conrad M. (1979). Organization of the therapeutic milieu in the partial hospital. In R. F. Luber, *Partial hospitalization: A current perspective*. New York: Plenum Press. pp. 47–70.

Chapter 26

Day School for Emotionally and Behaviorally Disturbed and Learning Disabled Children and Adolescents

Burton Lohnes, Ph.D.

INTRODUCTION

Education is the primary work of children and adolescents, intertwined in all other aspects of a child's and adolescent's life. A school program must, therefore, be part of the woven fabric that makes up any successful day treatment program serving children and adolescents. Philosophically, a school program should be part of the overall clinical treatment program, not an appendage.

Special education is defined by our government as "...specially designed instruction, at no cost to parents or guardians, to meet the unique needs of a child with a disability..." (Individuals with Disabilities Education Act of 1990, P.L. 101-476). Many of the children and adolescents who attend psychiatric day programs are educationally handicapped and in need of special education services as well as having a psychiatric disorder. The mere presence of a psychiatric disorder does not guarantee that an individual would also be found to have an educational disability. For many day patients, education is a strength, and their psychopathology has not interfered with the acquisition of knowledge.

In the case of an adolescent anonymously called "Tom," there is a clear interplay between the educational process and a psychiatric disorder but without an observable negative impact on his education. In Tom's case, he did very well at school by everyone's standard but his own. As a high school student, he received excellent grades, made the honor roll, and was involved in extracurricular activities at school and in the community. Tom's standards for himself were unrealistically high. He collected perceived insults, unnoticed by anyone except himself. A grade of "A" was not sufficient in a particular subject, since he did not receive the highest grade in the class. Having a major part in the school play did not measure up, since it was not the lead role. One after another, year after year, Tom collected the perceived insults as if adding a small pebble to his backpack each time, until the weight, in its cumulative form, overwhelmed him. Tom attempted suicide, was admitted to a general hospital in a comatose state, was stabilized, and admitted to a psychiatric inpatient unit. As part of Tom's transition home, he was stepped down to a day treatment program.

Tom's case illustrates the difference between a psychiatric disorder, which he clearly has, and an educationally disabling condition, which he does not manifest. Tom's psychopathology, which almost caused his death, did not exhibit its symptoms in school or impact his grades or social skills. For an individual to be identified as severely emotionally disturbed (SED)—i.e., educationally disabled—the psychopathology along with other criteria must be of a type "...which adversely affects educational performance" (Programs for Students with Disabilities, 1991). The criterion which requires that there be an adverse impact on educational performance for a student to be identified as severely emotionally disturbed is the standard cited most often when denying a request that an individual with a psychiatric illness be identified as educationally disabled. If someone cannot be identified as educationally disabled, he or she is not entitled to special education services or special education funding while attending a day treatment program.

The issue of whether or not a particular child or adolescent is eligible for special education services and/or funding, although very important, obscures the main issue at times. The point is that school is the work of children and adolescents, and we must provide an education program that encourages and facilitates the continuation of a student's normal developmental activities. A secondary school student simply cannot miss a month or more of instruction while he or she is attending a day treatment program. This is especially true for building block courses, such as upper-level math and science courses. If a student misses a month or more in these subjects, he or she is usually lost for the remainder of the school year.

Thus, the overriding question for an educator when a student is admitted to a day treatment program is: What does this *individual* student need educationally? Is this patient admitted for a short-term stay and thus in need of an itinerant home and hospital teacher to keep up with the subjects in the home school? Is the child or adolescent going to be with the day program school for a month or two so that the program becomes the school of record and needs to provide and coordinate all the activities leading toward grade advancement and/or graduation? Is the individual a previously identified special education student who comes with an individual education plan that the day program school must implement? Or is the student coming from a regular high school program and, most likely, returning to the same program? Some adolescents come to day treatment after they have already dropped out of school. In such a case, it is possible that the dropout attend class, work toward a *General Education Developmental tests* (GED) (Maryland State Department of Education, 1988), or formally re-enroll in school.

Each question has its infinite variations depending upon the history, strengths, and weaknesses of the student. Each student is unique. The answers to the above questions, along with the requirements that govern secondary schools in this country and the student's wishes and desires, dictate an individual education plan for each child or adolescent.

MODELS

Separate, stand-alone models are good for the sake of theoretical comparison but do not reflect the practice in the field. Patients who attend day treatment programs do not come as if punched out by cookie cutters. Students present themselves representing many themes and infinite variations on those themes. Their educational needs are distinctly varied and individualized, not completely fitting smoothly into model X, Y, or Z. In reality, most schools in day treatment programs are hybrids, offering elements of two or more of the following models because of the different programmatic needs of the population they serve.

Self-Contained Classrooms

A self-contained class is defined as a group of students spending most—or all—of the school day with the same teacher, or teacher and aide. A teacher certified to teach special education is expected to instruct the students in all major subject areas. The students may go to other specialty teachers periodically during the week, such as physical education, art, or music and practical arts, if the program is large enough to warrant their existence. The main focus, however, is their home-base, self-contained classroom. Self-contained classrooms at the elementary school level are appropriate for all populations. Self-contained classrooms at the middle and high school levels are normally found where there is a high concentration of low-functioning students.

Advantages Self-contained classrooms are easy to administer and organize. Communication lines are simplified, with clinical staff needing to deal with only one classroom teacher per patient instead of five to seven teachers. Behavioral programs are easier to design and monitor, with students working with one teacher instead of many. The chances of splitting staff are also decreased.

Disadvantages Students at the middle and high school levels are not taught by subject-certified teachers. Material presented does not have the breadth or depth of classes taught by subject-certified teachers. This model is not appropriate for middle and secondary students who are on or near grade level.

Departmentalized Classrooms

Departmentalized classrooms at the middle and secondary school level are normally found in many larger programs, especially where a high percentage of students are operating at, or near, grade level. Students rotate between classes as in a normal middle or high school, seeing five to seven different teachers each day. Each teacher instructs the students in the subjects in which they are certified.

Advantage Departmentalized classrooms offer superior academic instruction to middle and high school students by subject-certified teachers. This model replicates the educational reality of what most patients will return to upon discharge and offers the best chance for students to keep up with their regular school classmates.

Disadvantages Communication lines are complicated, with clinical staff needing to interface with five to seven classroom teachers. Behavioral programs are more difficult to design and administer. The chance of splitting is markedly increased, as more teachers are working with students on a daily basis.

Home and Hospital Instruction

Home and hospital teaching usually occur when, for example, a student is hospitalized with a broken leg or short-term psychiatric illness or is at home recuperating from a similar experience. Local boards of education, according to the Individuals with Disabilities Education Act of 1990, must provide instruction in institutions and hospitals as part of their continuum of alternative placements. Typically, a local board of education sends one or more teachers to the home or hospital to instruct an individual student on a one-on-one basis for a few hours per week. The minimum number of home and hospital instructional hours per week required by the state of Maryland is six (Programs for Students with Disabilities, 1991). Unfortunately, the minimum six hours of instruction per week routinely ends up being the maximum number of hours provided.

Advantages   Home and hospital instruction is productive when the length of stay is very short and the student is going to return to his or her regular school placement. The home and hospital teacher(s) involved can coordinate the educational activities presented in the day treatment program with what is going on in the patient's normal school setting. The teachers are usually provided and paid for by the local board of education. The hospital needs only to provide a quiet space, conducive to the educational process, and a contact person to facilitate the communication process.

Disadvantages   The number of instructional hours per week is insufficient to help a patient keep up with his or her regular school program for very long. This is especially true of the higher-level courses for which home and hospital teachers are usually not properly trained. A single teacher cannot adequately instruct in all the subject areas a student normally carries.

Continuation Program

This is a recently developed hybrid model (Educational Programs in Nonpublic Schools and Child Care and Treatment Facilities, 1993) which falls between a home and hospital instruction program and a full-day school model, either self-contained or departmentalized. It continues all of a student's regular school course work compressed into a three-hour school day with the remainder of the treatment center's time devoted to more traditional clinical group activities. The continuation model bridges the gap of time a student misses from his or her regular school setting. It is designed to continue the exact instructional program a student would receive in his or her regular school.

Advantages   Somewhat similar to a home and hospital instructional program, the continuation model is appropriate when the length of stay is up to 60 days and the student is going back to the home schools. This type of program is designed to keep a student current with the subjects he or she would be taking in the regular school setting. There is much less disruption in a student's school career as an attempt is made to follow the home school curriculum.

Disadvantages   Communication and coordination are more difficult in this model. Ideally, the textbooks and assignments utilized by the student's home school teachers will be obtained by the parents or the special education school staff. Educational programs for the patient, of necessity, are very individualized to the student's home school curriculum.

The inability to obtain the student's home school textbooks necessitates maintaining a large inventory of various subject textbooks.

Public School Placements

Placing children and adolescents attending day treatment programs into public schools is an infrequent result, in part, of the need for close supervision. Students have been included in regular public school classrooms for as little as 10 minutes per day initially, gradually working up to a full day. Another option would involve placing a student into a public school during his or her last days of treatment as a transition or as a trial placement before discharge.

Advantages   Including a day treatment patient in public school classrooms gives the student a chance to try out newly acquired coping and social skills while still having the backup and support of a day treatment setting. The public school classroom can also be the same class the patient will attend once discharged. This helps the transition while lessening the stigma attached to a stay in a psychiatric setting.

Disadvantages   Public schools cannot provide the constant close supervision needed by most children and adolescents who attend day treatment programs. The communication process can be somewhat cumbersome, especially if a student has many different teachers. The issue of transportation can be highly problematic depending on the ability of the local school system, day treatment program, or parent to be a reliable resource.

A review of the five models demonstrates advantages and disadvantages to each; in general, there is no absolutely right or wrong model. In practice, it is often necessary to use segments of each model to meet the varying needs of a treatment center's population. Each student's needs must be evaluated individually and programmed for on an individual basis, often using parts of more than one model.

As an example, a bright high school student whose major academic courses could be easily programmed entered the day school program. The student, however, was taking an advanced computer course. At that point the day school had just started offering beginning computer courses. To provide for the advanced computer course, the day school contacted the local home and hospital teaching program which provided a qualified teacher who came to the day treatment program, used the school's equipment, and provided the appropriate instruction to the student. Parts of two models were simply used together to provide a program that made sense for the student in question.

EDUCATIONAL PROGRAM

This section describes the educational program as it proceeds from day of admission, through treatment, to discharge. To keep matters simple, it focuses on the school program. It is worthwhile to keep in mind, however, that the operation of the school program is intimately intertwined with the overall day treatment program.

Intake

During the admission process, records are requested from all the previous schools attended by a student. The request includes copies of any special education program requirements, transcripts or all previous report cards, results of standardized tests, immunization history, and any anecdotal information available. Once all the necessary information is gathered, the diagnostic and prescriptive (D&P) teacher determines if any additional educational testing is required to place the child or adolescent in appropriate classes. If so, they are conducted by the D&P teacher. The D&P teacher remains available throughout the patient's stay to assist the classroom teacher(s) in understanding the individual's needs and to help the teacher(s) successfully program for the patient. The D&P teacher is also available to conduct further evaluations as conditions warrant.

Courses

Five classroom teachers provide the instructional program offerings in our continuation model which services both day and inpatient students. There are two self-contained elementary classrooms, two departmentalized middle/high school (MS/HS) classrooms, and a physical education (P. Ed.) teacher who serves our entire K–12 population. The two departmentalized classroom teachers who serve the MS/HS students each teach two subjects. The math teacher also teaches science and the English teacher instructs the history/social studies classes.

The MS/HS classes run for 36 minutes each, one in each of the four major subjects and P. Ed. for a total of three hours of instruction per school day. The elementary school (ES) classrooms are self-contained except for 36 minutes of P. Ed., for a total of three hours of instruction per school day. The state education agency has defined a three-hour school day as being appropriate for short-term students (Educational Programs in Nonpublic Schools and Child Care and Treatment Facility, 1993). The instruction is highly individualized for each patient depending on the course work they are taking in their home school. The patients interact with two or three teachers per day instead of five to seven, which diminishes the potential for communication problems or splitting of staff.

Many adolescents who are in need of psychiatric day programs have a history of missing segments of their formal education for various reasons. They often lag behind their peers in their credit standing and need to make up course work to graduate on time. Our program includes a 35-day summer session in an attempt to offer an opportunity for students who are behind to catch up with their classmates.

Children and adolescents who are nearing their discharge date may be mainstreamed into their local public school or an alternative that is located in the community adjacent on the day treatment program. Courses are offered to support those students who are working toward a GED.

Support Services

The resource room is the focal point of the behavioral intervention services provided to the students. Students who are experiencing behavioral difficulties in class are usually referred to the resource room by their teachers. Students also refer themselves when they are experiencing some emotional turmoil. The resource room accommodates three to six students comfortably with the intent of returning them to their classrooms as soon as possible. The resource specialists provide academic help to students who need extra attention and maintain the highly structured environment needed to get most of our patients through a typical school day. It is the center where many of the minute-to-minute decisions are made. Most of the communications that occur during the school day between the school and the day program are funneled through the resource room. Material that cannot wait until the more formal written communication is passed on at the end of the school day is expeditiously transmitted as needed.

A program coordinator and a secretary round out the support staff. The program coordinator is the program supervisor and also functions as the liaison between the public schools and the day treatment school program, funneling information in both directions. The coordinator also functions as the primary contact for the day treatment program as problems serving this population continually crop up. A full-time secretary is assigned to this relatively small, 48-student program in an effort to speed up the flow of information, especially that coming in from the public school sector. The acquisition of school information is vital to a program with such a short length of stay.

Discharge

As soon as a patient is admitted to the day program, the planning process for his or her school placement after discharge is begun. This is particularly important because the average length of stay, currently 19.7 days, has decreased sharply in recent years. The benefits of a psychiatric day program would be potentially diminished if a child or adolescent were discharged to a good living arrangement only to sit at home during the day for lack of an appropriate school placement.

The special education identification, funding, and placement process is cumbersome and time-consuming. This is especially true if placement is being sought in a residential treatment center and a local board of education is being asked to pay the entire bill, not just the school portion. If a particular student has never been identified as needing special education services, it can take many months to complete the screening, assessment, identification, and placement process. Nothing is lost by starting the process as early as possible. Parents can always stop the process whenever they like if plans change or if the avenue of exploration does not prove fruitful.

POTENTIAL PITFALLS

All intensive psychiatric day programs create an environment in which a number of built-in problems exist. Communication between school and clinical staff and the timing of team meetings/staffings are critical issue which must be addressed and solved to run a successful day program. If only there were 26 hours in a day and the extra two hours were added after our patients went home, the timing and communication issues would be easily resolved.

Communication

Successful communication is the life blood of a day treatment program. There are two phrases, two concepts, which must be indelibly inscribed in the brain of each individual who works with a psychiatric day treatment population from the day they are first employed. They are the word *communication* and the phrase *consistent, predictable environment*. The hallmarks of a successful day treatment program must be excellent communication and the provision of a consistent, predictable environment for the children and adolescents we serve. The two concepts actually feed into each other with excellent communication being a prerequisite for a consistent, predictable environment and a consistent, predictable environment enhancing the chances of excellent communication patterns.

When staff members state that three people have already passed on a particular bit of information, that should bring comfort to the program director. Too much communication, however potentially wasteful and inefficient the management engineers may deem the practice, is far preferable to poor communication or no communication at all. A high-pressure environment, such as a psychiatric day treatment program, only intensifies the problems created when players are left out of the communication loop. The children, and especially the adolescents, we serve force us to be good communicators, as they are usually so adept at splitting adults. Good communication becomes a necessary survival skill. Communication must be a way of life for everyone for a day program to succeed.

Collaborative Meetings

Team meetings, staff meetings, and case conferences need to take place when all or most of the staff can be present. Problems arise when specific segments of the staff need to attend a meeting at the same time that they are programmatically responsible for the patients. This occurs, for example, when teachers are needed for meetings, but the meeting is scheduled during the school day when they are in classrooms. If enough staff is available to cover a classroom or group activity, a teacher or group care worker would be available for meetings. The amount of time a group care worker or teacher is missing from his or her primary assignment in a given week is always a concern that must be kept in mind.

Competing Activities

Most schools that are part of day treatment programs are relatively small and enroll between five and 20 students. Many offer only one section of various subjects, such as algebra I, sociology, or biology, which would dictate when a student must attend that specific class. Seniors are a special group who cannot miss a substantial amount of school without putting their graduation at risk.

At the same time school is in session, there are various groups, therapies, and evaluations to be scheduled that are competing for the same prime time slots. The problem is more pronounced with short-term lengths. Everyone would like to work 8:30 a.m. to 4:30 p.m., Monday through Friday, but this is not possible given the demands of our job.

The patient's clinical team, including the classroom teacher, must decide what combination of therapeutic activities meet the patient's needs at a given time. For some patients, this means a full school program; for others, it does not. Many times, various therapeutic groups are more critical to a patient's recovery effort than his or her immediate classroom experience. The mixture of therapeutic efforts for a particular patient must be decided on an individual basis.

Academically, a student cannot miss more than one class period in a given subject per week and still expect to pass the course. The rule of thumb within our MS/HS program is: A student may be taken out of a given course for only one class period per week. In this manner, students can make up the work missed, hopefully without falling behind.

Parental Concerns

All parents have been through school to one extent or another. They have also lived through their children's educational experiences and have opinions of what should be done educationally for their offspring once they have entered a day treatment program. For some parents, school presents an arena where one can concentrate energies and concerns while denying the reason their child or adolescent entered a day treatment program. It becomes a smokescreen, in most instances and effort to hide from the truth. In some cases, parents refuse to allow contact with the previous school in an attempt to keep the psychiatric illness a secret. Students are not admitted to a psychiatric day treatment program because they need the specific educational services associated with a particular day program. An excellent school program will, however, attract admissions to one day treatment program over a mediocre one in another setting.

The closer a school program replicates the academic offerings of a public school, the more accepting parents tend to be of the program. This is easier to do with adolescents who are in a high school program. The same course requirements that are mandated by a given state also govern public schools and nonpublic schools that serve students with educational disabilities.

Integration of Programs

A school calls the education plan for a student in Individual Education Plan (IEP); in the day treatment program, this is called an Individual Treatment Plan (ITP). Laws and regulations govern psychiatric day programs and schools somewhat differently regarding formats and wording. Both plans contain different names, different emphases, but the same goals and objectives, especially the behavioral ones.

It is the communication process between the school and the day treatment program that is critical in aligning the goals and objectives for an individual child or adolescent. A teacher/advisor system is one method for keeping the channels open. The teacher/advisor transmits the information from the school to the day treatment program and from the clinical component to the school. This person attends both the team meeting(s) in the school and on the inpatient unit, transmitting information in both directions. Other devices used to keep the lines of communication open are point cards and homework sheets. Both devices can be utilized with an individual child and adolescent as needed. The patients carry the card(s) to school each day, where each individual teacher records points earned, comments, and/or nightly homework assignments. The information is transmitted to the day treatment program staff at the end of the student's school session. The system needs daily monitoring to minimize the splitting in which adolescents especially are so prone to engage.

CONCLUSION

The integration of educational programs into traditional psychiatric day treatment programs is an evolving process. With the average length of stay on inpatient units diminishing and the proliferation of various types of day programs we have experienced in recent years, states are propagating new regulations to govern day school programs with short lengths of student enrollment. Our patients clearly cannot simply miss two or three weeks of school when they are attending a day treatment program. Yet, they would not benefit from a drastic change to a completely different school curriculum offered by most comprehensive special education schools. The hybrid continuation model offers the promise of providing a quality educational experience for patients within day treatment programs while enabling the individuals to keep up with their educational program from their home school.

REFERENCES

Educational Programs in Nonpublic Schools and Child Care and Treatment Facilities, Code of Maryland Regulations § 13A. 09.10.11 (March 1993).

Individuals with Education Disabilities Act, 20 U.S.C. § 1401 (1990).

Maryland State Department of Education (1988). *The Maryland high school diploma by examination* (Maryland School Bulletin, Vol. 36-3), Baltimore, MD: the Author.

Programs for Students with Disabilities, Code of Maryland Regulations § 13A.05.01 (October 1991).

Part 6

Other Community-Based Programs

Chapter 27

Mental Health Services in Schools: Expanding Opportunities

Mark D. Weist, Ph.D.

Traditionally, mental health services in schools have been assessment-oriented and limited to youth in special education. However, in the United States, comprehensive mental health services of assessment *and* treatment services for youth in special *and* regular education are being developed in more and more schools. This national movement to develop a full range of mental health services from primary to tertiary preventive for youth in schools is part of a broader effort to bring health services to schools which began in the 1970s and gained considerable momentum in the past decade. The purpose of this chapter is to provide historical background and overview of administrative and clinical issues for these "expanded" school mental health services, which are providing new practice, program development, and research opportunities for mental health professionals.

HISTORICAL AND THEORETICAL BACKGROUND

Limitations in the Youth Mental Health Service Delivery System

Among mental health providers, planners, and policy makers, there is increasing recognition of the numerous barriers that prevent youth from receiving mental health services in typical community settings such as community mental health centers and private offices. Barriers operating at the family level, such as poor knowledge, stigma, transportation, and financial problems exist along with barriers in community clinics such as long waiting lists, insurance obstacles, lengthy intake procedures and staff turnover to impede the connection between youth with emotional/behavioral disturbances and needed mental health services. Related to these barriers, up to 20 percent of youth who need mental health services do not receive them (Office of Technology Assessment, 1991).

Perhaps more concerning is evidence that the dominant method of treating emotional and behavioral disturbances in youth with once a week outpatient visits may represent a questionable construct. Weisz, Weiss, and Donenberg (1992), in a meta-analytic review of psychotherapy outcome studies with children and adolescents, found only limited evidence for the effectiveness of such treatment as commonly practiced with clinical samples in applied settings.

Related to these increasingly obvious limitations in the mental health service delivery system for youth, there have been a number of efforts to restructure the way such services are provided (e.g., Child and Adolescent Service System Program [CASSP]; Day & Roberts, 1991). The increased placement of comprehensive mental health services in schools is one of these more prominent efforts. The most significant benefit of providing mental health services to youth in schools is greatly enhanced access to services. Particularly for youth who present internalizing disturbances of depression and anxiety, placing mental health services in schools increases the likelihood that they will reach those in need. For example, in our work in the Baltimore City schools, we have found that more than 80 percent of youth referred for significant presenting problems have had no previous contact with the mental health system (Flaherty, Weist, & Warner, in press). Further, there have been numerous cases where students with life-threatening disturbanaces have not received prior care following acute crises such as serious suicide attempts.

The other side of this issue is the common disappointment experienced by school-based clinicians when they refer youth for outside mental health services who often do not receive these services, or the services are very brief and limited.

Service Delivery Models for Expanded School Mental Health Services

There are many forms of expanded school mental health (SMH) services. In some programs, the emphasis is on consultative services, maximizing the number of students exposed to mental health interventions. For example, in an approach espoused by Adelman and Taylor (1993), mental health professionals or "specialists" (social workers, psychologists, psychiatrists) serve as "catalytic agents" within schools, assisting them in developing programs that will have the broadest impact given available resources. In this model, professionals prioritize resource development, improving connections to available community resources, and providing supervision with direct clinical assessment and treatment services viewed as a lower-order priority.

Other SMH programs place more emphasis on the provision of direct services. The more effective programs involve collaboration between schools and community agencies, with the latter taking primary responsibility for the development and implementation of the services (Dryfoos, 1994). For example, our school mental health program represents a partnership between the Department of Psychiatry of the University of Maryland School of Medicine and the Baltimore City Public Schools. In our program, clinicians provide focused mental health evaluation, psychological and psychiatric consultation, individual, family, and group therapy, and referral of students for more intensive services like medication and/or inpatient treatment in 14 Baltimore City schools.

The program also provides a number of preventive services. These include a range of support groups for youth who may not present frank emotional/behavioral disturbances, consultation with teachers and school health staff, and mental health educational activities for students. Similar programs are in place in a number of U.S. cities, including Dallas, Texas, New Brunswick, New Jersey, New Haven, Connecticut, and Minneapolis, Minnesota. In essence, these programs represent a shifting of primary mental health care from community mental health centers and private offices into the schools in areas where there are documented problems in access to mental health services for youth such as certain inner cities and very rural localities (Weist, in press).

Impact of School-Based Health Centers A major factor in the development of expanded SMH services has been the growth of school-based health centers (SBHCs). The mission of SBHCs is to bring needed health, and, recently, mental health, services to youth "where they are" (Dryfoos, 1994). Primary care health services in SBHCs include physical examinations and medical screening, treatment for acute illnesses and accidents, immunizations, family planning services, and a range of health education programs. After their beginnings in the 1970s, SBHCs have grown dramatically in the 1980s and 1990s from about 150 in 1987 to over 600 in 1994 (Dryfoos, 1988; Schlitt, Rickett, Montgomery, & Lear, 1994).

The development of SBHCs has been a major impetus behind the burgeoning interest in mental health services in schools. Staff in SBHCs complain of being overwhelmed by the number of youth presenting emotional and behavioral disorders, and in programs that have mental health staff, SMH services are either the highest or second highest utilized (Dryfoos, 1994). Given this intense need, SBHC staff are clamoring to develop mental health services. While some progress has been made, gaps remain. For example, a recent survey of SBHCs (Advocates for Youth, 1994) found that around 80 percent of SBHCs offered mental health services; however, only a small percentage of programs used mental health professionals to provide these services. I now turn to discussion of administrative and program development issues important to the devlopment of comprehensive school mental health services.

ADMINISTRATIVE AND PROGRAM DEVELOPMENT ISSUES

Funding

Any discussion of clinical programs should begin with the issue of funding. While it is beyond the scope of this paper to review the many issues germane to SMH funding, I will highlight a few. Most funds for expanded SMH programs are from state and federal sources as channeled through local agencies. For example, in Baltimore, the majority of SMH programs have been funded by Medicaid, which is controlled and allocated at the local level by various agencies including the public schools and the city health department. These agencies bill federal Medicaid for services rendered across schools and across providers. In the early 1990s, there was considerable growth in these funds, supporting a substantial increase in the number of Baltimore schools providing expanded mental health services, from around 20 in 1991 to over 60 in 1995. However, in the past two years managed care companies have enrolled increasing numbers of families with Medicaid, using "aggressive strategies" (School Health Policy Initiative [SHPI], 1993). These companies have consistently been unwilling to authorize school-based mental health services, resulting in a marked decline in revenue for SMH programs. To address this problem, more and more programs are forming relationships with managed care companies, and some of these companies are even funding SBHCs. In addition to this strategy, considerable activity is needed in this area to ensure stable funding for SMH services to not only survive, but thrive.

Planning of Services

After obtaining funding for a SMH program, careful planning for the development of services is essential. Such planning involves analysis of the local system of mental health care, its strengths and weaknesses, and gaps in service delivery. Unfortunately, such careful pre-planning of school mental health services is not the norm. For example, Adelman and Taylor (1993), assessing mental health services in Los Angeles schools, highlighted their "piecemeal" and disorganized qualities. This is congruent with experiences in Baltimore, where expanded mental health services are usually developed in schools based on the interest of the principal, or chance factors such as school staff "hearing about" mental health services available in other schools. Rarely are school mental health services developed based on a systematic assessment of the relative needs of youth who attend the school and considering variables such as the size of the school, the percentage of students receiving reduced-cost or free lunches, or socioeconomic and crime statistics in the surrounding community. This results in some small (student population of 400) and relatively advantaged schools having more than a full-time equivalent of clinical coverage, and other larger (population of 2,000) and relatively disadvantaged schools having no mental health services available other than academic/vocational guidance, and minimal assessment services for youth in special education.

Further, in Baltimore, we have observed a pattern of avoidance by planners and administrators of school mental health services for some of the more troubled schools. This appears to be related to factors such as concern for the safety of staff, poor office space in the school, and administrative staff in the school being overwhelmed to the point that adequate support for the mental health program is functionally impossible. These factors result in more advantaged schools devloping better and more comprehensive health and mental health services, while the environment in the more disadvantaged schools gets worse.

Integrating School and Community Services

A very serious problem is the failure of most SMH programs to be integrated with local systems of mental health care. As such, school-based services are disconnected from community mental health centers (CMHCs), leaving SMH providers with few if any options for more seriously disturbed youth requiring psychotropic medication or inpatient treatment. Conversely, community mental health providers often have difficulty following youth in schools. Hence, failure of these two systems to communicate precludes their ability to cooperate.

Optimally, SMH and community-based services should be integrated, so that youth experience a relatively seamless system of care. This is the vision for our program, where administrators and clinicians from 14 schools work closely with staff from three CMHCs, with specific relations between schools and CMHCs varying on specific catchment area. Staff from the school programs regularly refer youth to one of the CMHCs for more intensive evaluative services such as psychiatric and psychological evaluations, psychopharmacological services, inpatient treatment, and additional case management and treatment services dependent on the intensity of presenting problems. In turn, staff from the CMHCs regularly request on-site ancillary services by school-based clinicians for additional supportive counseling for school-related issues, classroom observations, and attendance at special education assessment meetings.

Coordination of Services Within Schools

As significant as ensuring that SMH services are integrated into local systems of care is ensuring they are coordinated with other school-based health and mental health services. As reviewed earlier, many schools contain health services, ranging from individual school nurses to comprehensive SBHCs. It is essential for mental health staff to form collaborative relationships with health staff. We have found that school nurses and nurse practitioners are highly attuned to psychosocial stress and emotional/behavioral difficulties in youth. Particularly in relation to internalizing disturbances such as depression and anxiety, school nurses can serve an important role in identifying youth in need of mental health services (Weist, in press). Also, nurses can augment supportive services for students in crises by scheduling "check in" visits on days when mental health professionals are not at the school. In turn, mental health staff can use school nurses and nurse practitioners for health screening, treatment, and referral for more intensive medical services. In addition, there are many other avenues for productive collaboration between health and mental health staff, including developing psychosocial interventions to address health risk behavior, and working together in addressing the multiple needs of youth who use school health services intensively and who are at risk for emotional/behavioral difficulties (Weist, Proescher, Freedman, Paskewitz, & Flaherty, 1995).

A second level of coordination involves working collaboratively with related mental health staff in a school. These staff commonly include guidance counselors, school social workers, and school psychologists. There is variability in roles of these professionals across schools, but a common arrangement is for guidance counselors to provide academic and career guidance to large numbers of students; school social workers to provide crisis intervention, case management, and administrative services primarily for youth in special education; and school psychologists to provide assessment and consultative services for youth being assessed for, or placed in, special education.

Clinical staff who enter schools to provide more intensive services (i.e., assessment *and* treatment services available to *all* students) must coordinate their activities with services provided by these "traditional" mental health staff. Most commonly, clinical staff are licensed social workers and clinical psychologists, and to a more limited extent, psychiatrists and members of other disciplines including counseling psychology and psychiatric nursing. It is important for clinical staff not to view their services as supplanting existing services; rather, expanded services should be meshed with existing services to be complementary of those provided by mental health staff hired by the educational system (Weist, in press).

Regardless of the scope of mental health services in a given school, staff hired by the educational system and staff hired by the collaborating community agency should work closely together. One mechanism to promote coordinated activity between these professionals is to create a team focused on addressing mental health issues in the school. The team is usually comprised of guidance counselors, school social workers and psychologists, the clinical therapist, and others, for example, substance abuse specialists. Functions of the team include: a) working together to ensure that services are not duplicated across providers, b) assessing and addressing gaps in available services for students, c) planning and implementing mental health education programs, and d) mounting school-wide programs to address pressing problems including violence, sexuality, and others.

In the Baltimore high school in which I work, the "Mental Health Team," which includes the disciplines noted above, has developed a crisis intervention plan, conducted a series of presentations on violence, developed a peer counseling program, conducted a survey of student mental health needs, and developed a range of group therapies to address student-identified needs (e.g., focusing on bereavement, and teen dating relationships). Not only has this team improved mental health services, but camaraderie and mutual social support has developed among team members. My view is that clinicians in such teams should act as equals, without preconceived notions of superiority of one discipline over another (see Conoley & Conoley, 1991). Such a stance can serve to circumvent the development of "turf" issues, wherein educational mental health staff often develop resentment toward clinicians from collaborating community agencies, based on the perception (or fact) that the clinicians get to perform the more preferred tasks such as treatment (Dryfoos, 1994).

Developing Relationships with Education Staff

In addition to coordinating efforts with school health and other mental health staff, clinicians entering the schools need to develop working relationships with administrative and teaching staff. Principals are often supportive of mental health services in their school, but may not know a great deal about them. However, because of the ever busy schedules of both the clinicians and principals, it is usually difficult to develop truly collaborative relationships. Related to these factors, and to employment by an outside agency, clinicians may receive less than adequate support for their efforts, and it is not uncommon for clinical staff to operate without phones, in poorly furnished and nonprivate offices, and to be unable to access administrative support services of the school such as secretaries, copy machines, and fax machines.

To decrease the likelihood of this scenario, we have found it useful for clinicians to diplomatically persist in their efforts to meet with school principals and other administrative staff to keep them apprised of mental health efforts. In this process it is useful to share reports of clinical activity, and highlight benefits to the school by documenting service effectiveness in relation to such factors as school grades and absences. We have also found joint planning with principals to bring additional resources into the school, for example, through collaborative completion of grant applications which goes a long way toward solidifying the relationship, by "showcasing" pragmatic skills of clinicians.

Developing solid relationships with teachers is yet another important, and often difficult, process. As mentioned, it is becoming increasingly common for health and mental health services in schools to be provided by collaborating, community agencies. Since practitioners are not hired by the educational system, they may be viewed as "outsiders" by other school staff. Another issue is that teachers and others may associate mental health services with stigma, and in some communities there is low tolerance for emotional/behavioral disturbance in youth, often associated with a "pull yourself up by your bootstraps" mentality. An additional side of this problem is that teachers are especially likely to refer acting out youth to mental health staff. Unfortunately, these youth may be the most likely to be absent from school or classes making it difficult for the clinician to have any impact, and may be the least amenable to change. Teachers often desire very fast, if not immediate, results when referring youth for SMH services, and are consequently disappointed when acting out youth do not change after referral.

One method to improve relationships with teachers, and to assist them in developing realistic expectations for mental health services, is to hold a series of didactic, interactive, and lively presentations throughout the year on mental health problems and interventions. An additional important focus of these presentations is to assist teachers in identifying behavior patterns that may signal internalizing emotional disturbances in youth, leading to enhanced detection of these problems, and subsequent referral. Schools represent the best site for mounting preventive interventions for youth; training teachers to detect expressions of emotional disturbance and to identify behavior problems early is a critically important function that offers vast potential for improved detection of these problems in youth.

Addressing Stigma and Ensuring Confidentiality

Mental health practitioners working in schools often confront stigma and poor understanding of their services by teachers, and this problem is particularly true for students. In general, students have little idea what the titles, "psychiatrist," "psychologist," or even "social worker" mean. Even the title, "therapist" is misunderstood by many youth. Two titles that seem more understandable are "doctor" and "counselor," and therefore we use these titles in our work in the schools, in spite of their ambiguity since "counselor" is the same title used by guidance counselors. However, our experience has been that no matter how careful the clinician is, word often gets out to the student body about his or her role. Some students do not wish to be associated with the clinician, for fear of being labeled "crazy." This speaks to the need for additional precautions to maintain stidents' privacy in their contacts with the school-based therapist by scheduling student arrivals to, and departures from, the counseling office to occur in between classes.

In addition to these privacy issues, there are unique confidentiality issues in school-based practice. In schools, there is usually a fairly open exchange of information about students between teachers and administrative staff, and frequently these staff members will query the clinician for information about referred students. In handling these requests, our policy has been to attempt to gain permission from the student before talking to a staff member, or limiting information given out to observations of the student (versus verbal content of sessions), or on the process of treatment (e.g., whether the student is attending appointments or not). We keep our records separate from educational and school health records in locked and secure file cabinets, and will only release information with appropriate consent by the student and parent.

Family Involvement in Services

Another major issue is the difficulty clinicians encounter in involving families in SMH efforts. Unlike CMHCs, where some level of ongoing parental involvement is often necessary (e.g., to register youth for treatment, transport them to sessions), school-based clinicians may see youth with minimal, if any parental involvement beyond providing consent for services. In our program, parental consent for services is routinely obtained for youth under 16 years, and most of the time for youth 16 and older. However, Maryland law indicates that youth 16 and older may independently consent for services, and in many cases, such independent consent is obtained. Usually, in these cases, there is noteworthy family pathology, and a goal of treatment is to help the adolescent develop functional barriers between himself or herself and disturbed family members, while pursuing a plan to become independent.

However, even with younger children, we often encounter difficulties in involving family members, which impedes assessment and treatment efforts. Limited family involvement in SMH services is a particular problem. Economically disadvantaged families confront numerous obstacles to being involved in SMH services, including elevated life stress, transportation difficulties, and child care problems. The functional impact of this is that many times the therapist's involvement with families is limited to phone calls and occasionally home visits. The problems of limited family involvement in SMH services is receiving increased attention, and programs are beginning to develop proactive strategies to bring parents to schools, for example, by providing support groups, and child development/management classes to parents on site.

AN INSIDE LOOK AT CLINICAL PRACTICE IN THE SCHOOLS

In CMHCs, a common scenario is for seven or eight children to be scheduled per day for each therapist, and, in reality, only three to five 50-minute sessions are actually held because of high noncompliance. Mental health services usually have a discrete beginning and end, and, with managed care, services are often limited to six or less sessions. Children require clear diagnoses to be seen, and if they do not present clear diagnoses, they are either "creatively" fit into a diagnostic category or not seen. After termination, the therapist is unlikely to see the child again. Although this may reflect a stereotyping of children's outpatient mental health services, it begins to capture the reality of such services for most therapists.

Mental health services provided in schools are often dramatically different from the previous picture for CMHCs. In most school-based programs, children do not require diagnoses to be seen. Following intake sessions, whcih may run 50 minutes, students are seen for briefer therapeutic periods of time, such as 30 or even 15 minutes. Many of these sessions are scheduled, others are impromptu, with students stopping in for a brief problem-solving session, or to share some news with the therapist. Given that the therapist is where the children are, there is no reason for down time in his or her schedule; if one student does not show for an appointment, usually another one can be quickly scheduled. The school therapist has contact with students not only in the therapy office, but in the hallway, at school-wide events, assemblies, athletic games, and in the cafeteria. Given these environmental factors, it is not uncommon for school-based therapists to see 10 to 12 children in a seven-hour day. Over the course of a 10-month academic year, a full-time clinician may see 150 students, and have over 800 clinical contacts for assessment or treatment.

Moreover, relationships with students do not have to be "terminated," often lasting from the 6th through 8th, or 9th through 12th grades. Sometimes, youths are seen for longer periods, as they drop into the neighborhood school to fill the clinician in on developments in their life. In such long-term relationships, at times clinicians are providing traditionally conceived therapy services, but at other times when there are no clear presenting problems, the therapist becomes more of a mentor to the student, providing encouragement and practical support. This transitioning back and forth from the role of therapist to mentor is neither possible, nor feasible, in community mental health clinics or in private practice.

To highlight what it is like to provide mental health services to youth in schools, I recently tracked all clinical activities during one randomly selected late winter day in a Baltimore high school in one of the more improverished and crime-ridden sections of the city, where I have worked for five years. In the following, I emphasize clinical problems presented to me on that day not including discussion of my interventions:

8:45 a.m.–9.35 a.m. Individual session with a 17-year-old girl who has a history of severe family instability, abuse, and neglect, and who is currently homeless related to a conflict with her boyfriend. She presents with major depression with vague suicide ideation.

9:45 a.m.–10:16 a.m. Intake session with a 14-year-old girl who was referred by one of the clinic nurses related to reported depression and grief over the death of her grandmother six weeks ago. The student's grieving appears normative, and she is doing well otherwise, maintaining good grades and involved in a number of school clubs.

10:17 a.m.–10:30 a.m. Drop-in visit by an 18-year-old girl with whom I have worked intensively. She is doing remarkably well as a candidate for 12th grade valedictorian, after presenting with major depression and suicidal ideation two years prior following her *14th* foster placement secondary to her mother's serious addiction to cocaine and inability to provide for her family. She excitedly informs me of her positive living situation in an independent living program and her college plans.

10:31 a.m.–11:17 a.m. Intake session with an 18-year-old girl who reports extreme life stress of raising her 1-year-old daugther, severely conflicted family relations, working 30 hours per week, and doing poorly in school, with symptoms of depression, anxiety, and nervousness.

11:21 a.m.–11:35 a.m. Drop-in visit by a 16-year-old boy whom I have seen for around a year. He meets diagnostic criteria for conduct disorder and substance abuse using marijuana multiple time per day, admits to stealing cars, is probably dealing drugs and carrying weapons, and will likely fail the 9th grade for the second time.

11:36 a.m.–11:50 a.m. Waiting for an 11:30 a.m. appointment who does not show, I meet in the hallway a 16-year-old girl with whom I have been working with for about a year, and invite her into my office. She has a grossly disfiguring medical condition that has been essentially neglected since birth related to her mother's polysubstance addiction. Currently, she has a highly conflicted relationship with mother related to the substance abuse, which has resulted in the student becoming homeless. Child protective services has been involved with the case based on my initiation, but the home situation remains unchanged.

12:05 p.m.–12:37 p.m. Drop-in visit by a 15-year-old boy whom I have not seen for around one month related to school absences. He meets criteria for Post-traumatic stress disorder related to the chronic and severe violence he has witnessed and experienced such as being "stuck up" twice and "banked" (beat up by a group) three times in his drug-infested neighborhood. He is often absent from school related to fear and avoidance of violence. He is doing very poorly in school and will likely fail the 9th grade. He reports that his father and three brothers are incarcerated for homicide and drug charges and "every other boy" he knows in his neighborhood is in some way involved with drugs.

12:42 p.m.–1:05 p.m. Brief individual session with a 15-year-old boy who is receiving poor grades and is frequently absent from school related to the severe taunting that he experiences from other students. Cruelty toward him by other students appears to be related to his physical handicap from cerebral palsy, his very short stature, and significant problems with vision and hearing.

1:05 p.m.–1:46 p.m. Intake session with a 15-year-old girl who is frequently absent from school related to not having "enough clothes to wear." She describes erratic behavior by her mother that suggests a psychotic condition, she feels confused and distressed about her mother's behavior, and is unable to focus on her schoolwork when she attends.

1:50 p.m.–2:42 p.m. Group session with five of seven members of a support group that has been meeting since the beginning of the past academic year. The group contains girls who are either sophomores or juniors in an accelerated college preparatory track. Each has experienced past and/or current family trauma and dysfunction, including sexual abuse, functional neglect, and parental substance abuse. All five girls are doing reasonably well today; we discuss problems that two of them are having with their boyfriends, and that one is having with her parents' marital conflict.

To summarize, in this intense but fairly typical day, 14 students were seen during school hours. Because of the demand and my limited time in the school, I usually do not take a lunch, which is consistent with the practices of many other school-based clinicians. I had nine individual sessions, three of which were intakes, and one group therapy with five students. These students were contending with serious problems such as homelessness, family deaths, family conflict, incarceration of family members, family mental illness, violence, abuse and neglect, exposure to substance use and dealing, taunting from other students, and physical problems. In relation to these conditions, students reported emotional difficulties including depression, anxiety, and nervousness, and behavioral problems including cutting classes, skipping school, stealing, fighting, and using drugs. This snapshot of one day of clinical practice in the schools highlights key elements of such practice, including the clinical intensity, flexibility in scheduling and seeing students from 15-minute, to more standard 50-minute sessions, enhanced accessibility to the therapist with three drop-in visits, and the improved capacity for long-term relationships with students.

CONCLUSION

Three issues stand out as needing immediate attention for SMH services to advance. First is the development of quality assurance guidelines for SMH programs. Beginning guidelines have been formulated for school health programs, as they have been for child mental health programs; but as yet, guidelines for SMH services are lacking. Second, SMH programs need to document treatment effectiveness. Although there have been a handful of studies assessing the treatment outcome of these programs (e.g., Weist, Paskewitz, Warner, & Flaherty, in press), very few programs have systems in place to monitor the impact of ongoing clinical services. Educational systems are particularly interested in documenting academic and school-related (e.g., attendance rates) benefits of SMH services, and such eveluation should be prioritized.

Third, *stable* funding mechanisms need to be pursued. As reviewed earlier, managed care is having negative impacts on SMH programs, to the point that some have closed down. Issues pertaining to funding for SMH programs in the managed care environment need to be resolved, and other innovative finding strategies must be explored, such as the example of the State of Massachusetts which funds school health programs through an excise tax on tobacco (Schlitt, Rickett, Montgomery, & Leer, 1994). These three issues stand out because they affect the survival of SMH programs, with each issue logically leading into the next. That is, high-quality programs should prove to be effective; documenting effectiveness should assist in procuring stable funding.

Beyond issues relating to the survival of SMH services, there are innumerable need areas. These include:

- forming better linkages between mental health services within schools, and between schools and outside agencies
- developing standardized assessment measures and databases across SMH programs in different localities and states
- identifying differing SMH needs for youth of various ages, cultural backgrounds, and geographic regions
- forging better links between education and mental health staff, and developing strategies to assist teachers in identifying youth with emotional/behavioral disturbances

- developing a broader array of preventive services, increasing SMH services in elementary levels, and extending them to preschool programs, and
- developing SMH specialization guidelines for the disciplines of psychology, psychiatry, social work, and psychiatric nursing.

Fortunately, efforts are underway to address each of these need areas, including: a) recent federal funding for two technical assistance centers at the University of Maryland at Baltimore, and the University of California, Los Angeles focus on advancement of SMH services, b) initiatives of the Psychosocial Services Section of the newly formed National Assembly on School-Based Health Care, and c) the development of task forces and working groups aimed at expanding and improving SMH services in professional organizations such as the American Psychological Association, the American Psychiatric Association, the American Academy of Child and Adolescent Psychiatry, and the National Association of Social Workers. However, these efforts just scratch the surface of the groundswell of activity in the United States to expand SMH services. Opportunities for clinical involvement, program development of, and research in, school-based mental health services are limitless.

Appreciation is extended to Lois Flaherty and Beth Warner for ideas generated in an earlier paper. Supported in part by project #MCJ24SH02-01-0 from the Maternal and Child Health Bureau (Title V, Social Security Act), Health Resources and Services Administration, U.S. Department of Health and Human Services.

REFERENCES

Adelman, H. S., & Taylor, L. (1993). School-based mental health: Toward a comprehensive approach. *Journal of Mental Health Administration, 20*, 32–45.

Advocates for Youth. (1994). Unpublished survey of school-based and school-linked health services. Washington, DC: the Author.

Conoley, J. C., & Conoley, C. W. (1991). Collaboration for child adjustment: Issues for school- and clinic-based child psychologists. *Journal of Consulting and Clinical Psychology, 59*, 821–829.

Day, C., & Roberts, M. C. (1991). Activities of the Children and Adolescent Service System Program for improving mental health services for children and families. *Journal of Clinical Child Psychology, 20*, 340–350.

Dryfoos, J. G. (1988). School-based health clinics: Three years of experience. *Family Planning Perspectives, 20*, 193–200.

Dryfoos, J. G. (1994). *Full-service schools*. San Francisco: Jossey-Bass.

Flaherty, L. T., Weist, M. D., & Warner, B. S. (in press). School-based mental health services in the United States: History, current models, and needs. *Community Mental Health Journal*.

Office of Technology Assessment, United States Congress. (1991). *Adolescent health*. Washington, DC: U.S. Government Printing Office.

Schlitt, J. J., Rickett, K. D., Montgomery, L. L., & Lear, J. G. (1994). *State initiatives to support school-based health centers*. Washington, DC: Making the Grade.

School Health Policy Initiative. (1993). *Ingredients for success: Comprehensive school-based health centers*. Bronx, NY: the Author.

Weist, M. D., Paskewitz, D. A., Warner, B. S., & Flaherty, L. T. (1996). Treatment outcome of school-based mental health services for urban teenagers. *Community Mental Health Journal, 32*, 149–157.

Weist, M. D., Proescher, E. L., Freedman, A. H., Paskewitz, D. A., & Flaherty, L. T. (1995). School-based health services for urban adolescents: Psychosocial characteristics of clinic users versus nonusers. *Journal of Youth and Adolescence, 24*, 251–265.

Weist, M. D. (1997). Expanded school mental health services: A national movement in progress. In T. H. Ollendick & R. J. Prinz (Eds.), *Advances in clinical child psychology*. pp. 319–348. New York and London: Plenum Press.

Weisz, J. R., Weiss, B., & Donenberg, G. R. (1992). The lab versus the clinic. *American Psychologist, 47*, 1578–1595.

Chapter 28

Finding Our Way Home: Home- and Community-Based Care

Charles Oseroff, M.D., Michael Longo, M.A., and
Ilene Joseph, L.C.S.W.C.

INTRODUCTION

As we approach the end of the 20th century, it appears that the pendulum of treatment system design has begun to swing in a new direction. The effect of system reform on psychiatric service delivery has been to challenge the existing approach to care with the belief that the best treatment is that which occurs in the natural setting, that good "intensive care" is possible in community-based settings, and that services must be organized to respond consistently to the ever-changing needs of young patients. Essential program components include creating partnerships with families and bringing services to the home and community, supporting the strengths of the child and family within the context of familial, institutional, and cultural systems, and having a range of flexible services and a case management approach that allows for the continual individualization of care. Care is defined as unconditional, meaning that the approach to unsuccessful care is to change the structure of the care rather than eject the child. The principles of cultural competence are applied to the system of care as well. The basic processes outlined to accomplish these goals include interagency collaboration, case management and coordination, provision of individualized wraparound services, and a flexible funding stream where dollars follow the child instead of vice-versa (England, 1992; Katz-Leavy, 1992).

In practice, this has led to the creation of a variety of programs whose staff meet with the identified patient and family in their home and other community sites and provide an array of creative and community-based supports and treatments including crisis intervention, psychiatric hospital diversion, out-of-home respite care, individual therapy, psychopharmacological treatment, intensive family therapy, case management, extended family and community outreach, parent education and training, advocacy, one-to-one staff assignments during and after school, and homemaker services. In most programs services can be accessed 24 hours a day, seven days a week and are generally delivered over a one- to six-month period with up to 20 hours a week of face-to-face contact in the home provided in some models. The treatment approach may be psychoeducational, behavioral, cognitive, strategic, or systems-oriented. Regardless of the program or its philosophical orientation, meeting families where they live can have a substantial impact on the treatment.

The Intensive Family Treatment Program in Baltimore, Maryland, had referred to it a 16-year-old patient who had had 10 psychiatric hospitalizations since finding her mother shot to death when she was 5 years old. It was starkly revealed to the first care providers to ever visit the home that not only had the deceased mother's bedroom become the patient's bedroom, but nothing inside or outside the house had been changed, maintained, or repaired since the mother's murder. As the case progressed with numerous meetings in the home and the clinic, unresolved feelings and unrealistic expectations of the caretaking grandparents were clarified. As the family's grief issues and the struggle over protection were illuminated, the nature of their relationships, the child's behavior, and even the house began to take on a new appearance.

OUTCOME ANALYSIS

Follow-up data suggest that home-based services are here to stay. Most programs report high rates of success in providing concrete services, stabilizing crises, and providing alternatives to out-of-home placement. For example, the Family Preservation Initiative of Baltimore City, which uses the Homebuilders Model and wraparound services, reports that 90 percent of children referred to them at imminent risk for removal were maintained in their homes for one year after the initiation of service (Hyde & Woodworth, 1994). The Family Services Research Center at the Medical University of South Carolina describes high rates of treatment success in a series of replicable, controlled studies with adolescent substance abusers and juvenile delinquents using a family-based, multisystemic approach (Henggeler, 1990, 1996). Both programs work intensively with children and their families in their homes, their schools, and wherever necessary in their communities to establish supportive and therapeutic linkages.

INQUIRY

There is considerable debate within the field, however, regarding how to interpret the generally positive findings. Program quality and design and the complicated relationship of intervention to long-term aftercare are difficult to quantify. Global outcome measures have not been standardized nor have control groups been used in the majority of studies. There is also active debate as to the cost-effectiveness of in-home intervention which has been addressed in a only a small number of studies, although alternatives to out-of-home placement appear to be less costly in the short-run (Nelson & Landsman, 1992; Rivera & Kutash, 1994; Santos, 1995).

At this point in the development of in-home intervention there are a series of questions that need to be asked to begin to place both enthusiasm and accomplishments in perspective. As many of the successful in-home programs are tied to progressive systems of care which offer significantly more resources, options, and case management, what positive effects can we attribute to in-home treatment, and what to overall systems reform? How is imminent risk for removal defined and operationalized consistently across a broad population of children, communities, and treatment systems? How do we really know that a given child would not have gone into care without provision of the designated service? How can we sort out the mobilizing effects on the family and the system of simply not removing a child? What is the impact of kinship care on placement prevention statistics? How do we assess which family is best matched with which kind of service? How is it determined which children should be placed out of their homes? Would it be more effective to place those children immediately and redefine service delivery for them? Is this current system of children and families needing to fail in the least restrictive educational and treatment placement to receive more intensive services in fact undermining those we seek to help? In supporting the delivery of services that are not quickly effective are we not creating obstacles for children and families that are increasingly difficult to overcome? Additional questions need to be asked as we look at the relationship of system reform to the existing systems of care and the issue of funding. What is the relationship of an in-home program to other care providers and social service institutions? Who defines the relationship? How is the relationship understood in terms of the developmental status of the family, the community, the society, and the providers? How does the family understand the relationship of service delivery to its own developmental struggle with dependency and autonomy? What are the risks and benefits to the family and the community for each type of in-home service? How do in-home services, their implementation, and their development impact on family competency and system reform?

MANAGED CARE

Questions about in-home treatment programs and their value are seen most clearly within the context of managed care. To be funded in both public and private managed care environments, in-home treatment programs will need to demonstrate significant clinical and cost effectiveness. This has been less of an issue to date in the public sector and with grant-funded programs because of their unique funding streams and the impact of projected savings from out-of-home and out-of-state placement diversions. However, public sector funding has shifted in many states from grant-based to managed care contract-funded such as with the Medicaid waiver. Whatever the funding source, treatment programs will undoubtedly evolve into more sophisticated provider networks that offer a greater variety of services. There may one day very soon be a single point of entry into the service delivery system and, ultimately, case management will be tied more closely to outcome measures and the efficiency of service delivery.

HOSPITAL DIVERSION: A SYSTEMIC APPROACH

An interesting debate in the shift to in-home or community-based treatment has been whether or not children should be kept in their homes specifically at the time of crisis. Traditionally this is a time when out-of-home placement risk is high. We will describe an innovative approach to in-home intervention, crisis intervention, case management, and psychiatric hospital diversion that proposes a clinically effective and cost-effective way to manage risk in crisis situations. This approach was first developed in Boston, by Longo and Tolomiczenko (1991), as a pilot project for the Massachusetts Department of Mental Health. The initial program succeeded in reducing inpatient admissions by over 90 percent for a population of children who had previously averaged over 100 days of inpatient care. This model utilizes the principles of narrative therapy, an approach to treatment that focuses on the family's language and the story of their relationship to the presenting problem (White & Epston, 1989; White, 1988, 1989). The treatment focuses on the relationship between the family, those trying to help them, and the effort to create change. Rather than looking primarily at the client's presenting crisis, a team of experienced family therapists focuses on broadening their work to include the language and the story of the crises of the child, the family, and everyone involved in the effort to provide help.

The task of the therapy team in this model is to understand in people's own words both the presenting crisis and its relationship to a second-order pattern of crisis which includes the failure, frustration, and worry that has become part of previously unsuccessful attempts at change. Uncovering the second-order crisis, the pattern of failure and frustration, is the first step in a conversation in which new understanding may emerge. Families and treatment providers must "step back" and look at the process of their working together and the second-order crisis that is imbedded within it so they may begin to redefine the problem, look more realistically at their relationships, and then reshape their work together. For treatment to be successful, the manner in which everyone involved approaches the attempt to help and the wish for change must shift.

This approach to treatment can be utilized to divert hospitalization, assist in hospital stepdown, or for case consultation. Treatment is voluntary and sessions are held in the home, the hospital, or other community settings. Therapists are available around the clock for consultation or intervention. Case management services, brief respite care, and psychiatric consultation are provided as needed.

Currently, Choate Health Management and Arbour Health Systems in Massachusetts use family teams as part of a continuum of managed care services. In Baltimore, the Intensive Family Treatment Program (IFT) at the Children's Guild serves children who had previously been admitted to the Carter Center, the state-run psychiatric unit for latency-age children, and in Delaware, the State Department of Children, Youth and Families at the Terry Children's Psychiatric Center is applying systemic narrative therapy to case management and hospital diversion. To date, these programs have been successful in treating between 85 percent and 95 percent of their high-risk clients in the community without the need for psychiatric hospitalization (Fassler, Hanson-Mayer, & Brenner, 1996).

THE SYSTEM AS THE CLIENT

Many clients referred for treatment have a history of multiple problems, multiple treatment providers, and long-standing treatment failure. Many times there is a family history of substance abuse, trauma, and multisystem involvement. Carefully looking at the larger pattern of crisis can help uncover the reasons for treatment failure. Exploring familial patterns over generations may highlight new and helpful aspects of the presenting crisis. The extended family and significant community members are included in the telling of the family story. Similarly, current and past treatment providers are interviewed to hear what it has been like to work with the family and to be experiencing the treatment crisis.

The following case exemplifies the importance of understanding the different beliefs about change of those involved in a treatment crisis:

During a brief consultation at the family's request about the need to hospitalize a 12-year-old female client who was oppositional and staying out at night, it became clear that the adoptive mother, daughter, and therapist each had different ideas about what it would take for things to change. Each saw the other as resistant. The mother held a religious-based idea of change; that her adoptive daughter would wake up one day and have "seen the light" and no longer misbehave. The therapist believed in weekly family therapy in which change would take place slowly. The daughter believed that her mother was the one who needed to change and that she would be changed by the therapist setting her straight.

Everyone was frustrated with each other and the effort to create change. The consultation focused on a conversation about how much patience true change required, that is, what kinds of change were worth waiting for. Following the intervention the group decided to spend more time talking about their expectations for each other, the pace of their work together, and the different supports each of them needed as part of the change process. The child's acting out behavior decreased and she remained in the home.

SAFETY CONCERNS

Risk management for in-home work in this context has several aspects. The first is that the team must determine quickly whether or not there is serious danger of injury or harm without hospitalization. To do this, as with any therapy, the team must assess the ability of the family and the treatment system to tolerate the anxiety generated by the crisis in order to bring to light the underlying beliefs, expectations, and assumptions that have put a lock on the group's power to change. Safety concerns are addressed at the level of the therapy team and the larger program team in consultation with the child psychiatrist.

The psychiatrist functions as a full team member and looks both at the child through the eyes of the team and at everything that surrounds the child at the level of the family, the system, and the family team. Safety can be effectively monitored and planned for as long as the team's conversations with the family, the treatment system, and each other are understood in the context of the team's ideas about the second-order crisis. The psychiatrist may interview the child directly or participate in a family or systems meeting if more information is needed.

In practice, the impact on the family of meeting the therapeutic team, the therapeutic interviewing approach to the crisis taken by the team, and the on-demand availability of the therapists and respite care change how the family experiences the crisis. This positively affects their ability to use help and manage the situation safely. In the context of this kind of user-friendly, therapeutic interface, families are empowered to understand themselves and the pattern of crisis and respond to both in new and helpful ways. The involvement of an ongoing treatment provider is crucial. The catalytic effect of the team's work occurs in the context of the existing treatment.

THE TEAM

The use of a team of cotherapists is crucial to the success of this kind of intensive therapy. Most cases are extremely complicated and demanding and tend to pull treatment providers in a certain direction or generate intense feelings of frustration, anger, or resentment. With this model the therapy teams are able to function in a thoughtful and helpful way, even under extraordinary circumstances. With the lead therapist asking questions and eliciting the family story, the cotherapist is able to look at and reflect on other aspects of the family story and the help-giving process. The team's clinical performance is predicated upon being able to explore continuously their reactions to the family and the family's treatment story during team meetings and even during sessions. The team members must be committed to sharing their personal and emotional experience of the work with each other, and oftentimes with the patient, family, and other providers. It is important that the team members have permission to question their own and each others' assumptions, beliefs, and struggles concerning change. This commitment is based on the belief that each team member's inner experience and the struggles between team members mirror patterns within the family and the treatment failure that need to be understood and externalized for treatment to proceed. The question needing to be asked to track hidden issues and potential treatment impasses is what is the team's relationship to any unspoken conversation? This team process becomes the vehicle which drives case reviews, treatment planning, interventions, and case management.

A family who presented for treatment because of the aggressive acting out behavior of their son appeared to be struggling with longstanding grief over the death of several extended family members. However, they were unable to talk about how they felt, and they could not see the impact of that on their son's behavior. The team therapists were able to share the family's profound sense of sadness and loss with each other during their twice weekly case review and move past their initial feelings of anger and frustration over the family's resistance to treatment. One team therapist was particularly moved by the family's experience. The child's mother appeared most connected with the same team member. In an extended family meeting the therapist shared her feelings and the cotherapist helped the family members verbalize and compare how they felt once the feeling had been planfully introduced. Subsequently, they were able to respond more realistically to the child's behavior.

CASE EXAMPLE

The following case is an example of a presenting crisis that has over time become embedded with a sense of treatment failure. J., a 15-year-old female patient, had been hospitalized six times in the past year for behavior suicidal threats, superficial cutting, running away, and threatening classmates in school. In each of J.'s hospitalizations, it was felt that her depression and how she expressed her anger needed to change. J.'s family had a two-generational history of alcohol abuse and trauma. Her paternal uncle committed suicide five years ago and her father was currently drinking, though struggling to stop. The family had been in treatment with a family therapist for one year. Her parents described themselves as "at the end of their rope." They were not sure that J. could live at home any longer.

The therapist believed that the family did not want to participate in treatment because, "... they don't really say anything." In response to the current crisis the school social worker believed that J. must be sent to residential treatment. The therapist and the social worker both believed that J. was depressed and had a major problem with control and they questioned whether she had a personality disorder. The school teacher felt "ineffective and scared." The social worker summarized the situation by saying, "we cannot provide any stability during these crises, the managed care company will not allow us enough treatment to be effective. Between the family not wanting treatment and the managed care company not allowing it we're stuck."

Creating a Conversation   Though J. was the identified patient, the team believed that her family and her treatment providers were also in crisis and in search of help. Rather than feeling responsible for changing J. and feeling compelled to take her and the responsibility for treating her away through hospitalization, the team worked quickly to create a conversation with the family and their treatment providers about their feelings and their worries.

Team Therapist: How does the fear you have heard the family therapist and school (to mother) talk about compare to the fear your husband is struggling with?

Mother: It's the same.

Team Therapist: How does being surrounded by fear affect your ability to go on? (to mother)

Mother: I don't know whom to turn to for strength. I always believed I could do it on my own. Now I'm not so sure.

Team Therapist: If you were more certain about where you could find strength, how would it affect your ability to face the fear that has invaded your family's life?

Mother: If I was stronger I could face anything.

Team Therapist: What is it like to hear that mother would face anything if she had (to family therapist) the strength?

Family Therapist: It's encouraging. I was not sure that you wanted to (to mother).

Team Therapist: How does your strength compare to your wife's? (to father)

Father: It's almost the same, a little less.

Team Therapist: When you feel you cannot take it anymore, who do you look to? (to social worker)

Social Worker: I call the insurance company.

Team Therapist: Who else?

Social Worker: I'm not sure.

Team Therapist: What is it like for J. to have the adults in her life not sure where they can (to father and mother) find the strength they need to face the difficulties that have invaded your family?

Father: It's terrible. She must believe we're giving up on her. She's afraid of being sent somewhere.

J.: (in tears) I guess so.

This case illustrates how a family and their helpers can be helped to look at hidden obstacles to treatment success. In this case the team was able to illuminate an immobilizing feeling of fear in the family and their treatment providers and highlight their shared belief that there was no one to turn to. This is an example of a second-order crisis. It was clear that the way the system responded to the presence of fear increased feelings of frustration and hopelessness which in turn undermined the work. In this case, as in many, the request for acute services was based on the lack of treatment success.

Team Therapist: If mother was able to find the strength that she was looking for (to social worker) and finally face the fear that has been part of the family for some time, what would that be like for you?

Social Worker: I would begin to feel more confident.

Team Therapist: If the confidence of the professionals in your family began to grow, how would it (to father and mother) affect the two of you?

Father: Finally we would feel that we were getting somewhere.

Mother: Yes.

Team Therapist: How would it affect your work if your colleagues became more confident? (to teacher)

Teacher: I would know that I could count on someone. I'd be less afraid to set limits on J.

Re-Storying the Treatment   Inviting family and treatment team members to become curious about each other's experience relative to the team's informed questioning creates meaningful and moving conversations about real family and treatment events and relationships. Instead of experiencing their therapists and other helpers as trying to correct a problem they have all become too familiar with, they experience a collective effort of generating new descriptions and understanding the meaning that these new descriptions hold for everyone involved. The treatment providers often move from a position of failed experts who have no answers to that of energized collaborators with feelings, questions, and new ideas. Help is experienced as a creative and expansive process rather than a reductionistic, problem-solving one as in a more dependency-based model where treatment is prescribed and alternative possibilities are limited. Being genuinely curious about people's experience allows these new descriptions to unfold into new treatment stories in which family and treatment provider struggles are seen in a different light. Relationships become strengthened in the process and new ideas about what can change, what needs to change, how things could change, and what change would mean emerge.

Team Therapist: When did you first come to believe that confidence was an (to mother) important ingredient in your life?

Mother: When I was 11 years old. My father would drink and then I would hear my parents fighting. I was scared but I looked out for my younger brothers and sisters. One night I heard my father hitting my mother. I ran downstairs and started screaming until he stopped. I promised myself that this would never happen to my family.

Team Therapist: You found the confidence to face what you were most afraid of, to make a stand.

Mother: Yes.

Team Therapist: How did you face your brother's suicide? (to father)

Father: With difficulty. I was close to him. We used to go fishing all the time. Now I think about the times we spent together.

Team Therapist: You have managed to remember the good times even in the face of your brother's death.

Father: Yes.

Team Therapist: Did you know that mother was able to face the violence (to social worker) to her family even though she was afraid?

Social Worker: No. I never heard this before.

Team Therapist: Did you know that father had the ability to hold onto something good even when (to family therapist) things around him feel really bad?

Social Worker: I hadn't heard that before either.

Team Therapist: If they made a decision once again to face the fear and violence that threatens their family, and hold on to something good would you join them?

Social Worker: Yes, I would try.

Family Therapist: Yes, finally we could get somewhere.

Team Therapist: What's it like to hear that the social worker and the family therapist (to mother and father) are prepared to face these things with you?

Father: It gives me hope.

Mother: Yes.

In this case, as in many, the loss of hope had everyone turning to J. with the expectation that there was something within her that was broken and needed to be fixed. What kept the cycle of hospitalizations intact was the second-order crisis, the unresolved struggle by the adults with their reactions to J. and her behavior. The family story of the struggle to be confident, and their forgotten success in facing disaster with confidence shifted the nature of the treatment and the expectations for change. The system's struggle to remain confident mirrored the problem within the family. By creating a supportive context and taking the time to bring the family and the treatment providers together to explore the story of her treatment, it was possible after a five-session series of interventions for J. to remain at home and at school and for the family to continue their work with the family therapist. It is by this establishment of a process-oriented rather than a problem-oriented collaboration between families and their community of helpers that safety can be restored quickly.

Six months later J. continued in her school placement and had required neither additional crisis intervention by the team therapists nor out-of-home placement. Though her behavior was still challenging at times, the suicidal threats, gestures, and running away behavior had stopped. Her parents, the teacher, and the school social worker collaborated frequently by telephone and in meetings on how best to handle J. J.'s father stopped drinking two weeks after the crisis intervention meeting. Though father and mother were still fighting with each other about what was best for their children, they were no longer thinking about placing J. out of the home.

CONCLUSION

From a clinical perspective, the concept of unconditional care may well be the driving force behind the intensive system reform of the past several decades. The problem is no longer defined as the need to find a disposition for children, but, rather, as a need to challenge ourselves and our institutions to design flexible, comprehensive, and powerful systems which meet their changing needs where they live. Home-based and community-based services are in an exciting developmental stage. They are filled with promise. Their application changes the systems within which they function. Ultimately, clinical and cost effectiveness will determine the shape and design of these services in the 21st century.

A narrative approach to second-order crises in systems work has helped clarify that many times within the helplessness and hopelessness of treatment and system failure there exist the energy and the ability to change. The change process is most helpful when there is collaborative participation. In this model the system is seen as needing to function as it grows and to grow as part of its function. This is particularly important as the funding paradigm shifts to one of managed care in both public and private sectors.

At its worst managed care is feared as a rationalization for giving limited, poor care. At its best it can serve the function of raising the expectations and standards we have toward our work both individually and as a diverse, collaborative network. Until a seamless system of care exists with a wide range of easy-to-access therapeutic services and sophisticated, clinically based case management, in many cases quality of care will depend on experienced therapists and therapist teams who tackle the problems of their clients and the systems within which they are imbedded, with a therapeutic and process-based focus.

We wish to acknowledge and thank the clinicians who have participated in the development of the hospital diversion programs described in this chapter. Special thanks to Laura Fertig, Allison Obioha, and Charmaine Simms from Baltimore, Maryland; Anthony Irsfeld and Katherine Theobold from Boston, Massachusetts; and Sarah Chenkin, Sam Blumberg, Richard Cruz, and all of the clinicians from the Terry Children's Psychiatric Center in Delaware. We also wish to thank Stanley Mopsik from Baltimore; Julien Taplin, Anita Amurao, and Jean Dunn from Delaware; and Marcia Hoch, Roy Ettlinger, David Fassler, and Stuart Koman from Boston whose leadership made these programs possible.

REFERENCES

England, M. J. (1992). Building systems of care for youth with serious mental illness. *Hospital and Community Psychiatry, 43*, 630–633.

Fassler, D., Hanson-Mayer, G., & Brenner, E. (1996). Home-based care. Chapter in press. Boston: Choate Health Management, Inc.

Henggeler, S. W. (1990). *Family therapy and beyond: A multisystemic approach to treating behavior problems of children and adolescents.* Pacific Grove: Brooks/Cole.

Henggeler, S. W. (1996). Eliminating (almost) treatment dropout of substance abusing or dependent delinquents through home-based multisystemic therapy. *American Journal of Psychiatry, 153* (3), 427–428.

Hyde, K., & Woodworth, K. (1994). *Reforming services to children and families. The Family Preservation Initiative of Baltimore City, Inc., FY 1994 annual report.* Baltimore: Family Preservation Initiative.

Katz-Leavy, J. W. (1992). *Individualized services in a system of care.* Washington: CASSP Technical Assistance Center.

Longo, M. A., & Tolomiczenko, G. (1991). *Research project.* Boston: Massachusetts Department of Mental Health.

Nelson, K. E., & Landsman, M. J. (1992). *Alternative models of family preservation: Family-based services in context.* Springfield, IL: Charles C. Thomas.

Rivera, V. R., & Kutash, K. (1994). Crisis services. In V. R. Rivera & K. Kutash (Eds.), *Components of a system of care: What does the research say?* (pp. 101–114). Tampa: The Research and Training Center for Children's Mental Health.

Rivera, V. R., & Kutash, K. (1994). Case management services and individualized care. In V. R. Rivera & K. Kutash (Eds.), *Components of a system of care: What does the research say?* (pp. 115–139). Tampa: The Research and Training Center for Children's Mental Health.

Santos, A. B. (1995). Research on field-based services: Models for reform in the delivery of mental health care to populations with complex clinical problems. *American Journal of Psychiatry, 152* (8), 1111–1123.

White, M. (1988, 1989). The externalizing of the problem and the re-authoring of lives and relationships. Adelaide, Australia: Dulwich Centre Newsletter, Dulwich Centre Publications.

White, M., & Epston, D. (1989). *Literate means to therapeutic ends.* Adelaide, Australia: Dulwich Centre Publications.

Chapter 29

Therapeutic Nursery

Robinson J. Munoz-Millan, M.D. and Noreen J. Herbert, R.N.

HISTORICAL BACKGROUND

Nursery schools, the antecedents of therapeutic nurseries, were first established in England at the beginning of this century. Their goal was to offer preschoolers services to facilitate their social, emotional, and intellectual development. When transplanted to the United States, the model was enhanced by the importance attached to the participation of parents in the school program. Many nursery schools were developed in collaboration with universities and some contributed significantly to the understanding of child development. Nursery schools flourished in North America following the Depression and during the Second World War (Shonkoff & Meisels, 1990).

Of particular interest are therapeutic nurseries developed in the United States during the 1950s. One classical model is the nursery school developed by Dr. Anny Katan under the auspices of Western Reserve University (Furman & Katan, 1969). This program was conceived following psychoanalytic concepts and its tasks were to enhance psychosocial development and treat specific pathological conditions. The goals of the therapeutic nursery were the development of healthy personalities, the facilitation of the child's full use of innate potentials for work, play, and constructive relationships, and to assist in the satisfactory progression through age-appropriate developmental stages. The therapeutic nursery program had educational and therapy components.

The educational component focused on the milieu at the nursery. The therapeutic milieu offered a supportive structure with sensitive attention to daily living activities such as dressing, eating, toileting, and napping. Verbalization of feelings was encouraged as a means to enhance the ego's capacity for control of impulses and emotions and to facilitate the ego's capacity to differentiate reality from wishes and fantasies.

The therapy program included classical psychoanalysis and "therapy via the mother." This later form of treatment engaged the mother as therapist under the guidance of an analyst. The treatment was psychodynamic and used interpretation as the main therapeutic intervention. This innovative form of treatment delivery stemmed from the work of Freud with Little Hans, where the father was the actual therapist of the child.

While reviewing these historical precursors of today's therapeutic nurseries, it is relevant to see multiple antecedents of current practices and concepts. In this retrospective view, current practices may appear less new and less innovative. The goal of enhancing the social, emotional, and intellectual development of the child is as valid now as it was at the turn of the century. The participation of the parents in the design and implementation of the educational and therapeutic program has undergone many revisions but continues to be a fundamental pillar of our current model for delivery of services just as it was in the past.

Like those of the 1950s and 1960s, our current therapeutic nurseries' aim is to prevent the consolidation of risk behaviors into maladaptive patterns and to treat emotional-behavioral disorders. The contribution of the last quarter of the century is most apparent in two areas. One is the understanding in transactional (Sameroff, 1993) and ecological terms of development, the origin of behavioral and emotional disorders, and the application of these perspectives in the design of preventive and remedial interventions. Two, a corollary of this change in perspective is the shift in locus of service from the professional office to the community, including schools and the home.

HEAD START AND UNIVERSITY COLLABORATION

This chapter describes one model of mental services delivery to preschoolers. The model represents the collaboration between a Head Start setting, the Coldspring Family Development Center, and the Center for Infant Study, a program of the Department of Psychiatry of the University of Maryland at Baltimore (UMAB). The Center, dedicated to the treatment of infants and young children up to the age of five years, established a therapeutic nursery at a local Head Start center. The purpose was to offer expertise and services to the Head Start children and their families in a setting that would be familiar, accessible, and more significant to the clients than a clinic in another part of town would be.

THERAPEUTIC NURSERY PERSONNEL

The staff of the therapeutic nursery consists of a child and adolescent psychiatrist who is also the medical director, a nurse program coordinator, a clinical psychologist, and a development specialist. With the exception of the nurse program coordinator, the staff is part-time and each person dedicates eight hours a week to the nursery. The therapeutic nursery is part of the Center for Infant Study, an agency of the Division of Community Psychiatry, Department of Psychiatry, University of Maryland at Baltimore (UMAB). The child psychiatrist and the clinical psychologist are part of the faculty of the Department of Psychiatry, UMAB and they are responsible for the supervision of fellows in child psychiatry and psychology interns from the Division of Child and Adolescent Psychiatry, UMAB during their year-long rotation through the nursery. Therefore, the staff of the nursery reports to the Division of Community Psychiatry regarding clinical and administrative issues, and to the Division of Child and Infant Psychiatry regarding training issues.

All the therapeutic nursery staff is involved in consultation, diagnosis, and treatment of the referred students. Some division of labor does occur, with the child psychiatrist being in charge of the mental status examinations, the clinical psychologist overviewing the psychological testing, and the nurse program coordinator being involved in the outreach program. The nurse program coordinator also overviews general functioning of the nursery, coordinates clinical functions, interfaces with Head Start staff regarding referrals and treatment, and carries out quality assurance and utilization reviews.

The therapeutic nursery is funded in part by a grant from Baltimore Mental Health Systems. The program is also eligible for reimbursement by third-party payers for clinical services rendered. However, no child or family is denied services because of inability to pay or lack of medical insurance. In addition to the funds already mentioned, the program is applying for extramural grants to fund clinical research.

Physical Plant

The therapeutic nursery has space located in the administrative and multipurpose floor of the Head Start Center on the campus of the Pimlico Elementary School in Baltimore, Maryland. The overall space measures 500 square feet and consists of one large room with an area dedicated to an office and another equipped as a playroom. There is a small play area separated from the rest, which is used for individual therapy and private conversation. The therapeutic nursery shares with Head Start the use of a conference room and other multipurpose rooms, which are engaged for psychological testing, interviews with parents, and group and other meetings. Clinical work with children is carried out mostly in the classrooms.

The objectives of the therapeutic nursery overlap to a great extent with those of the Head Start program (Piotrkowski, Collins, Knitzer, & Robinson, 1994). Those shared objectives are to:

• promote emotional, cognitive, and social development in children, leading to their increased social competence.
• provide families and staff with pertinent information about child development to facilitate child rearing practices that enhance health and development.
• prevent consolidation of emotional and behavioral difficulties by early detection of risk indicators and the implementation by families, Head Start staff, and mental health professionals of programs that decrease risk behaviors and enhance coping with the environment.
• detect early symptomatic behavior, diagnose emotional-behavioral disorder, and facilite remediating interventions. These interventions are to be implemented by parents, Head Start staff, and mental health professionals acting in coordinated partnership.

Underlying Principles

Current models of service delivery propose the desirability of integrated programs in which the needs of children and their families are addressed comprehensively, without the artificial divisions and fragmentations imposed by different professional identities and practices. When the needs of the child are seen as organically interrelated and indivisible, the classical boundaries between education and health appear counterproductive and the need for close collaboration between disciplines becomes self-evident. A corollary of this view is the conviction that comprehensive interventions cannot be focused only on the individual child, but support and services must also be directed to the family (a two-generation program strategy), because the family represents the basic and essential context for the child's development (Halpern, 1990).

Current models of service delivery also propose the need to offer services that are ecologically oriented, emphasizing the adaptation of natural environmental factors to strengthen coping patterns and behaviors. In practical terms, this concept implies that the resolution of difficulties is not something that the professional does to and for the patients, but, instead, such resolution stems from enlisting resources and competencies in the child, the family, and the social group toward a more desirable relationship with the environment. In this model the mental health professional plays the role of catalyst and consultant (Piotrkowski, Collins, Knitzer, & Robinson, 1994). A corollary of such an approach is the necessity of providing the services in the natural context of the child and family—that is, their home, school, and community. In the same line, the use of normative activities which are self-reinforcing reduces the use of artificial rewards.

THERAPEUTIC NURSERY FUNCTIONS

The mental health professional brings to the team a specific quantum of expertise involving knowledge of (a) current concepts of child development, (b) the assessment of development and of behavior and emotional difficulties, and (c) up-to-date interventions to prevent and to treat emotional and behavioral symptoms and disorders.

Consultation Services

Consultation services on developmental issues are offered by the therapeutic nursery to Head Start parents and staff. Therapeutic nursery staff is available for consultation with Head Start parents regarding issues of development, child rearing, and the best way to optimize the child's use of his or her abilities and potentials. These consultations can be informal with one parent who wishes to discuss specific issues, or can be more structured in the form of group discussions around specific parenting issues. The therapeutic nursery organizes a series of group discussions throughout the year, focused but not limited to parenting information sharing. When successful, these group discussions touch on all areas of concern to the Head Start parents. These group discussions move from purely information sharing to truly supportive interactions where the expertise and experiences of parents are shared creatively.

Therapeutic nursery personnel are available on a daily basis to Head Start staff (e.g., teachers, family coordinators) to examine with them questions and issues that may arise from the observation of specific behaviors of the students. These issues may concern individual students or group phenomena in the classroom. In the case of specific students, whatever the concern (i.e., particularly intense separation anxiety, changes in the behavioral pattern, unusual behaviors such as compulsive rituals), the teacher, family coordinator, or other Head Start staff bring the observation to the therapeutic nursery staff for informal discussion. The goal is to put the behavior of concern into an understanding in terms of developmental expectations and of current environmental events that may precipitate or shape it. From this discussion several conclusions may be reached: the behavior can be recognized as within the normative range for that specific child, or it can be determined to be at variance from expectations and a working hypothesis is established regarding possible precipitants and antecedents. If the issue is considered relatively benign and restricted to a narrow area of functioning, interventions at the classroom level can be designed and the outcome assessed. Therapeutic nursery staff will be equally available to the parents for similar discussion and planning for parental interventions in the home. If the behavior is considered more serious and of a more complex nature, the issue is brought to the parents with the recommendation for further evaluation at the therapeutic nursery.

Assessment and Diagnosis

The mental health professional coordinates and participates in developmental assessment and diagnosis of behavioral-emotional difficulties.

The assessment of 3- and 4-year-old children has been discussed previously in this book (see chapter 5). Psychiatric assessment includes evaluation of the child's verbal, motor, and social competencies and of temperamental variables. This component may also include psychological testing, speech and hearing testing, and medical consultations when pertinent. Psychiatric assessment also includes an evaluation of the parent-child (caregiver-child) interaction both in terms of actual behavior and of the internal meaning that the child represents for the parent. It includes an evaluation of the family in terms of the role played by each parent regarding the actual caregiving. It also evaluates the support (or hindrance) that a parent may represent for the child rearing functions of the other parent. The role of siblings is evaluated and a review is undertaken of the environmental and social factors that impinge on the family and the child, either enhancing development and growth or representing risk elements. A global rating of the degree of vulnerability or resiliency is included.

When there are actual symptoms and the child meets criteria for a given *DSM-IV* diagnosis, this diagnosis is given. However, as important as diagnosis for the design of intervention and treatment is, the understanding of all factors impinging on this specific child and family. Factors from biological, psychological, and social systems are integrated into a coherent, dynamic, and coordinated formulation. This formulation aims at noting how these factors interact and the multiple forces that impinge upon the family, either supporting or detracting from positive interaction with the environment. This formulation is the consolidated outcome of the input from the child, the family, and staff from Head Start and therapeutic nursery. This formulation is the essential blueprint for all further interventions. The degree to which it is accurate and sensitive to social nuance will reflect on the success of the interventions.

Prevention and Treatment

The mental health professional applies up-to-date knowledge of therapeutic interventions to prevent and to treat emotional and behavioral difficulties. The preventive and actually therapeutic interventions intertwine, yet for the purposes of exposition they will be presented separately.

Prevention   Preventive interventions consist principally of a series of programs directed to all the children in a classroom and to their parents. These universal interventions address three specific behaviors: aggressive, shy/withdrawn, and inattentive behaviors. These clusters were selected because of their disruptive effect on the learning process and because of the undesirable long-term outcomes with which they are correlated (Yoshikawa, 1994). The child engaged in aggressive behavior does not attend to teachers' directions or the activities at hand. Consequently, aggressive children are less successful at participating in classroom activities and interfere with the effective classroom participation of all other children present. Aggressive behavior observed in the school is generally present in the home as well, disrupting family processes and preventing the family from maximizing the child's development in an atmosphere of nurturance and harmony.

From a long-term perspective, aggressive behavior in young children is a strong predictor for adolescent school dropout, alcoholism, drug abuse, and juvenile delinquency.

This predictive power is supported by significant and multiple research evidence (Kellam, Brown, Rubin, & Ensmiger, 1983; Loeber & Dishion, 1983; Rutter, 1982). This negative outcome is exponentially augmented when early childhood aggression presents in association with shy behavior and it predicts higher levels of delinquency and drug use in adolescence than does aggressive behavior alone (Kellam, Brown, Rubin, & Ensminger, 1983). On the other hand, children with attention deficits are particularly prone to be noncompliant, to engage in physically and verbally aggressive behaviors, and to disrupt the behavior of others. Prospective, longitudinal studies suggest that such children demonstrate a higher proportion of antisocial behavior and/or delinquency as adolescents. (Barkley, Fischer, Edelbrook, & Smallish, 1990; Farrington, Loeber, & Van Kamen, 1990).

Child-Focused Preventive Interventions   The ominous predictive correlation of these behaviors led to their selection as targets for preventive interventions. These interventions include a behavioral management program and social skills training. These programs are directed to all children in a classroom and are implemented by teachers and therapeutic nursery staff.

The behavioral management intervention is an implementation of a modified version of the Good Behavior Game (GBG), developed by Barrish, Saunders, and Wolf (1969). This protocol has been designed to be used in elementary school classrooms and adjusted to meet the needs of preschoolers. The GBG is a behavioral management strategy that promotes adaptive behavior by rewarding teams that meet specific standards. The children are divided in heterogenous teams and points are given to the teams for "good" behavior and taken away for disruptive behavior. While the game is in progress, the teacher assigns a checkmark on the blackboard next to the name of the team whenever one of its members displays a desirable behavior, and removes a mark whenever a disruptive behavior is displayed. The team that has more marks wins and obtains rewards such as stickers or erasers. Initially, the GBG is played for short periods of time (10 to 15 minutes) on two to three days a week. The duration and frequency of the games is increased progressively.

The social skills training includes the administration of the Interpersonal Cognitive Problem Solving program designed by Spivak and Shure (1982). This consists of a variety of sequenced games, discussion, and group interactive techniques organized in short daily sessions. Pictures, puppets, and role-playing are used extensively to explore interpersonal conflicts and devise nonaggressive resolutions.

Parent-Focused Preventive Interventions   The preventive interventions directed to the Head Start parents include parenting training and conflict resolution training, both in group format. The parenting program consists of 12 weekly group discussions during which parenting issues are explored and discussed. While topics are suggested by the leaders, the emphasis is on discussion of actual problems that the participants are currently having in the care of the children. The leaders use interventions such as reflection, summarization, reframing, confrontation, reinforcement, and support to facilitate the process. Videotaped vignettes (created by staff at the Center for Infant Study) and role-playing are used extensively. The aims are twofold: to increase positive reinforcement and decrease coercive discipline, and to attune permissiveness to an adaptive level and increase monitoring of child behaviors.

A second component of the program directed to the parents parallels the children-focused social skills training with the goal of increasing in the parents adaptive interpersonal communication; nonaggressive, verbally organized conflict resolution, and improved affect and impulse modulation. The format of this component is similar to that of parenting training.

Treatment   Parallel to the preventive interventions already described, children and families with specific needs receive therapeutic interventions which can be directed either to the child, jointly to the caretaker and child, or to the caretaker separately.

Child-Focused Treatment Interventions   The child-focused therapy can include classroom and home behavioral strategies implemented by the teacher, the parent, or the therapeutic nursery staff. The child-focused therapy can also include individual therapy with staff from the therapeutic nursery.

Behavioral interventions in the classroom address maladaptive behaviors observed in that setting. Often, they represent specific case application of the principles discussed in the universal preventive interventions. Labeling of feelings, expression of negative emotions verbally, discussion of alternative (nonaggressive) resolution of conflict, practice in techniques for better modulation of emotions and impulses, encouragement to overcome shyness and the propensity to withdraw—all represent strategies to facilitate successful participation in the classroom activities. These strategies can be initiated by the teacher, the parent, or the therapeutic nursery staff. The mental health professional can facilitate the process, designing the program with teachers and parents, and can assess the partial outcomes of the program by keeping track of the frequency and intensity of behaviors and discuss ongoing adjustment according to progress.

Ideally, a parallel program can be applied in the home by the parents and caregivers, consisting of equivalent interventions adjusted to the home circumstances. The advantage of these interventions is that they occur in the actual natural settings of the child's experiences. Further, a consonant approach in the home and classroom will facilitate the generalization of responses to all settings. A specific module of interventions for children with attention difficulties has been developed. This module includes having children make eye contact while receiving instructions, having children repeat directions they have just received, and having students summarize main points in a story, breaking down tasks in small components and using a timer to assist in sustaining attention for increasing periods of time.

Individual therapy with children is used in circumstances that do not allow this classroom behavioral approach and when individual exploration of private or inner experiences is necessary (e.g., in cases of physical or sexual abuse, depressive mood, or anxiety and phobias). In those cases, individual, expressive psychotherapy is carried out. However, because of the paramount importance of the parent-child (or primary caretaker- child) relationship, individual therapy is never conducted in the vacuum but correlated with interventions directed to the parent-child dyad. Depending on the case, the emphasis of treatment may be mainly on the dyad, or varied combinations of individual and joint therapies.

Interventions Addressed to the Parent-Child Dyad or the Parent Individually   Individual interventions with the caretaker are usually a result of parent-child dyadic work. These interventions are used when the parent needs to be instructed in the application of specific techniques to deal with a child (e.g., as in the case of handicaps or sensory deficits) or in circumstances when the parental perceptions of the child and his or her behavior are distorted and actively interfere with the interaction with the child. In those cases the working model of the child, an internal representation of the child, may be contaminated with parental experiences in his or her own upbringing that become reactivated vis-a-vis the child. This technique, which has been developed as dyadic work with infants and toddlers (Lieberman & Pawl, 1993), can be applied also to dyads with three- or four-year-old children with some modifications (increased opportunities for work with the adult alone).

Family-Focused Interventions   As stated earlier, a two-generations strategy is essential to enhance child development and modify behavioral and emotional difficulties. In addition to the preventive and therapeutic interventions already mentioned, it is necessary to institute case management in cases of multiple needs and in the presence of varied risk factors. The goals of these interventions are to decrease parenting stress, strengthen social support, facilitate access to needed medical or other services, and enhance education and opportunities for employment. These functions are obtained through interagency collaboration.

CONCLUSION

The therapeutic nursery and Head Start collaboration offers the opportunity to develop a program of education, prevention, and treatment of mental health issues in a comprehensive manner, in an ecologically sound setting, with a flexible and rich array of interventions.

REFERENCES

Barkley, R. A., Fischer, M., Edelbrook, C. S., & Smallish, L. (1990). The adolescent outcome of hyperactive children diagnosed by research criteria: An 8-year prospective follow-up study. *Journal of the American Academy of Child and Adolescent Psychiatry, 29*, 546–557.

Barrish, H. H., Saunders, M., & Wolfe, M. D. (1969). Good Behavior Game. Effects of individual contingencies for group consequences and disruptive behavior in the classroom. *Journal of Applied Behavior Analysis, 2*, 119–124.

Farrington, D. P., Loeber, R., & Van Kamen, W. B. (1990). Long-term criminal outcomes of hyperactivity-impulsivity-attention-deficit and conduct problems in childhood. In L. N. Robins & M. R. Rutter (Eds.), *Straight and devious pathways from childhood to adulthood*. Cambridge: Cambridge University Press.

Furman, R., & Katan, A. (1969). *The therapeutic nursery school*. New York: International Universities Press.

Halpern, R. (1990). Community-based early intervention. In S. J. Meisels & J. P. Shonkoff (Eds.), *Handbook of early childhood intervention*. Cambridge: Cambridge University Press.

Kellam, S. G., Brown, C. H., Rubin, B. R., & Ensminger, M. D. (1983). Paths leading to teenage psychiatric symptoms and substance abuse: Developmental epidemiological studies in Woodlawn. In S. B. Guze, F. J. Earls, & J. E. Barrett (Eds.), *Childhood psychopathology and development*. New York: Raven Press.

Lieberman, A., & Pawl, J. H. (1993). Infant-parent psychotherapy. In C. H. Zeanah (Ed.), *Handbook of infant mental health*. New York: Guilford Press.

Loeber, R., & Dishion, T. (1983). Early predictors of male delinquency: A review. *Psychological Bulletin, 93*, 68–99.

Piotrkowski, C. S., Collins, R. C., Knitzer, J., & Robinson, R. (1994). Strengthening mental health services in Head Start. *American Psychologist, 49*, 133–139.

Rutter, M. (1982). Epidemiological-longitudinal approaches to the study of development. In W. A. Collins (Ed.), *The concept of development*. Hillsdale, NJ: Lawrence Erlbaum.

Sameroff, A. J. (1993). Models of development and development risk. In C. H. Zeanah (Ed.), *Handbook of infant mental health*. New York: Guilford Press.

Shonkoff, J., & Meisels, S. (1990). Early childhood intervention: The evolution of a concept. In S. J. Meisels & J. P. Shonkoff (Eds.), *Handbook of early childhood intervention*. Cambridge: Cambridge University Press.

Spivak, G., & Shure, M. B. (1982). *Social adjustment of young children: A cognitive approach to solving real-life problems*. San Francisco: Jossey-Bass.

Yoshikawa, H. (1994). Prevention as cumulative protection: Effects of early family support and education on chronic delinquency and its risks. *Psychological Bulletin, 115*, 28–54.

Chapter 30

Foster Care

Mohammad Haerian, M.D.

Societies have always had ways to care for children whom, for whatever reasons, were not being cared for by their own parents. Sometimes these arrangements were familial and almost tribal in nature. In other societies the church in its earliest forms was considered the responsible party or a caretaker of last resort.

The current American child welfare system has its roots in English Elizabethan Poor Laws which were designed to protect society from the poor, as being dependent was a sin. Our first efforts at caring for children therefore developed out of strong disapproval and rejection of the notion of dependency. Children who were homeless or whose parents could not care for them were forced to become as self-supporting as possible at an early age. The early American colonists provided services like workhouses, apprenticeships, and almshouses, although many children were kept in asylums and prisons with adults. Later, orphanages were developed as a more humane way of caring for children. In the early 19th century, with heavy waves of immigration and high unemployment, many parents were unable to care for their children. These children were either placed in orphanages or left on the streets to fend for themselves.

Reverend Charles Loring Brace developed a revolutionary plan of placing out children by sending groups of uncared for children on trains throughout the West to be cared for by farm families. Many of these children were adopted, others were simply kept indefinitely. The care children received ranged from being accepted as members of loving families to being exploited mercilessly. Between 1854 and 1929, over 150,000 children were placed into family homes by way of orphan trains (Terpstra & McFadden, 1993).

Orphanages continued to function well into this century. Gradually, public policy began to change as individual states started developing State Boards of Charities. The advent of the juvenile court in 1899 brought into the child welfare field the first legal process designed to serve the best interests of the child. In 1909 the first White House conference on children adopted a rather radical position stating that poverty alone was an "insufficient" reason to place children. This conference led to the establishment of the Federal Children's Bureau in 1912 (Young, R. unpublished paper).

Since then, the Children's Bureau has been responsible for developing policies for covering a wide spectrum of issues including health care, financial support, mental health, abuse and neglect, placement services, and adoption. The Bureau's efforts led to adoption of a public policy allowing payment to foster families as a matter of law. Along with these developments, child welfare gradually became more professionalized. Social work developed as a profession and became the primary base for child welfare with service, with a strong influence from psychiatry.

The increase in the number of infants entering care has been most striking. In 1983, infants comprised 16.3 percent of foster children, rising to 24.5 percent in 1993. In the past several years newborns have made up the largest share of infants placed in care. This trend is most likely a result of the epidemic of crack cocaine, which gained strength in the mid-1980s.

DEMOGRAPHIC DATA

In 1977, there were more than 520,000 children in care. With the passage of Public Law 96-272, escalating the cost of foster care and attempts at permanent placements, the number of children in foster care steadily declined to 275,000 in 1984 (Terpstra & McFadden, 1993). Since then, the number has begun to rise steadily. In 1993, a total of 657,000 children were in foster care. A one-day count of children in foster care in 1993 showed 445,000 children in foster homes—an increase of about two-thirds over the one-day count 10 years earlier.

The Chapin Hall Center for Children at the University of Chicago, in its report, *Foster Care Dynamics 1983–1993*, confirmed large increases in foster care caseloads between 1986 and 1993 in five states. The five—California, Illinois, Michigan, New York, and Texas—together account for almost half of all children in foster care. A 1995 study by the U.S. General Accounting Office reports that spending on foster care has increased dramatically at all levels of government since 1983 in response to the growing number of children in care and the increasing needs of families. The increased federal, state, and local spending on foster care has left proportionately fewer resources for child welfare services. According to the GAO report, for every federal dollar spent on foster care in 1993, just 12 cents was spent on other child services compared with 40 cents in 1983.

REASONS FOR PLACEMENT

Foster care is viewed as an alternative living arrangement for children while their parents are unable to care for them. A distinguishing aspect of foster care is that it is designed to be a temporary arrangement, yet many children remain in care for a rather long time. Many children are never returned to their birth parents, nor are they placed in an adoptive home. Instead, they go from one foster home to another. The longer a child stays in foster care, the greater the likelihood the child will remain in care. The first few months of foster placement are highly critical to the outcome. In fact, most children who do go home are returned to their parents within the first year (Kadushin, 1977).

Recent empirical research from the United States and England suggests that minority and poor children are overrepresented in the foster care system and that adolescents constitute almost half of all children in care. Available information suggests that the reasons for foster placement for the overwhelming majority of children are "parent-based" rather than "child-based" problems and are more likely to include child abuse, neglect, and parental physical or mental illness. Most foster children come from families in which the parents do not live together at the time of the child's entry into care.

RISK FACTORS

Since the passage of adoption assistance and the Child Welfare Act of 1980 (PL 96-272), most states have been successful in reducing the number of children in foster care and the length of stay (Rosen, Fanshel, & Lutz, 1987). Within the past several years, however, this trend has begun to shift and the number of children in care has increased rather steadily. Data reported by Besharov (1990) shows a 28.6 percent increase in the number of children entering into care between fiscal year 1988 and fiscal year 1989. Besharov suggested that the major reason for the increase in the number of children in foster care is substance abuse on the part of one or both parents, "The communities hardest hit by crack addiction have experienced startling increases" (p. 23).

The National Black Child Development Institute (NBCDI) (1989) identified a number of factors that are associated with foster care entry. Many placements, according to NBCDI, are attributable to "environmental stresses caused by chronic poverty" (p. 37). Inadequate housing, mental illness, and substance abuse are named as major barriers to reunification among black families. The NBCDI report suggested that substance abuse is a contributing factor in foster placement in 36 percent of cases. Besharov's study (1990), however, suggested that drug abuse may be present in as many as 90 percent of the abuse and neglect reports in major cities.

Jellinek, Murphy, and Bishop (1990) reported that substance abuse is a contributing factor in 33 percent to 80 percent of the cases involving severe neglect, and that poverty was a risk factor in two-thirds of cases of abuse and neglect brought before the Boston Juvenile Court. Most of these families were headed by a single mother and more than half included a parent with a major psychiatric disorder.

Some of the risk factors contributing to foster placement—including financial problems, low self-esteem, single parenthood, lack of parenting skills, lack of child care, and teen parenthood—can be remedied. However, substance abuse by the parents is very resistant to intervention (Kowal, Kottmeier, Ayouh, Komives, Robinson, & Allen, 1989). In a study of foster children in Baltimore, Slaght (1993) found that 37.2 percent of the children were placed because of parents' mental illness and 45.7 percent of placements were as a result of parental substance abuse.

In reviewing the literature, Pardeck (1985) identified the following risk factors contributing to foster care failure: older child, white child, being in care for an extended time, child having emotional or behavioral problems, and a child who is poorly socialized in terms of empathy and maturity. Risk factors attributed to the child's biological family include parental alcoholism, parents not living together, and parents' neglect or abuse of the child. Pardeck suggested that high caseworker turnover, caseworker's inability to establish rapport and limited contact with the child and foster family, foster parents' lack of training for working with the child having emotional and behavioral problems, and low motivation to be a foster parent also contribute to placement failure. The child's maltreatment in foster care is another reason for multiple placements. Psychological and physical characteristics of the child, foster parents, and home characteristics and agency practices all play a role in the child's maltreatment in the foster home. Attempts to develop predictive models to identify maltreating families have been unsuccessful.

In a study of 185 foster children five years after placement (Lawder, Poulin, & Andrews, 1986), Lawder found that 61.7 percent of the children returned to their families. Of those discharged, 80 percent went to their parents, with most going to single-parent homes. Almost 18 percent of the children were returned to their extended families. Sixteen percent were placed for adoption and 18 percent were still in foster care after five years.

Overall, 34 percent of the children left care within three months. Within one year from the time of placement 56.2 percent had been discharged and about 70 percent of the children were in care two years or less. In this study, overall, 93 percent of the children studied had one or two placements. Only 13 of the 185 children had more than two placements. Of 70 children discharged from the Treatment Family Program of Catholic Charities in Baltimore between January 1, 1993 and July 31, 1996, 29 percent were reunited with a parent or a relative, 34 percent were adopted by their foster parents, and 16 percent required residential placement (Haerian, unpublished manuscript).

The frequency of visits between the child and birth family members, and the severity of the child's behavioral problems seem to be the strong predictors of length of stay. Other predictors are related to reasons for placement. These factors include family crisis or emergency, parental mental health problems, parental neglect, and teenage parent. Regardless of the reason for foster placement, the continued contact with birth parents is the single most important factor predicting length of stay. Children with behavioral problems, those born to teenage mothers, and children placed in foster homes because of neglect tend to remain in care longer. Parental mental illness is another predictor of longer length of stay. Children placed in care because of a family emergency or crisis tend to return home sooner.

TREATMENT FAMILY PROGRAMS

These programs, also known as therapeutic or specialized foster care, are designed to serve the hard-to-place and behaviorally challenging youth. The development of treatment family programs (TFP) can be traced to regular foster homes and residential treatment centers (RTC). The route from foster homes followed a progression from free homes, boarding homes, and homes dealing with hard-to-place children. The 1961 amendment to the Social Security Act provided cost sharing for caring for difficult children and payments to programs organized to recruit, train, and pay foster parents to provide treatment for behaviorally challenging youth. The emergence of treatment family programs from residential treatment centers dates back to the early 1960s when the RTCs started to develop treatment foster homes to supplement their services or provide step-down placements for those children who no longer need residential treatment, yet their families were not ready to take them back (Hudson, Nutter, & Gallaway, 1994).

Like regular foster homes, the treatment family programs provide care within a family setting. They differ with regular foster homes in several important aspects however. The treatment family programs are targeted to children and adolescents who would otherwise be in more restrictive settings. The foster families are recruited and trained to provide care to children who have special physical but more often emotional problems. The programs provide different psychiatric therapies—for example, individual, group and family therapy, psychiatric assessment, and follow-up—in home service intervention and emergency services. Many programs provide the foster parents with ongoing training and education. Depending on the legal status of the child, the programs may work closely with biological parents, especially if the goal is to return the child home.

In a survey of 321 Treatment Family Programs operating in the United States and Canada in 1992, Hudson et al. found that the majority of these programs were small and privately owned. On the basis of data provided by 185 programs on over 1,600 former clients, they found that the vast majority of the recently discharged children and youth had been placed for severe emotional and behavioral problems. As the children got older at the time of placement, however, admission to a TFP was more likely made for criminal rather than psychiatric or emotional reasons.

After discharge 54 percent of the children went back to their parents' home, a home of their own, or other permanent living situations. Thirty-seven percent were discharged to other treatment settings. Many more children (ages 0 to 11 years old) than adolescents returned to their parents.

FAMILY REUNIFICATION

In recent years there has been a renewed attention to reunification of children in out-of-home care with their families of origin. In 1986, 103,000 (or nearly 59%) of the 176,000 children who left care were discharged to their biological families (Tatana, 1989). A substantial number (approximately 35%) of these children who are returned to their families, however, sooner or later re-enter some form of out-of-home placement (Maluccio, Walsh, & Pine, 1993). Maluccio suggested that "families as well as service providers need to recognize that reunification represents a continuum of outcomes from return home to other appropriate forms of contact with parents" (p. 9).

Family readiness for reunification, parents' emotional readiness, and re-entry into a changed family system contribute to the outcome of reunification. For reunification to be successful a careful assessment of the family's and child's willingness to reunite, the parents' skills, their ability to meet the child's changing needs, their capacity for conflict resolution and problem solving—all are essential. Many of the families to which children return are often crisis-ridden and in need of services in many areas such as housing, health, and income assistance. Family reunification programs consequently need to provide more comprehensive and longer periods of service for these families.

PSYCHIATRIC PROBLEMS

Behavioral problems of foster children may be attributed to a number of factors including difficulties in their biological families (e.g., family dysfunction, parental mental illness), the child's own problems and internal conflicts, or the stresses of adjusting to foster care.

Psychological Development of Children in Foster Care

Of various samples of foster children studied, between 29 percent and 38 percent showed significant emotional and behavioral disturbance (Thorpe, 1980; Rowe, Hundleby, Cain, & Keane, 1984). These numbers are not easy to interpret, however, because of variations in the ages of the children at placement and the various reasons for placement. Rowe et al. (1984), for example, found that foster children have a higher rate of temper tantrums, stealing, and destructive and disruptive behavior.

The child's own difficulties including difficult temperament and disruptive behavior may be factors in his or her initial out-of-home placement. Considering the fact that a significant number of children are removed from home as a result of neglect and abuse, one could suspect a high rate of psychiatric problems secondary to trauma—that is, reactive attachment disorder, posttraumatic stress disorder (PTSD), dissociative disorder.

The stresses of the child's leaving his or her own family and adjusting to a new family are manifold. In addition to separation from parents and feelings of rejection and abandonment the foster child often experiences a strong ambivalence toward the foster parents.

Acceptance of the foster parents is often perceived by the child as betrayal of the birth parents. The uncertainty inherent in foster care and the ambiguous and ambivalent status of the foster child in terms of membership in both the biological family and the foster family are unique stressors experienced by foster children.

Uncertainty about the future deprives the child of being able to develop a sense of belonging. The foster child is usually forced to give up not only his or her place in his or her family, daily routine, and previous connections with family members, but also his or her sense of belonging to a neighborhood, school, and a community. According to Molin (1990), "Part of that sense of belonging and stability, even when in the context of a dysfunctional family, is a sense of continuity in time, an ability to make a temporal link between past and future...." This sense of predictability in time gives the child a suitable setting while undergoing development transition (p. 503). Children in foster care are often deficient in these areas. The lack of belonging and the sense of being an outsider to one's own family and community contribute to these children's difficulty in staying emotionally invested and attached in self and others. Their sense of identity gets compromised.

Leaving care for independence brings to the surface past deficits and unfinished developmental tasks. The problems for those emancipating from public care include poor educational attainment, poor health, poor self-image, low aspiration, poor social skills, limited social support system, increased risk of homelessness, and poverty (Aldgate, 1994, p. 26).

In a follow-up sample of 203 children placed permanently in foster care from infancy, Bohman (1990) found that these children were more maladjusted than their classmates. This proportion increased at the age of 15 years and some of the problems persisted into adulthood.

The Role of the Child Psychiatrist

Older children are placed because of their own behavior rather than parental failings. The children with behavioral problems who have been placed in foster care are older and more likely to be recidivist. The exceedingly high rates of psychopathology found in foster children (McIntyre & Keesler, 1986) are often attributed to circumstances surrounding and/or preceding placement—for example, neglect, abuse, abandonment, and deprivation. Some aspects inherent in foster care experience also have been proposed as contributing to the child's psychopathology and impeding healthy psychological development (Goldstein, Freud, & Solnit, 1979).

These explanations of the causes of psychopathology among foster children that attribute the problems solely to environmental factors before, during, and after placement, have not been empirically supported. For example, in spite of extensive investigation, Fanshel and Shinn (1978) failed to find any factor which predicted the child's clinical condition at the time of entering care or during placement. This may be caused by failure to take into account the children's own variables and own contributions to psychopathology including vulnerabilities, temperament, and prior experiences. Our experience in working with children placed in the Treatment Family Program of Catholic Charities in Baltimore (Haerian, unpublished manuscript) shows strong genetic loading for mental illness and a preponderance of difficult temperament among the children.

Regardless of the causative factors, many investigators have found that psychological disorders are very common among foster children. McIntyre and Keesler reported that 50 percent of their sample suffered from a severe psychiatric disorder (McIntyre &

Keesler, 1986). Rowe et al. (1984) found that foster children have a higher rate of temper tantrums, destructiveness, enuresis, destructiveness, and stealing. We have found the rate of psychopathology among children placed in specialized foster care to be much higher; for example, 75 percent of our children carry a diagnosis other than adjustment disorder. Most of these children suffer from mood disorders, disruptive disorders, and PTSD. The reason for the high prevalence of psychiatric disorders in this group is rather obvious, for these children have, as a rule, failed placement in conventional foster homes. Many of them have a history of psychiatric hospitalization and/or residential placement and more than 70 percent are on a psychotropic medication.

The role of the child psychiatrist working with this population is manifold. Children placed in regular foster homes often do not come to the attention of the child psychiatrist. Although between 30 percent and 50 percent of them suffer from serious psychological problems, a relatively small number receive any kind of psychiatric treatment. This treatment is usually provided by the social workers from the department of social services or in community mental health centers or outpatient departments of large general hospitals. The child psychiatrist may act as a consultant to the child welfare workers to help clarify the nature of parent-child relationships, family dynamics, possible need for direct evaluation of a specific child, and specific behavior management techniques. Occasionally, the consultant may become involved in educating and training foster families to recognize and manage children's behavior problems. In this role the psychiatrist may help with feelings of frustration or failure that the foster families may have because of their failure to deal with the problem on their own.

The work with specialized foster care programs is much more involved. Many of these programs require an initial evaluation by the child psychiatrist. As mentioned earlier, almost all specialized foster children carry a psychiatric diagnosis and the majority of them are on psychotropic medications. Therefore, these children need to be seen by the child psychiatrist at regular intervals for follow-up and medication management.

Other responsibilities of the consulting child psychiatrist may include helping the program with standard setting, policy making, client care monitoring, and quality assurance; supervising the social workers who provide individual and family therapy; and helping and educating foster parents about the child's mental illness and appropriate management techniques.

CONCLUSION

Over the past two hundred years the care for the poor, disadvantaged, and troubled children and youth in this country has gradually evolved from sending them to asylums and farm homes to placement in highly regulated foster homes and specialized foster care programs. The number of children in care has risen as well. The increase is attributed to the rise in family dislocation, poverty, and use of drugs by parents. Along with these changes there has been an increase in the degree of psychopathology of the children and youth placed in care. Many investigators support the idea that the reasons for placement of infants and young children are mainly a result of family discord, and foster placement for older children and youth are generally secondary to their own psychopathology. Surveys, however, suggest that regardless of the age at entering care, many of these youngsters are genetically predisposed to major mental illnesses.

In recent years there has been a move toward placing very troubled children and adolescents in specialized foster homes providing them with intensive psychiatric care.

With the advent of the specialized foster care programs, the role of child psychiatrists has changed as well because they are no longer merely a consultant to social agencies or workers. Child psychiatrists have become an essential component of the treatment team, providing psychiatric evaluation and medication management of children, supervising the therapist, and helping the programs design their treatment policies. These specialized treatment family programs have been successful in reducing the number of children in group homes and residential treatment centers. In spite of the advances in TFP and other specialized programs, significant work remains for primary prevention and early intervention.

REFERENCES

Aldgate, J. (1994). Graduating from Care: A missed opportunity for encouraging successful citizenship. *Children and Youth Services Review, 16* (3/4), 255–272.

Besharov, D. J. (1990). Crack children in foster care. *Children Today, 19,* 21–26.

Bohman, M. (1990). Outcome in adoption: Lessons from longitudinal studies. In D. Brodzinsky & M. Schechter (Eds.), *The psychology of adoption* (pp. 93–106). Oxford, England: Oxford University Press.

Fanshel, D., & Shinn, E. B. (1978). Children in foster care: A longitudinal investigation. New York: Columbia University Press.

Goldstein, J., Freud, A., & Solnit, J. A. (1979). *Before the best interest of the child.* New York: Free Press.

Hudson, J., Nutter, R. W., & Gallaway, B. (1994). Treatment foster family care: Development and current status. *Community Alternatives: International Journal of Family Care, 6* (2), 1–24.

Jellinek, M. S., Murphy, J. M., & Bishop, S. (1990). Protecting severely abused and neglected children. *New England Journal of Medicine, 323,* 628–630.

Kadushin, A. (1977). Child welfare: Adoption and foster care. In J. B. Tuerner (Ed.), *Encyclopedia of Social Work, 17th Issue.* Washington, DC: National Association of Social Workers.

Kowal, L. W., Kottmeier, C. P., Ayouh, C. C., Komives, J. A., Robinson, D. S., & Allen, J. P. (1989). Characteristics of families at risk of problems in parenting - Findings from a home-based secondary prevention program. *Child Welfare, 68,* 529–538.

Lawder, E. A., Poulin, J. E., & Andrews, R. G. (1986). *Child Welfare League of America, 55* (3), 241–251.

Maluccio, A. N., Walsh, R., & Pine, B. A. (1993). Rethinking family reunification after foster care. *Community Alternatives, International Journal of Family Care, 5* (2), 1–17.

McIntyre, A., & Keesler, T. Y. (1986). Psychological disorders among foster children. *Journal of Clinical Child Psychology, 15,* 297–303.

Molin, R. (1990). Future anxiety: Clinical issues of children in the latter phases of foster care. *Child & Adolescent Social Work, 7* (6).

Pardeck, J. T. (1985). A profile of the child likely to experience unstable foster care. *Adolescence, 20* (79), 689–695.

Rosen, S. M., Fanshel, D., & Lutz, M. E. (Eds.) (1987). *Face of the nation, 1987.* Silver Spring, MD: National Association of Social Workers.

Rowe, J., Hundleby, M., Cain, H., & Keane, A. (1984). *Long term foster care.* London: Batsford.

Slaght, E. F. (1993). Reexamining risk factors in foster care. *Children and Youth Services Review, 15,* 143–154.

Tatana, T. L. (1989). Characteristics of children in foster care. *Newsletter of the Division of Child, Youth and Family Services. American Psychological Association, 12,* 16–17.

Terpstra, J., & McFadden, E. J. (1993). Looking forward to new directions in foster care. *Community Alternatives: International Journal of Family Care, 5* (1), 115–134.

Thorpe, R. L. (1980). The experience of children and parents living apart: Implications and guidelines for practice. In J. Triseliotis (Ed.), *New Developments in Foster Care and Adoption.* London: Routeledge and Kagan Paul.

Index